THE

ENVIRONMENT

FOR

CHILDREN

ONE WEEK LOAN

THE
ENVIRONMENT
FOR
CHILDREN

Understanding and acting on
the environmental hazards that threaten
children and their parents

DAVID SATTERTHWAITE

ROGER HART • CAREN LEVY • DIANA MITLIN

DAVID ROSS • JAC SMIT

CAROLYN STEPHENS

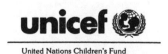

United Nations Children's Fund

EARTHSCAN
Earthscan Publications Ltd, London

First published in the UK 1996 by
Earthscan Publications Limited

A catalogue record for this book is available from the British Library

ISBN: 1 85383 326 6 Paperback   1 85383 321 5 Hardback

Typesetting and page design by PCS Mapping & DTP, Newcastle upon Tyne
Printed and bound by Biddles Ltd, Guildford and Kings Lynn
Cover design by Andrew Corbett

For comments or further information on this and other UNICEF projects, please
contact:

Mr Gourisankar Ghosh
Chief, Water, Environment and Sanitation Cluster
UNICEF
3 UN Plaza
New York, NY 10017, USA

For a full list of publications please contact:
Earthscan Publications Limited
120 Pentonville Road
London N1 9JN
Tel. (0171) 278 0433
Fax: (0171) 278 1142
Email: earthinfo@earthscan.co.uk
World Wide Web: http://www.earthscan.co.uk

Earthscan is an editorially independent subsidiary of Kogan Page Limited and
publishes in association with the WWF-UK and the International Institute for
Environment and Development.

The material in this book has been commissioned by the United Nations
Children's Fund (UNICEF). The contents of this book are the responsibility
of the authors and do not necessarily reflect the policies or the views of the
United Nations Children's Fund.

CONTENTS

List of Acronyms and Abbreviations

DALY	disability-adjusted life years
EU	European Union
FAO	Food and Agricultural Organization
IFAD	International Fund for Agricultural Development
IIED	International Institute for Environment and Development
NGO	non-governmental organization
OPP	Orangi Pilot Project
OECD	Organization for Economic Cooperation and Development
PEC	primary environmental care
UNDP	United Nations Development Programme
UNEP	United Nations Environment Programme
UNICEF	United Nations Children's Fund
WHO	World Health Organization
WCED	World Commission on Environment and Development

List of Figures, Tables and Boxes

FIGURES

TABLES

BOXES

About the Authors

Roger Hart is a Professor of Environmental Psychology in the PhD Psychology Program of the Graduate School and University Center of the City University of New York. He is also an Affiliate Professor in Developmental Psychology and Co-Director of the Children's Environments Research Group. He earned a BA from Hull University in England and a PhD from Clark University in Worcester, Massachusetts. His research has focused on children's development in relation to the physical environment. Much of his work has concerned the application of theory and research in child development to the planning and design of children's environments and to the environmental education of children. He advises UNICEF on their urban and environmental programs and has written two UNICEF publications: *Children's Participation: From Tokenism to Citizenship* (Innocenti Essays, ICDC, Florence, 1992) and *Children's Participation in Sustainable Development: Involving Citizens aged 4 to 14 in Community Development and Environmental Care* (published by Earthscan, London, 1996).

Caren Levy is a senior lecturer at the Development Planning Unit (DPU), University College London. She is also Director of the DPU Gender Policy and Planning programme. A planner by background, over the last 10 years her work has focused on developing and implementing strategies to integrate a gender perspective into the policies, programmes and projects of international agencies, government agencies and NGOs. This has included work with the European Union, NORAD, SIDA and UNCHS (Habitat), and with organizations in Brazil, Egypt, Mozambique, Namibia and Sri Lanka. She also works on environmental, transport and housing issues in urban areas.

Diana Mitlin is an economist working in the Human Settlements Programme at IIED with a first degree in economics and sociology (University of Manchester, 1979–82) and a masters in economics (Birkbeck College, 1986/7). Her current interests include NGOs, urban community development, sustainable development, housing finance for low-income groups and the use of participatory methodologies in urban areas. Recent activities include contributing to UNCHS, *An Urbanizing World: the Global Report on Human Settlements 1996*, (Oxford University Press); project leader of the ODA consultancy 'Local Initiatives Facility for the Urban Environment' and coordinator of an IIED research project on community environmental initiatives in Karachi and Manila. Recent publications she has co-authored include *Funding Community Initiatives*, Earthscan, 1994 and *Environmental Problems in Third World Cities*, Earthscan, 1992. For the last three years, she has been managing editor of *Environment and Urbanization* and has recently joined the advisory board of *Third World Planning Review*. She is also chair of the British charity Homeless International.

David Anthony Ross grew up in Nigeria before attending school and university in the UK. While studying medicine, he took a year out to do a Masters in epidemiology based on research of innovative community health systems in a rural area of Sierra Leone, and since qualifying from medical school in 1980 has continued to work as a research epidemiologist within the general area of public health in developing countries. He has been on the staff of the London School of Hygiene and Tropical Medicine (LSHTM) since 1983, where he is currently a Senior Lecturer within the Department of Epidemiology and Population Sciences. In the early 1980s he and colleagues initiated a programme of work at LSHTM on health problems in urban areas of developing countries. His main current interests include the health effects of vitamin A deficiency in both children and adults, the health of adolescents in developing countries, the potential for reducing health risks to young children associated with attending day care centres, and the ability of retrospective interviews of relatives to establish causes of death or of illness in young children. He is co-organiser of the Masters course in Public Health in Developing Countries at the London School of Hygiene and Tropical Medicine, and has previously spent one year (1984/5) living and working for Oxfam in the Horn of Africa, and almost four years (1988–92) in charge of the setting up and running of the Navrongo Health Research Centre for the Ministry of Health in the north of Ghana. The Centre conducted two large field trials of the effects of vitamin A supplementation on child mortality and morbidity during that time.

David Satterthwaite is Director of the Human Settlements Programme at the International Institute for Environment and Development (IIED) and editor of its journal *Environment and Urbanization*. He is also a member of the Board of IIED-América Latina in Buenos Aires and Associate Fellow of the Institute of Latin American Studies, University of London. Most of the work of IIED's Human Settlements Programme has been in collaborative research, with teams based in Africa, Asia and Latin America, mainly on issues of housing, health, environment, urban development and rural-urban linkages. Recent publications include *Environmental Problems in Third World Cities* (with Jorge E Hardoy and Diana Mitlin), Earthscan, London, 1992 and *Squatter Citizen: Life in the Urban Third World* (with Jorge E Hardoy), Earthscan, London, 1989. He was also the main author of UNCHS, *An Urbanizing World: the Global Report on Human Settlements 1996*, Oxford University Press, 1996 and advisor to the World Commission on Health and Environment and to the World Commission on Environment and Development (The Brundtland Commission).

Jac Smit is principal author of *Urban Agriculture: Food, Jobs and Sustainable Cities*, published by the United Nations Development Programme in February 1996. He is an agricultural scientist and an urban planner and he founded the Urban Agriculture Network. He has worked on urban agriculture in over 25 countries since 1990 and has advised UNICEF, UNDP, the UN Centre for Human Settlements, the UN Food and Agriculture Organization, CARE International, the World Bank and many other agencies involved in urban agriculture.

Carolyn Stephens is a lecturer in Environmental Health and Policy at the London School of Hygiene and Tropical Medicine, where she has worked since 1988. She holds a bachelor's degree in English Literature, a Masters in Health Planning and Financing and a PhD in Public Health Medicine. Her doctoral dissertation focused on inequalities in urban environmental health conditions in the South. She has worked extensively overseas – in Liberia, India, Tanzania, Ghana and Brazil. Her current research focus is on the urban environment, poverty and health in the South. Most recently she was principal investigator of a two country collaborative epidemiological study of urban differentials in environment and health in Accra and Sao Paulo. She has worked for the Overseas Development Administration on multi-sectoral slum projects in India and on environmental health perceptions of the urban poor in India and Tanzania. She has also advised several international agencies including WHO, the World Bank, UNCHS (Habitat) and the World Resources Institute. She currently holds a UK Economic and Social Research Council fellowship in Global Environmental Change related to the policy implications of urban environmental health research in cities in the South.

Preface

The intention in this book is to provide all those interested in environmental issues and in development with a review of the environmental hazards that threaten the life and health of infants, children and their parents and with some ideas as to how these might be addressed. This book also seeks to make explicit the influence of social, economic and political factors on why such environmental hazards occur and who is most affected by them. In part, *The Environment for Children* is to encourage those working in development to take environmental issues more seriously. In part, it is to encourage environmentalists to take a greater interest in environmental health; there are too many reports on 'the state of the environment' which ignore or hardly mention the environmental factors that cause or contribute to so much ill health, injury and premature death among infants and children, especially in the South.

There is also one particular area that this book tries to address but which I believe still remains ill-understood. This is the phenomenal difficulties that low-income parents face in trying to provide their children with a safe, healthy and stimulating environment when housing conditions are very poor, livelihoods precarious and all the infrastructure and services that are important for child health are lacking or inadequate – including safe and sufficient water supplies piped into the home, provision for sanitation, drainage and (where necessary) the regular collection of household wastes, schools, easily accessible and affordable health services, emergency services for serious accidents or sudden acute illnesses – and also safe, stimulating and easily accessible places where children can play. It is a demanding task for all parents to look after young children even with good quality housing, especially when they are sick. It is difficult to imagine how parents can cope when they lack such basic needs as spare clothing and bedding to use, if the child's bedding or clothing become soiled, readily available hot water for washing clothes and personal hygiene, emergency health services on hand if needed and the possibility of parents taking time off work to nurse sick or injured children and purchase medicines without a serious loss of income or assets. But a high proportion of the world's parents do not enjoy these advantages. It is also clear that children are seriously sick or injured much more often if they live in poor quality housing that also lacks basic services; so too are their parents.

In most instances, most or all of the burden of coping with sick or injured children falls on mothers or older girl siblings. This is certainly a burden that very few middle or upper class men have ever had to cope with. It may be a burden that relatively few researchers have had to cope with. Perhaps new qualitative research methods and more emphasis on participatory research may reveal how we greatly underestimate the human costs on children and on their parents of not giving a higher priority to ensuring children have safe, healthy and stimulating living environments.

This book began life as a paper prepared for the United Nations Children's Fund (UNICEF) at the request of R Padmini as part of UNICEF's preparation for the UN Conference on Environment and Development (also called the Earth Summit) in 1992. Parts of this were incorporated into a UNICEF report entitled *Environment, Development and the Child* published in 1992. With encouragement from Padmini and then from Deepak Bajracharya (who joined UNICEF as an environmental advisor) this was further developed into a longer background paper prepared for the UNICEF's Environment Unit for a workshop on primary environmental care (PEC) in Colombia in 1993 – but drawing not only on the work of my programme (the Human Settlements Programme) within the International Institute for Environment and Development (IIED) but also on the work of other programmes, especially the Forestry and Land Use, Sustainable Agriculture, and Drylands Programmes. After this workshop, it was agreed that the paper be developed into this book; and, with UNICEF's encouragement and support, that it would benefit from drawing on the knowledge of other specialists.

Roger Hart, Caren Levy, Diana Mitlin, David Ross, Jac Smit and Carolyn Stephens agreed to review the original paper but in doing so their role became much more than reviewers: new paragraphs were drafted, existing paragraphs rewritten, new themes introduced and other changes incorporated. Roger Hart also drafted the final chapter. As such, this book ceased to be my work, although the final responsibility for the text and for any mistakes or errors of judgement remain mine. Involving Roger Hart, Caren Levy, Diana Mitlin, David Ross, Jac Smit and Carolyn Stephens in this way also proved a great pleasure and a wonderful way to learn more about the complex interactions between the physical environment and children (and their parents). Although developing books collaboratively can be time consuming, and UNICEF were almost too patient and generous in the time they permitted us to do this, it allows the final text to reflect the knowledge and experience of people from different disciplines in ways that no book written by a single author can. This kind of collaboration appears particularly important when dealing with things like the links between environment, health and children which cross so many disciplinary boundaries.

This text also owes much to several other people – particularly Deepak Bajracharya at UNICEF, on whose work and enthusiasm it draws, Padmini, and Jules Pretty and Irene Guijt on whose work Chapter 6 draws heavily. It has benefited much from the suggestions and comments of Padmini, Deepak Bajracharya, Anjaly Bhansali and some anonymous reviewers within UNICEF and of Andy Inglis. It draws on my work with the World Health Organization and, as with our earlier publications, I am grateful to WHO staff in Geneva for their advice and their readiness to encourage non-health specialists such as myself to become involved in health issues. It also inevitably draws on my many years of work with Jorge E Hardoy who died in 1993 – but who would have so enjoyed working on this book (which he had planned to do). Jorge Hardoy had introduced the issue of children's needs and priorities into our work programme many years ago.

This book is the fifth in a series of Earthscan books published by IIED's Human Settlements Programme since 1989; details of the other four are given at the end of this volume. As with all previous books, we are grateful to Jonathan Sinclair Wilson at Earthscan for his enthusiasm and support for our writing and to Rowan Davies, Jo O'Driscoll and other staff at Earthscan for helping to publish it.

This book also owes a great debt to my father, not only as my father, but also as someone who worked tirelessly for many years to ensure that children in the UK had ready access to safe and stimulating play spaces and that national and local governments took seriously children's right to this. It was he who first took me to an adventure playground and explained how it worked and why it was important.

David Satterthwaite
International Institute for Environment and Development
June, 1996

1

The Environment for Children

THE MAIN ENVIRONMENTAL ISSUES

For more than half the world's children, their health and often their lives are constantly threatened by environmental hazards – in their home and its surrounds, in the places where they play and socialize and, for working children, in their workplaces. The *child crisis* – the 40,000 child deaths that occur each day from malnutrition and disease and the 150 million children a year who survive with ill health and with their physical and mental development held back – has somehow become separated from much of the discussion about the world's most serious environmental problems. Yet, it is pollutants or disease-causing agents (pathogens) in the child's environment – in air, water, soils or food – and poor households' inadequate access to natural resources (fresh water, food, fuel) which are the immediate causes of this child crisis. Given the importance of environmental factors to infant and child health (and survival), it is perhaps surprising that the relationship between children and the environment has not been given more attention. Environmental hazards also take a serious toll on the health of a high proportion of the world's parents and this, in turn, makes it much more difficult for parents to provide their children with a safe, stable and stimulating environment.

This book describes the environmental hazards that cause or contribute to most illness, injury and premature death among children below the age of 15 and how these can be acted on.* It concentrates on those hazards to which hundreds of millions of infants and children are constantly exposed in their everyday lives in both rural and urban areas. It does not cover in detail the particular and often horrific environmental problems faced by children in what UNICEF terms 'especially difficult circumstances' – for instance orphans and abandoned children living on the street. Although special programmes can reduce the environmental hazards faced by children of the street – for instance through ensuring they have facilities for

---

* Although the term 'children' is often used to include all those between 0 and 18 years of age, this book focuses mainly on infants and children below 15 years. In part, this is because less is known about the environmental risks that 15–18 year olds face. But it is also because it is more difficult to disentangle the influence of environmental factors on their health from other factors.

1

bathing, washing, defecation and laundry and access to health care – the problems these children face and the factors that led to their expulsion or desertion of their home need much more than this. It also does not consider the environmental problems faced by children living in hastily erected emergency camps or other places when they and their families are forced to flee from their homes, or children (and their households) living in regions in the midst of wars or civil strife when there is little or no effective civil authority and no public services. These deserve a more detailed consideration in their own right. But, perhaps more importantly, the environmental hazards these children face or the other environmental problems that such instability can generate are rarely resolvable with environmental action. This is much less the case for the environmental hazards to which children are exposed within their homes and neighbourhoods as, in most instances, these hazards or their health impacts can be eliminated, or much reduced, at relatively low cost.

This book also aims to raise the priority given to the environmental problems that underlie most illness, injury and premature death among children. These are rarely given much prominence in discussions, debates and publications about the environment – perhaps because they affect children most and because most of the illness, injury and premature death occur in the South.* The environmental concerns of the world's wealthier inhabitants, most of whom live in Europe, North America and Japan, still dominate the discussions of 'environmental crisis'. Here, most of the concern for the environment is related to chemical pollution in the air and water, damage to the natural environment and the scale of resource use and waste. There is also the growing concern about the loss of biodiversity, the depletion in the stratospheric ozone layer and the possible health and environmental implications of global warming.

However, there are two, more serious, environmental crises that are forgotten or their importance is downplayed. They are more serious because of their immediate impact on human health – and especially on the health of children. The first is the ill health and premature death caused by pathogens in the human environment – in water, food, air and soil. Each year, these contribute to the premature death of millions of people (mostly infants and children) and to the ill health or disability of hundreds of millions more. As the World Health Organization (WHO) points out,[1] this includes:

- the three million infants or children who die each year from diarrhoeal diseases and the hundreds of millions whose physical and mental

---

* In 1995, what this book terms 'the South' had 79.6 per cent of the world's population. The South is taken to include all of Africa and Latin America and the Caribbean, and Asia except Japan. Although the term 'the South' is inaccurate geographically in that many of the countries it includes are in the northern hemisphere and Australia and New Zealand are not part of 'the South', geographic inaccuracy is preferred to such terms as 'developing' or 'less developed' countries that imply that the countries so designated are inferior to 'developed' countries. An alternative would be to call them 'non-industrialized' countries but this is even more inaccurate than 'the South' as certain Asian and Latin American countries are among the world's major industrial producers and have higher proportions of their labour force in industry than North America and most of Europe.

development is impaired by repeated attacks of diarrhoea – largely as a result of contaminated food or water.

- the two million people who die from malaria each year, three quarters of whom are children under five; in Africa alone, an estimated 800,000 children died from malaria in 1991;[2] tens of millions of people suffer prolonged or repeated bouts of malaria each year.
- the hundreds of millions of people of all ages who suffer from debilitating intestinal parasitic infestations caused by pathogens in the soil, water or food, and from respiratory and other diseases caused or exacerbated by pathogens in the air, both indoors and outdoors.

There are very large differences between the disease burdens suffered by those living in the wealthiest and the poorest countries from pathogens such as these. For instance, the disease burden per person from diarrhoeal diseases acquired in 1990 in sub-Saharan Africa was around 200 times larger than in West Europe, North America, Japan, Australia and New Zealand[3*] – and virtually all this disease burden is preventable or curable at a modest cost. In this same year, the disease burden per 5 to 14 year old child in sub-Saharan Africa from infectious and parasitic diseases and maternal causes was nearly 100 times higher than that for 5 to 14 year olds in the world's wealthier countries.

The proportion of infants who die from infectious and parasitic diseases among households living in the poorest quality housing in Africa, Asia and Latin America is several hundred times higher than for households in West Europe or North America; all such diseases are transmitted by airborne, waterborne or foodborne pathogens or by disease vectors such as insects or snails. Of the 12.2 million children under the age of five who die each year in the South, 97 per cent of these deaths would not have occurred if these children had been born and lived in the countries with the best health and social conditions.[4]

The second 'environmental crisis' is the hundreds of millions of people who lack access to natural resources on which their health and/or their livelihood depend. The most common is no safe and convenient supply of water for drinking and domestic use. (Official statistics on water supply provision greatly overstate the proportion of the world's population with safe and convenient supplies; see Chapter 2 for more details.) But there are also hundreds of millions of households who depend for part or all of their livelihood on raising crops or livestock – and their poverty (and the malnutrition and ill health that generally accompanies it) is the result of inadequate access to water and fertile land. This lack of access to land and water for crop cultivation or livestock underlies the poverty of around a fifth of the world's population (see Chapter 4).

Although these two environmental crises – the life threatening pathogens in the human environment and the lack of access to natural

---

* This is the average current and future disease burden per person from new cases of diarrhoeal diseases acquired in 1990. The figure includes the disability-adjusted life days lost in later years that arose from diarrhoeal diseases caught in 1990. The final section of Chapter 2 describes these disease burdens in more detail.

resources needed for health and/or livelihoods – are often forgotten in the North, less than a century ago, diarrhoeal diseases, acute respiratory infections and other diseases spread by biological pathogens in the air, food or water were still the major causes of ill health and premature death in Europe, North America and Japan.[5] Large sections of the population in these countries or regions also lacked access to fresh water while many of their rural populations also had too little land to support themselves adequately. This can be seen in the infant mortality rates that existed only 100 years ago in what were then the world's most prosperous countries. Today, infant mortality rates (the number of infants who die between their birth and their first birthday per 1000 live births) in healthy, prosperous societies should be less than ten and can be as low as five. In such societies, it is very rare for an infant or child to die from an infectious or parasitic disease. Yet only 100 years ago, most prosperous European cities still had infant mortality rates similar to those in the poorest countries today, exceeding 100 per 1000 live births; in many, including Vienna, Berlin, Leipzig, Naples, St Petersburg and many of the large industrial towns in England, the figure exceeded 200.[6]

The fact that these two environmental crises have been tackled in the North in little more than a century shows the extent to which purposive human action can solve them. This is especially so for the pathogens in air, food, soil and water – either through environmental modification (for instance much improved housing and living conditions, including adequate provision for water supply and sanitation) or through protecting people from them or their health impacts. There are also many examples of countries in the South or particular states or regions within countries that have successfully tackled these environmental crises – and some have done so in a few decades. Most countries have made some progress in this, over the last 20 to 30 years. But much more could be done.

THE NEED FOR A SAFE ENVIRONMENT

The built environment in which an infant or child lives and the natural environment in which all settlements are located should be a safe environment. Environmental factors should not figure as major causes of infant and child deaths. The role of environmental factors in causing or contributing to ill health or injuries can be minimized. Indeed, the human environment should have a very positive role in promoting and supporting children's physical and mental development. *It is this book's contention that governments and aid agencies can do far more to improve the environment for children and greatly reduce the toll that environmental factors take on child health and development – and on the health of their parents or carers.* The cost of doing so is also, generally, not very high.

Many of the interventions to do this have not only very high social returns relative to costs but also high economic returns – for instance through the increased productivity of a healthy workforce and decreased expenditures on medicines and health care. Obviously, the greatest difficulties in funding such interventions come in the nations with the lowest

4

incomes and the least prosperous economies and in the villages or urban districts with the lowest-income inhabitants who have the least possibility of repaying the cost of the needed interventions. But there are many examples of successful interventions to reduce environmental hazards for children which required modest levels of external funding – including numerous examples of community-based initiatives which received some support from local non-governmental organizations (NGOs) or foundations (and sometimes from municipalities, government agencies or international agencies). Many also recovered most of their costs. These are considered in more detail in Chapter 6. There is also the fact, much stressed by UNICEF in its annual *The State of The World's Children*, that much child illness and death is preventable at low cost as in the vaccine preventable diseases and in addressing micronutrient deficiencies such as iodine, vitamin A, iron and zinc (for more details see Chapter 2). The cost of curing or controlling many of the infectious and parasitic diseases associated with poor quality living environments is also very low.[7]

This first chapter sets the context for the rest of the book by considering the environmental components of 'development', especially those that concern children, and the great variety of environmental and non-environmental factors that influence child health. It also locates this discussion of the environmental problems that children face in their homes and neighbourhoods within the social, economic and political context in which they occur – especially why it is almost always the children (and adults) in the households with the lowest incomes and least assets that suffer most ill health, injury and premature death from environmental problems. Chapter 2 describes the different kinds of environmental hazards that affect child health and development while Chapter 3 describes how and in what way these hazards affect the health of infants and children and how the scale and nature of environmental hazards change the older the child. Chapter 4 describes the links between children and renewable resources, although the main concern is how and under what conditions households obtain those natural resources on which their children's survival or development depends. It concentrates on rural and urban households whose livelihood depends in part or wholly on access to natural resources.

Chapter 5 discusses the meaning of 'sustainable development', especially for children, and how a concern for sustainable development fits within the concerns outlined in previous chapters. It also considers current patterns of consumption for non-renewable resources and the wastes arising from production and consumption, and what these imply for the achievement of sustainable development. It also questions the much published assertion that 'the poor' are a significant contributor to the depletion of the world's environmental capital. Chapter 6 describes a community-based approach to addressing environmental problems, termed 'primary environmental care', that can serve as the means through which groups of people (including children) can better manage their own environment while also addressing their own livelihood and health needs. Chapter 7 discusses the involvement of children in primary environmental care and in other environmental concerns.

LINKS BETWEEN THE ENVIRONMENT AND CHILD HEALTH

The early chapters in this book concentrate on describing the range of physical, chemical and biological hazards to which infants and children are exposed in their homes, settlements (and workplaces) and on highlighting those that take the largest toll in child health and survival. Box 1.1 describes how such hazards may arise independent of human action or as a direct result of human action – or through human action modifying the natural environment. The early chapters also describe how it is usually a combination of environmental and non-environmental factors that underlie high levels of ill health, injury or premature death among children.

Table 1.1 gives examples of some of the main causes of injury, illness and premature death among children in which there are links with the environment. These are placed under different categories to show how the strength and nature of the association between the environment and the health problem differs – as does the extent to which environmental modification can address the health problems. In some, environmental modification represents the most effective response. In others, there is a strong relationship between the disease and the environment but the best means to reduce the incidence or severity of the disease is through non-environmental means – for instance through immunization or rapid treatment. Table 1.1 is not a complete list and more details about these and other links between environment and health are given in subsequent chapters.

Although much of this book is dealing with health issues, its focus is on the impact of the human environment on children and on the households of which they are part, rather than the health status of children. The book highlights, but does not cover in detail, one very important aspect of the environment–child relationship – the ways in which the physical environment of the home, neighbourhood, creche/day-care centre, school, playground, and other areas used by children for play and other social activities can promote and support child development. It may also give too little attention to the importance of involving children in understanding and being able to influence their own physical environment; this is the theme of a companion volume to this book.[9] As Roger Hart, the author of the companion volume (and also a co-author of this book) notes, children have a valuable and lasting role in environmental issues, but only if their participation is taken seriously and supported with a recognition of their developing competencies and unique strengths.

> *We need children to become highly reflective, even critical participants in environmental issues in their own communities. We need them to think as well as act locally while also being aware of global issues.*[10]

Box 1.1 **The Environment**

Many different definitions are given to the term 'environment'. In some instances, it is a term given to all that is external to a person while in other instances, it is restricted to something more specific – for instance wilderness areas or the 'natural' environment. In this book, the concern is the environment in which children live that is made up of the built environment (ie a physical environment constructed or modified for human habitation) and the natural environment in which all human settlements are located. Thus, it focuses on the physical, chemical and biotic (of or relating to living organisms) conditions within this human environment and their implications for children's health and development and for their parents' capacity to adequately care and provide for them.

Environmental hazards for children may arise from:

- *physical, chemical and biotic conditions that exist independent of human action.* For some, human actions seek to modify conditions to reduce or eliminate the hazard – for instance the control or eradication of particular insects that are vectors of diseases. For others, human actions seek to protect the children from such conditions – for instance the construction of housing to protect against rain, disease vectors, dust and extremes of heat or cold.
- *physical, chemical or biotic conditions that have been influenced by human action* – for instance as human-induced environmental changes create new possibilities for disease transmission or disease vectors.
- *conditions or hazards created by human action* – for instance the introduction of hazardous chemical wastes into the human environment as these are dumped on land sites or into water bodies or the introduction of physical hazards such as motor vehicles into the human environment.

The influence of environmental factors on child health and development can be contrasted with influences arising from children's own human biology, 'lifestyle' (ie individual, household or societal decisions in regard to lifestyle) and the health care system.[8]

THE HOME ENVIRONMENT

The quality of the environment in which a child grows up has a profound, direct influence on their physical, intellectual, social and emotional development. Many children are fortunate enough to grow up in a safe, healthy and stimulating environment. For a significant proportion of the world's adult population, the environment in which they live and work, and in which their children develop, poses few serious threats to their health.

Table 1.1 *Examples of Important Links between Disease/Injury and the Environment*

Diseases	Notes
Strong relationship between disease/injury and environment	
Most insect borne diseases (including malaria, Chagas disease, dengue fever, yellow fever, leishmaniasis) and schistosomiasis	Modifying the environment to reduce the breeding, feeding or resting places for the vector is often a major part of disease control; in addition, for schistosomiasis, improved sanitation reduces the cycle of infection as schistosome eggs are no longer released into the environment
Most diarrhoeal diseases, cholera, hepatitis A, most intestinal worms	Adequate provision for water, sanitation, drainage and hygienic food preparation and storage can greatly reduce their incidence; overcrowded housing is also a risk factor
Most of the common eye and skin infections and louse-borne diseases	Large reductions in their incidence are possible through improved water supply (including provision for washing) and sanitation
Accidental burns, scalds and other injuries within the home and its surrounds, including those from road accidents	The incidence of such injuries is strongly associated with the size and quality of the home and the settlement or neighbourhood in which it is located
Diseases and injuries in the workplace	Most are related to toxic chemicals and/or dust in the workplace, and inadequate protection of workers from heat, machinery and noise
Important relationships between disease and environment but other factors also important	
Acute respiratory infections	Overcrowding, inadequate ventilation, dampness and indoor air pollution influence their incidence and severity; so do high levels of ambient air pollution
Tuberculosis; also meningococcal meningitis and rheumatic fever	Overcrowding and poor ventilation increase the risk of disease transmission
Many psycho-social disorders	There is a strong association with poor quality housing and stressors associated with it, although many non-environmental factors are also important

Relationship between disease and environment but other factors more important

Maternal and perinatal health	Most of the above health problems affect the health of mothers but improved health care and provision for safe delivery are more important in reducing maternal and perinatal deaths

Important relationship between disease and environment but most cost-effective means of addressing it is through non-environmental means

Measles and pertussis	Both are transmitted through aerosols with increased transmission in overcrowded dwellings but immunization against them is much the most cost-effective way of reducing their health impact
Tetanus	Often caused by an accidental injury as the pathogen enters the human body through any cut or wound; rapid treatment and immunization against it are the most effective means to control it as the pathogen that causes it cannot be controlled through environmental modification
Certain forms of under-nutrition eg those linked to iodine, iron and vitamin A deficiency	Iodine and vitamin A deficiency are particular problems in regions where foods rich in iodine and vitamin A are limited; provision of supplements, fortification of food and, for vitamin A and iron deficiency, dietary modification are the most effective ways of preventing these deficiencies

Perhaps a third of the world's population fall into this category.[*] For these people, the last hundred years or so have brought remarkable progress in improving housing conditions that also reduce environmental hazards. The change to much safer, more healthy and (generally) more spacious housing has been rapid, but such housing has qualities that are so taken for granted by those that have them that their role in improving health and reducing environmental hazards (especially for children) is often forgotten. Within such housing, the health impact on infants and children of pollutants, pathogens and physical hazards has been enormously reduced. Box 1.2

---

[*] This is no more than a rough guesstimate of the proportion of the world's population who have living and working environments where life-threatening environmental hazards have been greatly reduced. In virtually all nations, a proportion of the population live in homes and neighbourhoods where environmental hazards for infants and children have been greatly reduced. The proportion of the population in this group must vary between a few per cent (in the poorest nations) to over 90 per cent in some of the wealthiest nations. There will be a strong correlation between the wealthiest households and the households in this category in most nations, although in some of the wealthier nations, substantial progress has been made in ensuring that life threatening environmental hazards have been much reduced for most low-income households.

summarizes the differences between the homes of the wealthiest third or so of the world's population and that of the rest of the world in terms of water supply, sanitation, space heating, lighting, kitchen facilities and quality and size of the building. It emphasizes how little improvement has been made in the home environment of a large proportion of the world's population over the last few decades, despite the fact that the size of the world's economy has increased many times (in real terms) since 1950.

The wealthiest third or so of the world's population not only enjoys homes with adequate provision for water, sanitation, space and the other characteristics noted above but most also live in neighbourhoods where household wastes are collected regularly, so there is no problem of garbage and other wastes covering the places where children walk and play. Such neighbourhoods have provision for storm and surface-water drainage so flooding and waterlogged paths and open spaces are not a problem. The efficient removal of garbage and waste water also eliminates virtually all the problems of disease vectors such as mosquitoes that breed in standing water or flies and cockroaches that so often breed or feed on garbage. Most such neighbourhoods have schools with safe environments – where, for instance, there is sufficient space, school equipment, and provision for washing, defecation and the hygienic preparation and consumption of food.

Most such neighbourhoods also have an effective health care service, so rapid treatment is available when environment-related diseases or injuries occur. Such health services include an effective 'preventive' component by being accessible and convenient and ensuring all children receive immunization against the vaccine-preventable diseases. These people can also rely on an emergency service that provides rapid expert medical attention if one of their children has an accident or a sudden illness – with doctors, paramedics and ambulances able to quickly reach their home if needed. Of course, their home can always be reached by motor vehicles because of paved roads. Although further improvements are needed in these homes and neighbourhoods to protect and promote children's health – perhaps most especially in further reducing accidents in the home and from road vehicles and in ensuring much greater variety and accessibility of areas for recreation and play for children of all ages, especially in lower-income inner city areas – the very low levels of infant and child mortality in these areas compared to 50–100 years ago show the progress that has been made.

Most of the population in West Europe, North America, Japan and Australia enjoy home environments with these qualities. But only a minority of the population of Africa and of most Asian and Latin American countries do so. As is summarized in Box 1.2, this two thirds of the world's population generally have:

- homes that do not have water piped into their homes (and even where they do, its quality is often very poor and water is only available for a few hours a day). By 1991, according to official figures, only half of the urban population and less than 10 per cent of the rural population in the South had a water supply piped into their home.[11] At least 350 million urban dwellers and one billion rural dwellers have no water supply where some attempt is made to ensure it is uncontaminated

Box 1.2 **A Comparison of Home Environments**

This wealthiest third or so of the world's population generally have home environments characterized by:

- Water of drinking quality piped into the home and available at all times, hot and cold running water available in kitchens and bathrooms, toilets connected to sewers (or other sanitation systems that are as convenient and hygienic) and baths (or showers).

- In climates where space heating is needed, homes with heating equipment that does not require open fires or stoves.

- Electricity supplies which eliminate the need for kerosene lamps or other forms of lighting that often cause accidental fires.

- Homes made of building materials that do not readily burn, and housing designs that make provision for escape in the event of a fire.

- Kitchen facilities that make it easy and convenient to prepare and store food safely – including sinks with running hot and cold water and refrigerators. They allow food and drinks to be prepared and stored for infants and young children with very little or no danger.

- Sufficient space for children to have their own bedrooms and to have space for play within the house.

The less wealthy two thirds or so of the world's population generally have home environments characterized by:

- No water supplies piped into the home (and even where they do, its quality is often very poor and water is only available for a few hours a day) and no toilets with connections to sewers or to septic tanks.

- Open fires or stoves for cooking (and, where needed, heating) usually within relatively small houses made of flammable materials which are a major cause of burns and scalds for children and of accidental fires. Indoor air pollution from such fires or stoves may also have a serious health impact, especially on women and children.

- No electricity supplies, so kerosene lamps or other forms of lighting are used that often cause accidental fires.

- Homes made of flammable building materials – for instance wood, cardboard and thatch for roofs.

- A lack of space and facilities for the safe and convenient preparation of food and for washing eating and cooking utensils and clothing. No electricity generally means no refrigerators and thus great difficulty in storing food safely.

- Between a fifth and a twentieth of the space per person, compared to the norm in wealthy nations. A high proportion of households in both rural and urban areas live in one room.

and of reasonable quality. The remainder has what their governments claim is 'access to safe water' but, for a high proportion of such households, this is a water supply that is inconvenient and inaccessible – for instance from public standpipes shared with dozens or even hundreds of other households and with all water needed in the house having to be carried considerable distances. (It is often assumed that water supplies within 100 metres of a house are 'adequate' yet it is very time consuming and laborious to fetch and carry enough water for a household from 100 metres away.)

- homes that do not have adequate provision for sanitation. Official statistics suggest that at least a third of the South's urban population and around half its rural population are unserved by sanitation and an even greater number lack adequate means to dispose of waste waters.[12] But a much larger proportion lack adequate provision for sanitation based on three criteria. The first is a toilet to which they have easy access; tens of millions of urban dwellers that governments claim have 'adequate provision for sanitation' only have access to shared toilets with so many people using them that access is difficult or even at times impossible. The second is a sanitation system that minimizes the possibility of human contact with human excreta; most do not do so – and most latrines have no running water and no basin to permit washing, after defecation. The third is a sanitation system that is easy to maintain and to keep clean; tens of millions of households rely on pit latrines which need to be emptied regularly but there is no efficient service to do so.[13]

- Open fires or stoves for cooking (and, where needed, heating) that are usually within relatively small houses. Many households with five or more persons live in one room. This combination of open fires or stoves that are usually at ground level and of small rooms with many people (and thus little chance of keeping children away from the fires and stoves) means that children are often burnt or scalded. Accidental fires are common. The health impact from burns, scalds and accidental fires are made much greater by the absence of emergency services that can rapidly treat those injured or tackle the fire.[14] As Chapters 2 and 3 will describe in more detail, indoor air pollution from such fires and stoves may also have a serious health impact, especially on women and children.

- No electricity supplies, so kerosene lamps, candles or other forms of lighting are used that often cause accidental fires. Poor quality lighting also restricts children's activities after dark, including studying and reading.

- Homes often made of flammable building materials such as thatch for roofs and the widespread use of wood. In many low-income urban settlements, widespread use is made of cardboard, plastic sheeting and wood as the inhabitants lack secure tenure of the land and are reluctant to build with permanent materials when they may be evicted from that land at any time. In many cities, a considerable proportion of the population live in overcrowded 'tenements' and cheap boarding or rooming houses within illegal or informal settlements which are also made of flammable building materials and where landlords have made little or no attempt to reduce the risk of accidental fires, or make provisions for escape when an accidental fire starts, or provisions to stop such fires spreading.

- A lack of space and facilities for the safe and convenient preparation of food, and for washing their eating and cooking utensils and clothing. No electricity generally means no refrigerators and thus great difficulty in storing food safely.
- Houses with between a fifth and a twentieth of the space per person, compared to the norm in wealthy nations. Among people with good quality housing, the amount of housing space per person is measured in terms of *rooms per person*; among the majority in Africa, Asia and Latin America, it is measured in *persons per room*. A large proportion of both urban and rural households live in one room – and often with five or more persons living and sleeping in that one room. It is not uncommon for there to be less than one square metre per person – whereas the average for housing in many cities in the North is for 30–80 square metres per person.[15]

The description by Ashraf of his home and daily life in Delhi in Box 1.3 gives some insight into what it is like for children to live in such an environment. The mother, father and five children live in two rooms whose total floor area is 12.5 square metres – the size of one small bedroom in a house in the West. Ashraf and his father defecate in the open in the morning as they would have to pay to use the local latrine. The household has to get water from a handpump at some distance from the house. Ashraf's description also brings out the extent to which his 12 year old sister Ayesha undertakes the housework – fetching water from the handpump, washing the family's clothes and undertaking much of the cooking and helping with other aspects of housework.

Most of this same two thirds of the world's population who live in poor quality housing also live in neighbourhoods that have no services to collect household wastes regularly. It is common to find garbage and other wastes covering the open sites, roads and pavements within the settlement – all places where children walk and play. Such neighbourhoods rarely have provision for drainage, so flooding and standing pools of waste water are a constant problem. Not surprisingly, there are often serious problems from diseases spread by disease vectors which breed or feed on garbage or breed in standing water. Most such neighbourhoods lack an effective health care service, so rapid treatment from a doctor or para-professional is simply not available when environment-related diseases or injuries occur. This also generally means that many or most children have not been immunized against the vaccine-preventable diseases.[17] Many settlements are at some distance from paved roads and are inaccessible by motor vehicles, at least for parts of the year, which further limits the possibility of any emergency service in response to acute illness or injury.

A considerable proportion of this two thirds of the world's population also have little or no security of tenure in the home they have built themselves or that they rent or have purchased. Both in rural and in urban areas,

Box 1.3 **Ashraf's Description of his House in Delhi**

Ashraf lives with his family in the ground floor of a very small house in what is known as 'the 12.5 sqm clusters' in Raghubhir Nagar, Delhi. This settlement was formed by people who were forcibly evicted from their homes in illegal settlements in Delhi in the aftermath of the Declaration of Emergency in 1975.[16] The settlement gets its name from the fact that each plot is only 12.5 square metres. Four fifths of all houses are one storey with 73 per cent having only one room. Only a very small proportion have a separate bathroom or kitchen. Ashraf's house is unusual in having three floors – but the family live only in the ground floor rooms.

Our house has three floors. On the first one (ground floor) there are two rooms. We use one room to cook and eat and we all lie down in the other room – my mummy, papa, two sisters and three brothers (including Ashraf). There is a small toilet for peeing and bathing. Two uncles and a cousin sleep in the middle room (first floor); they give rent of Rs 200 or 250 per month (about £4 or US$6 per month). There are two rooms above that (second floor); nobody lives there.

We had so many mice in our house, most of them in our kitchen. A friend of one of my uncle's told him that he could catch them all and give them to a place (laboratory) where 'they' (students) cut them before they learn to be doctors. A few months back, two friends of my uncle came, caught all the mice and sent them away. Now we have only a few in the kitchen.

I wake up in the morning at 7 o'clock and brush my teeth with toothpaste. I go to defecate with my father near the nallah. In the 'private' latrine, they take money only from men and boys. My mother goes with Ayesha (Ashraf's 12 year old sister) to the private latrine. Papa has a bath every night in the bathroom; I also bathe there every night.

There is a handpump near our house, but it brings up muddy water – we don't use it. For household work and bathing we get water from another handpump a little further away. We get drinking water in two pots and two tins from the 25 sqm area (the adjoining settlement, formed before the 12.5 sqm clusters, where plot sizes are 25 square metres). Sometimes I go to fetch water. Usually my mother or Ayesha go and sometimes one of my uncles.

We eat three times a day – in the morning at 7.30 we have a vegetable, roti and tea, in the afternoon also we have vegetable and roti, sometimes rice. At night (8 pm) all of us eat together – we have dal, rice, vegetable and sometimes roti. Ayesha cooks for everyone twice a day. She also cleans the utensils and sometimes cleans the house. Mummy sweeps and mops the floor and cleans the almirahs. When Ayesha has a stomach ache (implying her menstrual period), then mummy cooks the food. Ayesha also washes our clothes.

Source: TARU for Development, Giving Children back their Childhood? Habitat and the World of a Child, Prepared for Plan International, TARU, Delhi, 1994.

millions of people are forcibly evicted from their homes each year against their will, usually with little or no compensation or provision to rehouse them.[18] These include the people evicted from illegal or informal settlements in urban areas – as in the case of Ashraf and his family described in Box 1.3. Many low-income families in urban areas report that they have been forcibly evicted from their homes and settlements several times.[19] Millions of rural people are also evicted each year to make way for reservoirs and building works associated with dams or other 'infrastructure works' and farmers, pastoralists and hunter gatherers evicted from lands they traditionally 'owned' and managed.[20]

In most such evictions, the people evicted not only lose their homes but often their possessions, as little or no warning is given before the bulldozers destroy their settlement. They often lose touch with their friends and neighbours as they scatter in the search for other accommodation or livelihoods and thus lose the often complex reciprocal relationships which provided a safety net of protection against the costs of ill health, income decline or the loss of a job.[21] They often lose one or more sources of livelihood as they are forced to move away from the area where they had jobs or sources of income.[22] The direct and indirect impact of such evictions on children's health, education and sense of security must be very considerable.

The historical experience in countries which have sustained economic growth to become among the wealthier nations of the world shows how a new set of environmental problems come to prominence as a society becomes increasingly industrialized and/or urbanized. These include the chemical pollutants associated with industrial development and modern farming, and the ecological impacts arising from the unprecedented level of resource use and waste generation. In the countries which first underwent rapid industrialization and urbanization, while these may still have serious health impacts on women and men in particular age groups, income groups and occupational groups, overall the scale of the health impact of this new set of environmental factors has been considerably reduced. The one area where far less progress has been made is in ensuring that children have ready access to a diverse and stimulating environment. This access has deteriorated badly in the past 10–20 years for a high proportion of children in the North. This is especially so in urban areas where access to play space has deteriorated and where the risks from road traffic, crime and other hazards make parents reluctant to allow young children to play outside the house. This problem may show up less in health statistics, as parents or carers stop their children playing outside because of the dangers there. Chapter 3 will consider this issue in more detail.

UNDERLYING SOCIAL, ECONOMIC AND POLITICAL CAUSES OF AN UNHEALTHY ENVIRONMENT

Virtually all environmental problems have underlying social, economic or political causes which either led to the environmental problem in the first place or explain why it has not been addressed. This can lead to problems whose origin is essentially social or political being labelled as 'environmental'. Those with low incomes, few economic assets and the least political power are almost always those who suffer most from environmental problems because the lower the income, the poorer the quality of the housing that can be afforded and, in most instances, the more deficiencies there are in provision for water, sanitation, drainage and health care. Low-income groups generally have the least power to demand that governments provide them with basic services and protection from other environmental hazards.

The nature of any political system also strongly influences the priority given by governments to addressing environmental problems – and whose environmental problems receive priority. For instance, waterborne diseases may be 'environmental problems' as it is through contaminated water that human infection takes place. But, in most countries where waterborne diseases are major causes of ill health and premature death, this is not because of an absolute shortage of fresh water. It is much more the refusal of governments and aid agencies to give a higher priority to the supply of safe water, sanitation and drainage, especially to lower-income populations. City authorities or national agencies are usually pressured into giving more attention to the environmental problems that are the concern of the middle and upper income groups, even where these same groups are the ones who already benefit most from publicly provided infrastructure and services.

Poverty usually has important environmental dimensions – for instance a rural household's lack of fertile land on which to make an adequate living or a rural or urban household's lack of safe and sufficient water supplies. But in most countries, the underlying cause is not a shortage of a natural resource (land, fresh water) but the inequitable distribution of rights to own or use such resources. This inequity in access to natural resources or to basic services that reduce or eliminate environmental hazards is largely the result of inequalities in income and assets – although there are also many inequalities linked to ethnicity. It is also rooted in gender inequality, as women own a very small proportion of the natural resources and often face discrimination, when compared to men, in obtaining land, education, employment and housing. Virtually all governments and aid agencies could do much more to reduce current levels of ill health, injury and premature death arising from environmental factors, but not only through environmental actions but also through non-environmental measures such as improving the incomes or the size or quality of land-holdings for low-income households – especially for women – and through better health care that protects people from infection or provides rapid treatment. This makes it difficult to isolate the impact of environmental factors on child health and survival from political, social, economic and cultural factors.

While environmental modifications are often among the most effective ways to diminish the health impact of infectious and parasitic diseases, other factors need to be addressed. This can be illustrated by considering how best to reduce malnutrition and the role of environmental modifications in this. Malnutrition is one of the most serious health problems for more than a quarter of the world's population. This is largely the result of inadequate incomes or inadequate land holdings (ie not environmental hazards).

However, malnutrition may lower a person's immunity to communicable diseases such as diarrhoeal diseases (which are usually environment-related diseases arising from contaminated food or water), which then exacerbates the malnutrition. Intestinal parasites, which people generally pick up from contaminated food, soil or water, are another environmental hazard that often contributes to malnutrition. In addition, it is not only environmental modification that can address environmental hazards. Some are far more easily addressed by boosting the human immune system (as in immunization for the vaccine-preventable diseases) or rapid treatment (for instance, early diagnosis and rapid treatment of pneumonia would save hundreds of thousands of infants' lives each year) or ensuring increased incomes that allow low-income groups to choose to spend more to obtain more healthy accommodation and better health services.

The fact that most of the environmental problems that threaten the lives and health of children occur within low-income households and are heavily concentrated in nations with relatively low per capita incomes could imply that it is problems of poverty and inequality that should be addressed, not environmental problems. At household level, it is so often a lack of income or assets that limits households' capacity to pay for improved home environments and basic services while a lack of education (or literacy) limits knowledge about how to guard against environmental hazards. At national level, the capacity for governments to provide those basic services that greatly reduce environmental hazards or their health impacts depends much on the level of prosperity of the national economy – and, in general, the higher a country's per capita income, the higher the proportion of a nation's population with access to piped water, provision for sanitation and health care.

But a focus on poverty and inequality and on their consequences for child health and development often misses or underestimates the 'environmental' aspects of illness, injury and premature death among infants, children and their parents. Many studies on poverty do not give detailed consideration to health problems or to the many environmental aspects of the health problems of 'poor' groups. The criteria most commonly used for defining who is 'poor' are related to income and give no consideration to health status, living conditions or to access to basic services.[23] A focus on the economic and social aspects of poverty may underestimate or misunderstand the role of environmental modifications in addressing these health problems and the extent to which relatively modest levels of external support can help low-income households and communities to reduce life-threatening and health-threatening environmental hazards. It may underestimate the priority that many low-income households give to a safer home and neighbourhood environment and the many direct and indirect benefits this can bring to child health and development.[24]

A focus on the *environment for children* helps highlight aspects of deprivation among households with inadequate incomes or assets that many studies on poverty have neglected. It certainly highlights the immense difficulties that parents with inadequate incomes and assets have in providing a safe and healthy home environment for their children. It highlights the additional work burden placed on households (and within households usually on women and girls) when provision for water supply, sanitation, health care and, where needed, garbage collection services are inadequate. It highlights the tremendous health burden that infants, children and parents face in the absence of a safe and healthy home and neighbourhood environment. It also highlights the ways in which low incomes contribute directly or indirectly to increased vulnerability to environmental hazards.

A focus on the *environment for children* will also ensure that the environmental aspects of child health and development become a central concern among environmentalists – or among anyone interested in 'the environment'. This includes the need to promote a broader understanding of the links between the environment and health – especially the need to go beyond the idea that 'the environment' means forests and agricultural lands. There are still reports being prepared for countries that hardly mention the environmental factors that have the profoundest influence on child health and development. In effect, they are reports on 'the state of the natural environment' with little concern for 'the state of the human environment'. The same is true for many works on sustainable development where the main interest is sustaining the natural environment, with little or no consideration of the environmental or developmental needs of children (see Chapter 5 for more detail on this point).

ENVIRONMENTAL AND NON-ENVIRONMENTAL INFLUENCES ON CHILD HEALTH

Figure 1.1 illustrates the many linkages between environmental factors and non-environmental factors that influence child health. It shows the range of environmental, social, economic and political factors which influence the health (and chances of survival) of any child. Its purpose is to promote a broader view of the environmental hazards which threaten the life and health of children. It also seeks to show the many possible entry points to improve child health – although many specific, sectoral interventions may have little or no impact without other complementary interventions. For instance, an exclusive emphasis on hygiene education may achieve little in villages or squatter settlements where water supplies are inadequate and contaminated and provisions for sanitation, drainage and health care services are very inadequate, and where most parents are uneducated, have no title to the land they live on, and have to travel long distances to work each day, leaving their children unattended or inadequately cared for.

The factors listed in Figure 1.1 range from what might be termed the micro-scale factors in box C (the social, economic and environmental context of the household) and box D (on parental and child knowledge about how to avoid or cope with environmental hazards) through to box A which is the most macro scale of the international economic and political context. These international factors and the national factors listed in box B must be continuously kept in mind in considering the household's social, economic and environmental context (box C) since they provide so many limits and constraints on household and community action to address environmental problems. Although Figure 1.1 shows a linear progression from box A through to box E, obviously, the linkages between the different boxes is more complex than this. For instance, a household's social and economic context is much influenced by the level of infant and child health – as sick or injured children need treatment that has to be paid for and nursing that can cut down on adult time spent earning an income.

The Household

Figure 1.1 also shows how the concentration of this book, on the environmental context for children's daily lives and tasks (ie on the first half of box C) is only a part of the whole picture. It is so often national and international factors that are a primary cause or major contributor to the most serious environmental problems. However, except for the very small proportion of children born or brought up outside of a household, it is the environmental context of home, neighbourhood, school and (where relevant) place of work that has such an influence on their health and their development.

This environmental context is largely determined by the first four factors listed in box C. The *indoor environment* (at home, school, day-care and work) includes characteristics of the buildings (eg amount of space, extent of protection from the elements, extent of indoor air pollution) in which children live, study, play and work – and, where they work away from the home, the quality of that environment and the degree of protection from injury by machines, toxic chemicals etc. *Infrastructure and service provision* includes the quality and quantity of water, provision for sanitation and drainage, garbage collection/disposal, emergency services, health care, public transport etc.

The *immediate outdoor environment* covers the quality and ease of access to play space around the home or school and within the locality. Its impact on child health is both in terms of the extent to which it contains physical hazards and dangerous pathogens from excreta or wastes (especially for infants and young children) and its adequacy in terms of providing a stimulating environment for play and hence for physical, intellectual and social development. Some of the most common environmental hazards are animal and human excreta, faecal contamination of water and waste water, flooding and garbage if there is inadequate provision of the infrastructure and services noted above. The fourth factor is the *extent to which air, water, food, soil and noise pollution and other environmental hazards are controlled*. Within most cities, this includes the air and water pollution arising from industries and service enterprises, thermal power stations, intensive farming and motor vehicle emissions.

The social and economic context of the household are influenced by the bottom five factors in box C. The *quality and accessibility of health care* includes measures to prevent infection (eg immunization, health and nutrition education, provision of condoms or other measures to limit the spread of sexually transmitted diseases) or injury. It also includes the level of provision for accessible and affordable basic health services, including emergency services. The quality and extent of pre-natal, peri-natal and post-natal care and of provision for childbirth is obviously a very important

Figure 1.1 *The macro and micro context on which infant and child survival, health and development depend*

A The International Economic and Political Context
Nation's position within the world market and status in regard to development assistance agencies and the major economic powers/power blocs. This provides the international context for the national social, economic and political macro-context outlined below.

B The National Social, Economic and Political Context
1   The strength and prosperity of the national economy
2   Distribution of income and assets within the society by class, gender and ethnicity
3   National political and administrative structure and the capacity of national and local government to guarantee citizen rights and ensure equitable provision of basic services to all

Special relevance of:
•   The nature of the legal structure and the extent of protection for individuals from pollutants and occupational hazards and safeguarding of social, economic and political rights
•   The priority given to children (eg in health), to women (especially for reproductive health) and to environmental health

These set the context for the possibilities that parents have to obtain adequate livelihoods and the likelihood that government can (or will) ensure good environmental health, including the provision of infrastructure and services.

C Household's Social, Economic and Environmental Context
The environmental context is largely determined by:
•   The indoor environment at home, school, day-care and work
•   The immediate outdoor environment
•   Infrastructure and service provision within the residential area
•   Extent to which air, water, food, soil and noise pollution and other environmental hazards are controlled

The social and economic context is influenced by:
•   Quality and availability of health care provision
•   Income and access to resources for women and men
•   Ownership of assets or secure right to use them for women and men (eg land use rights)
•   Quality of educational services
•   Degree of community organization and support

(More details of each of these is given within the text)

Figure 1.1 *continued*

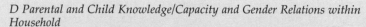

D *Parental and Child Knowledge/Capacity and Gender Relations within Household*

- Level of education and knowledge of child development and of health enhancing behaviour of adult women and men (especially carers) and children
- Knowledge of health enhancing behaviour among women and men at community level and level of community organization and solidarity (for instance in developing mutual support networks)
- Use made of health care system and other public services and facilities
- Knowledge of environmental hazards in and around the home so as to know how to avoid them or mitigate their effects
- Knowledge of the natural resources within the settlement/community which could be employed in child development and how to maximize use of these resources while maintaining ecological sustainability
- Gender relations which influence the proportion of income spent on children's needs and whether girl children are discriminated against

E *The Level of Infant and Child Health*

As indicated for girls and boys by:
- Physical, emotional, social and cognitive development including capacity to enjoy physical and social environment
- Frequency and type of ill health and nutritional status and disability
- Duration and severity of ill health and disability
- Levels and patterns of mortality

component. These should greatly diminish the toll taken by biological pathogens on the health of infants and of mothers during pregnancy and during and after childbirth. The second factor is the *income and access to resources for women and men* – and the kind of work available to different household members. In many societies, the level of income earned by mothers is more important for child health and nutrition than that earned by fathers, because a greater proportion is devoted to children's needs.[25] It is important to include not only income but also access to resources which allow food to be produced, collected or purchased, and time. For instance, the nutritional status of hundreds of millions of households is influenced by the extent to which low-income household members (usually women) can retain rights to open access and common property resources (cropland, water, forests, grazing lands, foraging rights) in the light of an increasing commercialization of resources. Certainly, one of the most damaging (but almost invisible) environmental problems is the increasing exclusion of millions of women from the resources to which they have long had access, as a result of such commercialization.[26] The time that different household members have to work to earn enough to maintain the household and the time taken getting to and from work are also important influences on the time that adult members have to prepare wholesome and nutritious food and to spend with children (including time spent playing with them and helping them learn). The income level and non-work time available to household members are also an important influence on the capacity of households to improve or extend housing and improve other aspects of the home and its surrounds.

The third factor is the *legal status* of land ownership (or use) for housing or for crop and livestock raising for women and men. This obviously influences the level of security that the household feels. An unclear or officially 'illegal' status obviously discourages household investments. A clear legal title also makes the land an economic asset and such assets have an important role in reducing the vulnerability of low-income households[27] and allowing credit to be obtained (or obtained more cheaply).

Fourth is the *quality and accessibility of educational services* which influence the level of literacy and education of parents and the education and physical and mental development of children. The educational level of parents is important for child health since the higher the educational level, the greater the possibility of learning about the protection and promotion of child health and development. The extent of provision for education, including provision for pre-primary school learning, also influences parents' (mainly mothers') income earning possibilities. The extent and quality of the education relating to health and the role of environmental factors and the ways in which environmental hazards can be avoided or their health impact prevented is also important. As Chapter 7 will outline, it is important for children's education but it is also important to involve children in research and action around environmental issues within their own community.

The final factor is the *degree of community support* – ie the extent to which parents can draw on the help of neighbours or on community organizations (formal and informal), when needed. This can be regarded as a resource, buffer or safety net. For instance, child health may be influenced by the degree of cohesion and mutual self-help within a low-income group – as a sick parent can turn to kin or friends or a community organization for help in looking after their children or for loans of food or money to help ensure the children are adequately fed and provided for when the income earners cannot work. This has particular importance where housing and living conditions and the provision of basic services are very poor. And as Chapter 6 will describe in more detail, it has great importance in influencing how much community or collective action can achieve in reducing environmental hazards and improving environmental quality.

There is also variety in the types of households, with different household structures having different implications for child health and survival. Single parent households are usually at a particular disadvantage, as only one adult has to combine looking after the children and maintaining the household with earning an income or producing or collecting the food to sustain household members. In addition, all households with children go through periods where costs are particularly high and income earning possibilities most constrained by the need for adult supervision of the children.

As box C within Figure 1.1 suggests, it is also difficult to separate a household's environmental context from its socio-economic context since the level of income and its distribution in any household will influence the quality of the housing (including the quality of infrastructure and services) and generally determine (or at least influence) the quality of health care to which they have access. The access that any household or individual has to a healthy physical environment (including safe and sufficient water, sanitation etc) is much influenced by their income level and/or their social status – although governments can greatly reduce the differences between the quality of the home environment of high-income and low-income households through efficient systems to provide piped water, sanitation, drainage, health care and other basic services to all households.

There are also the factors that influence the level of infant and child health that come between the micro-context of the household and the individual infant or child (box D in Figure 1.1). These include the parents' level of education and knowledge about health enhancing behaviour. One example of this is the level of education of a mother; infant and child mortality rates tend to be lower, the better educated the mother.[28] The precise reason for this may be difficult to ascertain but, given women's primary responsibility for child care in most societies, a mother's ability to read and to make use of health education materials which advise on how to prevent child illnesses and how to treat them is obviously an advantage.

Perhaps at least as important in this, however, is the increased status and self-confidence which education gives to a woman, and the fact that education usually alters the person's value and belief systems (eg by realizing that ill health is not a normal/universal state and that pathogens are responsible for many diseases). These more indirect influences of education on women have profound effects on her care for her children and the use that is made of the various official and unofficial support services in the community. The extent to which women have access to education is much influenced by the macro-context – for instance, the extent to which the society, at government, community and household levels, supports women's education, the level of priority given by the government to education and the extent to which the national economy generates the resources to allow this to be funded.

Children's health can also be strongly influenced by social and economic differentiation within households based on age and gender. This includes the differences in the roles that girls and boys are expected to take within households, which also means gender differences in the interaction of girls and boys with the environment and in their exposure to environmental hazards. It also includes differences in the way girls and boys are treated – for instance in attending schools and in use of health services, when they are sick or injured. In addition, gender relations affect the activities, knowledge and capacity of adult women and men themselves to ensure healthy environments for themselves and their children – for example, through differential access and control over income and its distribution in the household, and differential access to education. Since it is almost always women who take primary responsibility for feeding, clothing and looking after children, and seeking health care and medicines for children when they are sick, the proportion of household income on which women can draw has an important influence on the extent to which she can meet these responsibilities.

The Broader Context

A household's social, economic and environmental context is in turn influenced by what might be termed the national social, economic and political macro-context (see box B in Figure 1.1). This includes the distribution of income and capital assets as well as gender relations within the society. It also includes the national political and administrative structure, including its capacity and competence to respond to citizen demands and democratic pressures. The laws, codes, norms and practices of national, city and municipal governments, both in their form and in the way that they are enforced, obviously influence the context of households and their members. The priority given by a government to basic service provision is obviously one factor in its quality and coverage. The social and economic context is, for most households, also influenced by such factors as the level of prosperity within the national or regional economy.

Each nation's macro-context is in turn influenced by the international economic and political context, including the working of the international market (see box A in Figure 1.1). This international economic and political context has a strong influence on whether a particular government has the resources to allow it to become more effective at addressing environmental problems. It also influences the extent to which many individual households have the possibility of earning sufficient income. Consider, for instance, the case of the workforce in a particular factory in an Asian city which sells much of its output to Europe or North America. They may have their work hours (and wages) cut because of a fall in demand for that factory's product. This may in turn be the result of a protectionist barrier created by the European Union (EU) or the US government or the result of their own government's economic policy which increased the value of the national currency against that of their main export markets. Lower incomes for the workforce can mean poorer quality diets for their children who then become more vulnerable to diseases so that deaths from diarrhoea or measles, for example, may increase.

Consider, too, the impact of international policy. For example, structural adjustment has had many economic and social impacts on households – and a differential impact on different household members. It has resulted in the overexploitation of natural resources, either because of support to commercialization and privatization of land and forests or because of the reduction in subsidies for essential items such as kerosene. It has also increased the number of urban households with incomes below the poverty line and increased the intensity of their deprivation.[29] This affects adult women and men in the performance of their roles as producers, and women in their roles as home managers and mothers.[30] All have serious implications for the health of children in the household. Moreover, increases in the employment of girls and boys as part of households' survival strategy to cope with falling incomes and/or rising prices have also been recorded.[31] There is also the impact of structural adjustment on government-provided services like health, education and child care, which also has a direct impact on children and the capacity of parents to ensure their health and welfare. Among the parents, the burden from cuts in such services generally falls most heavily on women, given the gender division of labour in most societies.

MAIN CONSTRAINTS ON CHILD HEALTH AND DEVELOPMENT IN POORER NATIONS

For many of the nations with low per capita incomes, the main constraints to improved health (and a healthier environment) lie more in the national and international macro-context. If one reviews the list of what the UN terms the world's 'least developed nations', it is difficult to imagine how many of them can ever, under current conditions, achieve a level of economic stability and prosperity which allows the elimination of poverty and a continuous improvement in environmental health and health services. Many of these countries lack a stable, viable economic base to allow them to function effectively as nation states. If one takes an inventory of their resources and potential areas where some comparative advantage can be developed, they have very little that the world market wants that cannot be produced more cheaply in another nation. On the other hand, most lack the resources and trained personnel to provide adequate living standards for their citizens, using only their own internal resources.

The economic future for such nations (and in effect the health future for their children and other citizens) is bleak without a worldwide redistribution of resources in their favour and a more equitable deal from the world market (the main exports of most such nations are primary commodities whose price within the world market has fallen steadily, in comparison to manufactured goods).* In such nations, more can be done to improve health and the way environmental resources are used, but achievements will always be limited by economic constraints. It is also not uncommon for poor and unstable economies to experience political instability, from internal and/or external conflict and this greatly limits the possibility of available resources being used in the most effective manner for supporting child health and development. In such countries, the national and international context will always limit the level of health the population is likely to achieve.

This does not mean that a country's level of wealth is the sole determinant of the possibilities for health. In fact, there are very large differences in health indicators between countries with similar per capita incomes. Figure 1.2 shows that average life expectancy between nations generally increases with per capita income, but with significant variations. The outliers in this graph of the relationship between per capita income and life expectancy are

---

* The discussions in the mid 1970s about the 'New International Economic Order' sought to address this issue but with little success and with all such discussions virtually ceasing during the 1980s.

particularly interesting. Jamaica, Costa Rica, China, Sri Lanka and Cuba[*] have unusually high levels of life expectancy at birth, relative to their per capita income while the reverse is true for Congo, Gabon, Botswana, South Africa, Brazil and several oil-rich Arab states. Although some care must be used in interpreting this figure, in that several of the oil-rich Arab states which perform poorly in Figure 1.2 also had some of the world's most rapid improvements in average life expectancy over the last 30 years or so, what this figure shows is that there are variations of 10–15 years in the average life expectancy of people in nations with comparable per capita incomes – at least for countries with levels of per capita income below $12,500. For instance, in countries with per capita incomes of around $1000, average life expectancies vary from under 45 years to close to 60 years. In countries with per capita incomes of around $3000, the range is from under 55 to over 70.

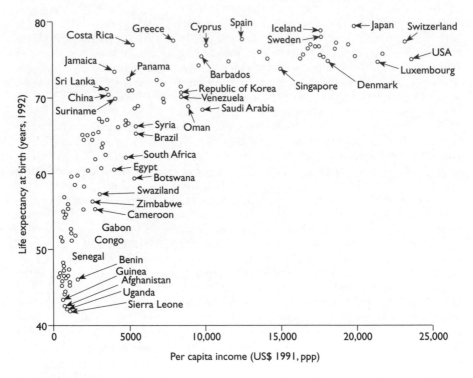

Figure 1.2 *Nation's average life expectancy at birth against per capita income*

Similar analyses to that shown in Figure 1.2 can also be done within countries, to highlight the extent to which life expectancy varies between the richer and poorer regions. In countries where there are large regional differences in per capita income and considerable differences among sub-national

---

* Cuba is also among the most outstanding performers in terms of life expectancy relative to per capita income, but Cuba is not included in Figure 1.2 because statistics for Cuba's per capita income were not included in the dataset on which Figure 1.2 draws.

(regional, provincial or state) governments in the priority they give to health and education, the differences in infant mortality rates or in life expectancy can be dramatic. For instance, within Brazil, life expectancy within the poor north-east is 17 years lower than in the much more wealthy south while in Nigeria, there is a 20 year difference in life expectancy between Borno State and Bendel State.[32] Among Brazil's major cities, average life expectancy varied by 22 years in 1988 with the city of Fortaleza having a life expectancy of just 51 years compared to 73 years in Porto Alegre.[33] Comparable differences in life expectancy exist between states in India where certain states (the best known of which is Kerala) have much higher life expectancies and much lower infant and child mortality rates relative to their per capita income than other states. Life expectancy in Kerala is 11–12 years higher than India as a whole.[34] This is also little related to per capita income; indeed, Kerala, the best performer in most social indicators, is not among the wealthiest states in India.[35]

Again at the micro-level, the quality of housing, living and working conditions are also much influenced by the broader economic context. A rapidly growing national economy increases the possibility that incomes for some poorer groups will rise and that more public resources can be devoted to improving water supply, sanitation, health care and other services, but in itself it is not sufficient; political and socio-economic structures limit the allocation of resources to this and often ensure that most of the benefits are concentrated in the hands of a small proportion of the population. By contrast, a stagnant economy will limit the possibility of improved health although there are examples of changes in government policies that improved the level of health for poorer groups, despite economic stagnation. For instance, in Brazil, provision for the supply of water and sanitation improved considerably during the 1980s, although the economic performance was much weaker than in the 1960s and 1970s. A study of 22 low-income countries found that the significantly positive relationship between life expectancy and per capita income disappears in a regression of life expectancy against poverty incidence, public health spending and average income. As the study notes: this does not imply that economic growth is unimportant in expanding life expectancy but that the importance of growth lies in the way that its benefits are distributed between people and the extent to which growth supports public health services.

'Average income matters but only insofar as it reduces poverty and finances key social services.'[36]

ENVIRONMENTAL PROBLEMS, POLITICAL SOLUTIONS?

It is easier to point to the environmental hazards that have the greatest impact on infants and children, as will be done in later chapters, than to state precisely the best means to reduce them. This and later chapters describe a whole range of environmental hazards for girl and boy children that can be identified in rural and urban settlements, but addressing them may depend as much on non-environmental factors (eg provision of schools and health services, increased income levels for lower income groups) as on environmental improvement. The wide range of environmental hazards to which many children are exposed in workplaces may be solved by environmental legislation but are more likely to be eliminated through households no longer needing to have under-age children working illegally as part of their survival strategy. Thus, addressing environmental problems cannot be separated from development goals, since the achievement of development goals can greatly reduce the environmental hazards which are the greatest risk to child health and survival. But increasing per capita incomes and the increases in urbanization and industrial development that usually accompany it also bring new environmental hazards and economic and social changes that can make households more vulnerable to such hazards.

Several developmental factors underpin a reduction in life and health threatening environmental hazards within the household and the living and working environments of different household members. Among the most important are: prosperous economies, a relatively equitable distribution of income and assets within a society and an effective, accountable government, spurred into action on environmental issues by an electorate. The role of government in environmental protection is at least threefold:

- to ensure that all sections of the population have access to safe and healthy homes (which include adequate provision for water, sanitation and drainage);
- to ensure that health care and educational opportunities are available and accessible to all and include those elements which limit environmental hazards or increase women and men's, girls' and boys' capacity to avoid or cope with them; and
- to ensure that pollution (and other environmental hazards) are controlled or reduced.

It might be suggested that the most serious, life and health threatening environmental hazards in any nation are best dealt with through increasing prosperity and internal political processes which demand a more equitable distribution of the benefits. An increasingly prosperous economy can permit a greater societal investment in improved living and working environments while increased purchasing power for poorer groups also permits a greater effective demand for piped water, sanitation, better quality housing and health care. But there are four reasons why the solution to environmental problems should not be left to *economic development*:

1 *Many nations are experiencing long term economic difficulties*, so it cannot be assumed that the environmental problems that take the greatest toll on child health will be resolved by increasing prosperity. What is needed within each country and neighbourhood is an internal process that identifies the range and relative importance of environmental problems there (and their causes) and reviews the priority they should receive in the use of

limited resources. There is still a tendency to dismiss environmental problems as something to worry about when an economy becomes increasingly urbanized and industrialized. This is largely the result of a very restricted view of 'the environment'; it certainly misses the toll taken on health by biological pathogens in the human environment and usually underestimates the current and future cost of soil, forest, air and water degradation.

2 *Conversely, many of the most serious life and health threatening environmental problems can be much reduced with relatively modest expenditures and without the need for a society to wait until it is 'prosperous'.* The monetary cost of substantially reducing some of the most serious environmental health hazards for infants and children by ensuring safer and more adequate water supplies, improved sanitation and drainage and safer and more healthy homes, schools and neighbourhoods is not very great. This has been demonstrated by many projects or programmes in Africa, Asia and Latin America, as can be seen in the examples given in Chapter 6. This chapter also shows how community-based, community-driven approaches often achieve remarkable cost savings, in comparison to conventional government or contractor implemented approaches. These need to be complemented by effective programmes of vaccination and measures to address micronutrient deficiencies and to ensure that medicines are readily available to treat the most common diarrhoeal and respiratory infections and intestinal parasites – and these are also not costly .[37]

Countries or regions do not need to reach income levels per person that are typical in West Europe or North America to greatly reduce the most serious life and health threatening environmental problems. But they do need a greater priority by governments and development assistance agencies to child health and development and to its social, economic and environmental underpinnings. WHO recently made a statement that extreme poverty was 'the world's most ruthless killer' and the largest cause of suffering on earth; it also stated that poverty is the main reason why mothers die in childbirth, babies are not vaccinated, clean water and sanitation not provided, and curative drugs and other treatments are not available.[38] This UN agency that is responsible for 'health' has long stressed the economic and social conditions that underlie so much disease, injury and premature death. But the analysis needs to go further since it is not so much poverty that underlies this but the fact that most governments and international agencies do not give a higher priority to reducing poverty and to reducing the health consequences of being poor.

3 *The growing health burden which will accompany economic growth, if provisions are not made to limit or eliminate them.* Most of the more prosperous and industrialized economies in the South now have serious problems with chemical contamination and other environmental hazards in workplaces, toxic/ hazardous waste management in urban centres, air pollution in their major cities and large numbers of the urban population living on sites at risk from landslides, floods or other natural hazards. Many of the most prosperous cities in the South also have increasing problems keeping up with demand for water. These problems could have been much diminished if action had been taken earlier in anticipation of such problems.

4 There are global limits to the level of resource use and waste generation world-wide. Underlying the assumption that economic growth is the solution to environmental problems in the South is a second assumption that it is feasible for the South to achieve levels of resource use comparable to the North. But there are serious doubts about whether planetary resources and waste-assimilation capacities can cope with a growing proportion of a growing world population coming to depend on levels of resource use comparable to those enjoyed by most people in the North today. But since stronger and more stable economies in the South will imply rising consumption levels, even where provision is made to use resources efficiently, this also requires cuts in levels of resource use and waste generation in the North. These global environmental limits will be discussed in greater detail in Chapter 5. The conclusion is that continued economic growth cannot be relied on to solve local environmental problems and alternative solutions need to be identified.

REFERENCES

1   WHO (1992), *Our Planet, Our Health*, Report of the Commission on Health and Environment, Geneva.

2   WHO (1992), 'World Malaria situation 1990', Division of Control of Tropical Diseases, WHO, *World Health Statistics Quarterly*, Vol 45, No 2/3, pp 257–66.

3   This figure is calculated from the tables in the back of the 1993 World Development Report – see World Bank (1993), *World Development Report 1993; Investing in Health*, Published for the World Bank by Oxford University Press, Oxford.

4   WHO (1995), *The World Health Report 1995: Bridging the Gaps*, WHO, Geneva.

5   See for instance Wohl, Anthony S (1983), *Endangered Lives: Public Health in Victorian Britain*, Methuen, London.

6   Wohl 1983, op cit; Bairoch, Paul (1988), *Cities and Economic Development: From the Dawn of History to the Present*, Mansell, London.

7   See WHO 1995, op cit for many examples.

8   For a discussion of this, see Lalonde, D (1974), *A New Perspective on the Health of Canadians*, Canadian Department of Health and Welfare, Ottawa; Howe, G M (1986), 'Does it matter where I live', *Transactions*, New Series, Institute of British Geographers, Vol 11, No 4, pp 387–411; and Foster, Harold D (1992), *Health, Disease and the Environment*, John Wiley and Sons, Chichester.

9   Hart, Roger (1996), *Children's Participation in Sustainable Development: The Theory and Practice of Involving Young Citizens in Community Development and Environmental Care*, Earthscan, London, 1996 – Chapter 7 in this book was written by Roger Hart to emphasize the links between the two books.

10 Ibid

11 WHO/UNICEF (1993), *Water Supply and Sanitation Sector Monitoring Report 1993*, Water Supply and Sanitation Collaborative Council.

12 WHO/UNICEF 1993, op cit; Sinnatamby, Gehan (1990), 'Low cost sanitation' in Jorge E Hardoy et al (Ed), *The Poor Die Young: Housing and Health in Third World Cities*, Earthscan, London.

13 See Cairncross, Sandy, *Sanitation and Water Supply: Practical Lessons from the*

Decade, Water and Sanitation Discussion Paper Series, DP Number 9, World Bank, Washington DC, 1992.

14 Goldstein, Greg (1990), 'Access to life saving services in urban areas' in Jorge E Hardoy et al (Ed) *The Poor Die Young: Housing and Health in Third World Cities*, Earthscan, London.

15 UNCHS (1996), *An Urbanizing World: Global Report on Human Settlements 1996*, Oxford University Press, Oxford.

16 Around 150,000 people were evicted from their homes in Delhi as part of a city 'beautification' programme between 1975 and 1977 – see Shrivastav, P P (1982), 'City for the Citizen or Citizen for the City: the Search for an Appropriate Strategy for Slums and Housing the Urban Poor in Developing Countries – the Case of Delhi', *Habitat International*, Vol 6, No 1/2, pp 197–207.

17 The number of children worldwide who die as a result of not being immunized against the vaccine-preventable diseases has been reduced very considerably since 1985, although in 1993, there were still some 2.4 million children under five years of age who died from such diseases – see WHO 1995, op cit.

18 See The Ecologist, (1992) *Whose Common Future: Reclaiming the Commons*, Earthscan, London, 1992, and Audefroy, Joël (1994), 'Eviction trends worldwide – and the role of local authorities in implementing the right to housing', *Environment and Urbanization*, Vol 6, No 1, April, pp 8–24.

19 See as one example Asian Coalition for Housing Rights (1989), 'Evictions in Seoul, South Korea', *Environment and Urbanization*, Vol 1, No 1, April, pp 89–94.

20 Ibid; The Ecologist 1992, op cit.

21 UNCHS 1996, op cit.

22 See for instance Audefroy 1994, op cit and Hunsley Magebhula, Patrick (1994) 'Evictions in the new South Africa: a narrative report from Durban', *Environment and Urbanization*, Vol 6, No 1, April.

23 See for instance many papers in *Environment and Urbanization* Vol 7, Nos 1 and 2 (1995) which consider different aspects of poverty, especially the editorials in both issues, Chambers, Robert (1995), 'Poverty and livelihoods; whose reality counts?' and Wratten, Ellen (1995), 'Conceptualizing urban poverty' both in *Environment and Urbanization*, Vol 7, No 1, April, pp 59–62.

24 Ibid.

25 World Bank 1993, op cit; see also Kanji, Nazneen (1995), 'Gender, poverty and structural adjustment in Harare, Zimbabwe', *Environment and Urbanization*, Vol 7, No 1, April, pp 37–55.

26 Lee-Smith, Diana and Catalina Hinchey Trujillo (1992), 'The struggle to legitimize subsistence: Women and sustainable development' *Environment and Urbanization* Vol 4, No 1, April, pp 77–84.

27 Chambers, Robert (1989), 'Editorial introduction: vulnerability, coping and policy', in *Vulnerability: How the Poor Cope*, IDS Bulletin, Vol 20, No 2, April, pp 1–7.

28 Caldwell, John C and Pat Caldwell (1985), 'Education and literacy as factors in health', in Scott B Halstead, Julia A Walsh and Kenneth S Warren (Eds), *Good Health at Low Cost*, Conference Report, Rockefeller Foundation, New York, pp 181–185.

29 Moser, Caroline O N, Alicia J Herbert and Roza E Makonnen (1993), *Urban Poverty in the Context of Structural Adjustment; Recent Evidence and Policy*

Responses, TWU Discussion Paper DP #4, Urban Development Division, World Bank, Washington DC. For specific examples, see also Kanji 1995, op cit and Latapí, Augustín Escobar and Mercedes González de la Rocha (1995), 'Crisis, restructuring and urban poverty in Mexico', *Environment and Urbanization*, Vol 7, No 1, April, pp 57–75.

30 Commonwealth Secretariat (1989), *Engendering Adjustment for the 1990s*, Report of the Commonwealth Export Group on Women and Structural Adjustment, London.

31 See for example Barrón, Anonieta (1994), 'Mexican rural women wage earners and macro economic policies', and Evers, Barbara (1994), 'Gender bias and macroeconomic policy: methodological comments from the Indonesian example', both in Isabel Bakker (Ed), *The Strategic Silence: Gender and Economic Policy*, Zed Books in association with the North–South Institute, London.

32 UNDP (1994), *Human Development Report 1994*, UNDP, Oxford University Press, Oxford and New York.

33 Mueller, Charles C (1995), 'Environmental problems of a development style: the degradation from urban poverty in Brazil', *Environment and Urbanization*, Vol 7, No 2, October, pp 68–84.

34 Sen, Amartya (1994), *Beyond Liberalization: Social Opportunity and Human Capability*, Development Economics Research Programme DEP No 58, London School of Economics, London.

35 Ibid.

36 Anand, S and M Ravallion (1993), 'Human development in poor countries: on the role of private incomes and public services', *Journal of Economic Perspectives*, Vol 7, No 1, Winter, pp 143–144.

37 See WHO 1995 op cit and UNICEF (1995), *The State of the World's Children 1995*, Oxford University Press, Oxford and New York.

38 WHO 1995, op cit, p 1.

2

The Links between Environment
and Health

INTRODUCTION

This chapter describes the different environmental hazards present in the human environment and the toll they take on health. Virtually all such hazards can be greatly reduced or eliminated or their health impact much reduced. Most are only there because of human action (for instance high levels of air pollution from industries, power stations and road vehicles) or human inaction (for instance the failure of governments to ensure residential areas have safe, protected water supplies and drains). Where possible, figures are given for the number of people who are disabled or die each year from each hazard, or are at risk. There is some overlap between this and the next chapter, but while this chapter concentrates on the environmental hazards, Chapter 3 concentrates on the infant and the young and older child and what makes them particularly vulnerable to environmental hazards.[*]

Both this chapter and Chapter 3 try to remain readable to people who are not specialists in child health or environmental health. Both chapters necessarily mention a long list of diseases where the disease causing agent (pathogen) is in the human environment and enters the human body through the air or through eating food or drinking water or via some disease vector (for instance through an insect bite). Many of the names of these diseases have become much less familiar to those living and working in the wealthier countries, as the incidence of such diseases and their health impact have been enormously reduced by improved housing and living conditions, better diets and the almost universal provision of piped water, sanitation, drainage, garbage collection and health care. For instance, typhoid, typhus and cholera spread by contaminated water or food were major causes of infant and child death in the North 100 years ago and are

---

[*] The reader who is primarily interested in the link between children and the environment might want to read Chapter 3 first, and use Chapter 2 more as a reference text on particular environmental hazards.

now almost unknown. Many diseases discussed in this chapter where infection is spread by bacteria or viruses in airborne droplets – for instance tuberculosis, measles, whooping cough, influenza and meningitis – are major causes of child death in many parts of the South but rarely cause child death in the North. Diseases such as pneumonia and influenza may remain common in the North but are rarely causes of infant or child death; they remain among the largest causes of child death in the South.

This chapter describes the hazards to health within the human environment under seven headings – see Box 2.1. Four have a direct bearing on health: biological pathogens and their vectors or reservoirs, chemical pollutants, a shortage of (or lack of access to) particular natural resources, and physical hazards. These are the four most pressing environmental problems in Africa and much of Asia and Latin America, in terms of their current impact on health (especially infant and child health).

Three others also influence health (although less directly): aspects of the built environment with negative consequences on psychosocial health, natural resource degradation, and national/global environmental degradation (including a rising concentration of greenhouse gases in the atmosphere and the depletion of the stratospheric ozone layer).

BIOLOGICAL PATHOGENS

Among the seven kinds of environmental hazard listed in Box 2.1, it is the biological pathogens in the human environment, in water, food, air or soil, that take much the greatest toll on health.[1] These pathogens can be classified according to the medium through which human infection takes place: foodborne, airborne and water-related. Not all pathogens fall into exclusive categories, since many can be ingested either through contaminated food or through contaminated water. In addition, some transmission is direct human-to-human – for instance faeces on hands to the mouth of another person.

Table 2.1 presents examples of the main water-related infections with estimates of morbidity, mortality and population at risk. These are grouped under headings which describe how infection takes place. Waterborne and foodborne diseases are caught from water or food contaminated with disease-causing bacteria or viruses from human or animal excreta, while water-washed diseases are those which diminish when there is sufficient water to be used for regular washing. Water-based diseases are ones in which the disease-causing agent spends part of its life in an aquatic animal, while diseases with water-related insect vectors are those in which the insect whose bite transmits the disease breeds or bites near water. Waterborne diseases are the second single largest category of communicable diseases contributing to infant mortality worldwide – after acute respiratory infections. Waterborne diseases account for more than three million deaths per year.[2] They are second only to tuberculosis in contributing to adult mortality, with one million deaths per year. In contrast, very few fatal cases of waterborne diseases are now recorded in Europe or North America. Diarrhoeal diseases account for most waterborne infant and child

Box 2.1 **Hazards to Health within the Environment**

1 *Biological pathogens and their vectors/reservoirs within the human environment* which impair human health – including, for instance, the many pathogenic micro-organisms in human excreta, disease vectors such as malaria-carrying mosquitoes, disease reservoirs such as plague-carrying rats, and airborne pathogens (for instance those responsible for acute respiratory infections and tuberculosis).

2 *Chemical pollutants within the human environment* – for instance chemicals added to the environment by human activities – eg industrial wastes or particulate matter in the air from fossil fuel combustion or pesticides.

3 *Inadequate quantity or availability of natural resources on which human health depends* – for instance food, water and fuel.

4 *Physical hazards* – including both those within the house (domestic injuries often figure as major causes of children's injuries and in some circumstances major causes of death) and the wider settlement (including road traffic hazards in the places where children play, and flooding, landslides and mudslides).

5 *Aspects of the built environment with negative consequences on psychosocial health* (eg inadequate protection against noise, poor design, inadequate provision of infrastructure, services and security, and inadequate provision for maintenance and supervision of common areas).

6 *Natural resource degradation* – including soil erosion and deforestation and the degradation of air, soil and water quality as a result of gaseous, liquid and solid wastes.

7 *National/global environmental degradation* with more indirect but long term impacts on human health. These include: the depletion of finite non-renewable resource bases; and wastes from human activities which contribute to possible threats to the functioning and stability of global cycles and systems; and the increasing frequency of extreme climatic conditions (eg greenhouse gas emissions and gaseous emissions which contribute to the depletion of the stratospheric ozone layer).

deaths and a high proportion of illnesses. Risk factors include overcrowding, poor sanitation, contaminated water and inadequate food hygiene.[3] As Chapter 1 noted, most of the urban and the rural population in the South lack homes with adequate provision for sanitation.[4]

Among the many water-based and water-related diseases, schistosomiasis, filariasis, guinea-worm (dracunculiasis) and intestinal worms (especially roundworm and hookworm), stand out for the debilitation they cause; only a small proportion of those with these diseases die from them but they cause severe pain and some disability to millions of people.[5] The infectious eye and skin diseases listed in the table such as impetigo, scabies and the different forms of conjunctivitis (especially trachoma) are also common and unpleasant – but their incidence is considerably reduced with

Table 2.1 *Most Serious Water-related Infections with Estimates of the Burden of Morbidity and Mortality they cause and the Population at Risk*

Disease (Common name)	(name)	Morbidity	Mortality (No of deaths/year)	Population at risk
1 Waterborne (and water washed;* also foodborne)				
Cholera	Cholera*	More than 300,000	More than 6000	
Diarrhoeal diseases	this group includes: salmonellosis,* shigellosis,* Campylobacter,* E. coli, rota-virus, amoebiasis* and giardiasis*	700 million or more people infected each year, 1.8 billion episodes a year	More than 3 million	More than 2000 million
Enteric fevers	Paratyphoid Typhoid	500,000 cases; 1 million infections (1977–8)	25,000	
Infectious jaundice	Hepatitis A*			
Pinworm	Enterobiasis			
Polio	Poliomyelitis	204,000	25,000	
Roundworm	Ascariasis	800–1000 million infected; 214 million with clinical symptoms	60,000	
Leptospirosis	Leptospirosis			
Whipworm	Trichuriasis	133 million cases		
2 Water washed				
(a) Skin and eye infections				
Scabies	Scabies			
Impetigo	Impetigo			
Trachoma	Trachoma	6–9 million people blind 13 million infected;	197,000	500 million
Leishmaniasis	Leishmaniasis	400,000 new infections/year		350 million

(b) Other				
Relapsing fever	Relapsing fever			
Typhus	Rickettsial diseases			
3 Water based				
(a) Penetrating skin				
Bilharzia	Schistosomiasis	200 million infected	Over 200,000	500–600 million
(b) Ingested				
Guinea worm	Dracunculiasis	Over 10 million infected		Over 100 million
4. Water-related insect vector				
(a) Biting near water				
Sleeping sickness	African Trypanosomiasis	20,000 new cases/year	55,000	50 million
(b) Breeding in water				
Filaria	Filariasis (lymphatic)	100 million people infected		900 million
Malaria	Malaria	267 million infections a year; 107 million clinical cases a year	2 million (more than half children under 5)	2100 million
River blindness	Onchocerciasis	18 million infected (over 300,000 blind)	35,000	85–90 million
Yellow fever	Yellow fever	200,000 new cases/year	30,000	
Breakbone fever	Dengue fever	Millions of cases each year with 500,000+ people needing hospital treatment	23,000	

Source: Adapted from WHO (1992), Our Planet, Our Health, Report of the World Commission on Health and Environment, *Geneva. The structure of the table was drawn from Cairncross, Sandy and Richard G Feachem (1983).* Environmental Health Engineering in the Tropics - An Introductory Text, *John Wiley and Sons, Chichester; and White, G F, D J Bradley and A U White (1972),* Drawers of Water: Domestic Water Use in East Africa, *University of Chicago Press, Chicago. Figures for morbidity, mortality and population at risk from WHO (1991),* Global Estimates for Health Situation Assessment and Projections 1990, *Geneva, April, with figures updated from WHO (1995),* The World Health Report 1995: Bridging the Gaps, *World Health Organization, Geneva.*

adequate provision for water supply and sanitation;[6] Trachoma is also one of the major causes of blindness worldwide.[7] By contrast, malaria, whose vector, the *anopheline* mosquito, breeds in water, causes two million deaths a year including hundreds of thousands of infant and child deaths as well as morbidity and debility, especially (but not only) in sub-Saharan Africa. An estimate for 1993 suggested that 940,000 children under age five died of malaria.[8] Malaria can also bring serious economic burdens as income-earners miss work; in a study of Sudanese households, each lost, on average, 40 working hours a year from malaria alone.[9]

Biological contaminants are the main causes of foodborne diseases and are responsible for a wide range of diarrhoeal diseases – see Table 2.1.[10] Cholera and hepatitis A can be transmitted by food, as well as water. Contaminated or undercooked food are also the cause of some of the most widespread intestinal worms such as ascariasis (roundworm), trichinosis (whipworm) and taeniasis (beef and pork tapeworm). Crowded, cramped conditions, inadequate water supplies and inadequate facilities for preparing and storing food greatly exacerbate the risk of food contamination. McGranahan notes that:

> *'microbially contaminated food contributes to a high incidence of acute diarrhoea in Third World countries and foodborne diseases including cholera, botulism, typhoid fever and parasitism … microbial activity generally contributes to food spoilage while unsafe chemicals may deliberately be added to retard or disguise spoilage … food contamination is intimately linked to the sanitary conditions of food preparation, processing and even production.'[11]*

In addition:

> *'within the home, there are likely to be numerous interconnections and interactions among water, sanitation, flies, animal, personal hygiene and food that are responsible for diarrhoea transmission.'[12]*

Acute respiratory infections are the single largest cause of infant and child death in urban and rural areas. An estimated four to five million infants and children die each year of these infections (mostly from pneumonia or influenza), most of them before their first birthday. However, despite a considerable increase in research on them within the past decade, their extent, their health impact and the risk factors associated with them remain relatively poorly understood.[13] In recent studies in Accra and Jakarta, mothers reported that respiratory infections were among the most common sources of ill health among their children and themselves.[14] The quality of the indoor environment has an important influence on the incidence and severity of respiratory infections – perhaps most especially through overcrowding, inadequate ventilation, dampness and indoor air pollution from smoky open fires or poorly vented and inefficient stoves used for cooking and/or heating that use coal or wood, dung or some other biomass fuel. Working children's susceptibility to respiratory infections may be increased by dust and other chemical pollutants in factories and workshops.

Household members who spend most time indoors, especially time spent close to the fires or stoves, are obviously most at risk. It is generally women and girls who are at greater risk than men and boys, because within the gender-based division of work, they generally take responsibility for most cooking and for maintaining and managing the household.

A recent WHO report summarized the problem:

> '*Acute respiratory infections tend to be endemic rather than epidemic, affect younger groups, and be more prevalent in urban than in rural areas. The frequency of contact, the density of the population and the concentration and proximity of infective and susceptible people in an urban population promote the transmission of the infective organisms. Poorer groups ... are much more at risk because of the greater proportion of younger age groups, limited health and financial resources, and over-crowded households in congested settlements with limited access to vaccines and antibacterial drugs. The constant influx of migrants susceptible to infection and possible carriers of new virulent strains of infective agents, together with the inevitable increase in household numbers fosters the transfer of nasopharyngeal microorganisms.*'[15]

The incidence of tuberculosis is also linked to overcrowded conditions. Tuberculosis alone is responsible for some three million deaths each year and is the single largest source of adult death[16] accounting for a quarter of all adult deaths.[17] Around 95 per cent of sufferers live in the South.[18] The highest incidence tends to be among populations living in the poorest areas, with high levels of overcrowding and high numbers of social contacts. In urban areas, a combination of overcrowding and poor ventilation often means that TB infection is transmitted to more than half the family members.[19] Its incidence has been increasing rapidly over the past decade or so, probably linked to the spread of HIV/AIDS.[20]

Rheumatic fever and meningococcal meningitis are among the other diseases transmitted by biological pathogens where overcrowded conditions increase the likelihood of transmission.[21] Both remain serious health problems in much of the South; their health impact in the North has been much reduced. Meningococcal meningitis (sometimes referred to as epidemic meningitis) is usually transmitted by airborne droplets. Its health impact in wealthy nations has been enormously reduced both by less crowded and better ventilated housing and workplaces, and also by immunization, but outbreaks are common in many low-income countries, especially in Africa with some epidemics causing hundreds or even thousands of deaths. For instance, epidemics in the Sudan in 1988 and 1989 involved at least 38,805 cases with 2770 deaths reported.[22] Overall, this disease is thought to cause around 35,000 deaths a year.[23] Rheumatic fever, which develops in a small percentage of cases of streptococcal infection, occurs most commonly in children of between five and nine years of age. In the North, its incidence has been much reduced, as the infection from which it develops has also been controlled by early antibiotic treatment of severe sore throats. However, in the South, its incidence can be up to 70 times that in countries in the North, among children living in populations with overcrowded living conditions.[24]

There are also links between communicable respiratory diseases and indoor air pollution (for instance smoke from coal-burning or wood-burning stoves) but the nature of the link between the diseases and environmental aggravation of symptoms remains poorly understood.[25]

Several important diseases are spread by airborne infection or contact, such as measles and pertussis (whooping cough). These two diseases are easily prevented by vaccination. However, a combination of overcrowded conditions and a lack of health care services which can implement effective immunization programmes help ensure that these remain major causes of ill health and infant and child death.

There is also a large range of disease vectors which live, breed or feed within or around houses and settlements. The diseases they cause or carry include some of the major causes of ill health and premature death – especially malaria (*Anopheles* mosquitoes) and diarrhoeal diseases (cockroaches, blowflies and houseflies). There are many other diseases caused or carried by insects, spiders or mites that also have significant health impacts worldwide. These include: bancroftian filariasis (*Culex* mosquitoes), Chagas disease (triatomine bugs), dengue fever (*Aedes* mosquitoes), hepatitis A (houseflies, cockroaches), leishmaniasis (sandfly), relapsing fever (body lice and soft ticks), scabies (scabies mites), trachoma (face flies), typhus (body lice and fleas) and yellow fever (*Aedes* mosquitoes).[26] Many of these vectors thrive when there is poor drainage and inadequate provision for garbage collection, sanitation and piped water. *Anopheles* mosquitoes breed in clean water. The sandflies which transmit leishmaniasis can breed in piles of refuse or in pit latrines, while the *Culex quinquefasciatus* mosquitoes which are one of the vectors for bancroftian filariasis can breed in open or cracked septic tanks, flooded pit latrines and drains.[27]

Leptospirosis outbreaks have been associated with flooding in Sao Paulo and Rio de Janeiro – the disease passing to humans through water contaminated with the urine of infected rats or certain domestic animals.[28] The link between house structure and Chagas disease is particularly strong; the blood-sucking insects which are the vector of the parasite rest and breed in cracks in walls. An estimated 17 million people suffer from it and 45,000 die from it each year in Latin America[29] with some 65 million at risk.[30] As noted already, malaria spread by the Anopheline mosquito remains one of the major causes of infant, child and adult death worldwide – see Table 2.1. This table also shows how river blindness, yellow fever and dengue fever – which are, like malaria, spread by insect vectors breeding in water – take a large toll on human health.

Tetanus remains a major health problem, as tetanus spores enter the human body through a cut or wound – and neonatal tetanus claimed the lives of more than 500,000 newborn babies in 1993.[31] However, it is addressed by immunization and early treatment (including immunization) as it is not substantially affected by improving environmental quality. Neonatal tetanus can be much reduced or eliminated by immunizing women of childbearing age and/or by good delivery hygiene.

Box 2.2 **Chemical Pollutants within the Human Environment which are Hazardous to Human Health**

Chemicals which can be found in food and water:
- lead (in food, in drinking water, especially where there is a combination of lead water pipes and acidic water);
- aflatoxins and other natural food toxicants;
- nitrates in drinking water (and their conversion into nitrites in the body);
- trace pollutants in water supply, many from agro-chemicals (for instance various halogenated organic chemicals);
- aluminium (food and drinking water);
- arsenic and mercury.

Chemicals commonly found in the indoor environment (home/workplace):
- carbon monoxide (incomplete combustion of fossil fuels);
- lead (paint – ingested by children);
- asbestos (usually from roofing insulation or air conditioning conduits);
- smoke from combustion of coal and wood (or other biomass fuel);
- tobacco smoke;
- potentially dangerous chemicals used without health and safety safeguards (by home-workers and in occupational setting);
- formaldehyde (mostly from insulation; also some wood preservatives and adhesives).

Chemicals found outdoors in urban areas in the air (ambient):
- lead (exhausts of motor vehicles using gasoline with lead additive, from external paint, some industrial emissions);
- sulphur dioxide, sulphates and smoke/suspended particulates (mainly from coal or heavy oil combustion by industries, power-stations and, in some cities, households);
- oxides of nitrogen (in most cities, mostly from motor vehicle emissions; also some industries);
- hydrocarbons (motor vehicles, petrol stations, some industries);.
- ozone (secondary pollutant formed by reaction of nitrogen dioxide and hydrocarbons in sunlight);
- carbon monoxide (incomplete combustion of fossil fuels, mostly by motor vehicles);
- VOCs (Volatile Organic Compounds): there is a considerable range of such compounds, that are, or may be, hazardous.

Chemicals which may contaminate land sites:
- cadmium and mercury compounds and other heavy metal compounds (industrial wastes);
- dioxins, PCBs, arsenic, organochlorine pesticides (industrial wastes).

Also in both indoor and outdoor settings:
- micro-pollutants;
- mixtures each at trace level (with possible additive effects).

Box 2.3 **Health Impacts from Indoor Pollution from Biomass Fuels**

Biomass fuels include wood, logging wastes and sawdust, animal dung and vegetable matter containing grass, leaves, crop residues and agricultural wastes. These have the potential advantage of being a renewable energy resource. In rural subsistence economies, wood is usually plentiful initially but, in the absence of replanting, demand can grow to exceed supply.

Nearly half the world's population rely mainly or exclusively on biomass fuels for their daily energy needs. It is usually burnt in open fires or in a simple clay or metal stove. The stove is often at floor level adding to the risk of accidents, especially burns to children, and jeopardizing food hygiene. Often there is no chimney. In cool regions (including high altitudes in tropical countries), the combination of open fires or inefficient stoves, absence of chimneys and poor ventilation leads to severe indoor air pollution which has several adverse effects on human health.[33]

The combustion of raw biomass products produces hundreds of chemical compounds including: suspended particulate matter, carbon monoxide, oxides of nitrogen and sulphur, hydrocarbons, aldehydes, acenaphthelene, benzene, phenol, cresol, toluene and more complex hydrocarbon compounds including polyaromatic hydrocarbons. Although indoor concentrations vary considerably, it is very common for health guidelines to be exceeded by several orders of magnitude. Using improved stoves with ventilation and exhaust chimneys can reduce indoor emissions of suspended particulate matter by up to 60 per cent, carbon monoxide by up to 8 per cent and aldehydes by up to 30 per cent.[34]

The most serious health risks are from burns and smoke inhalation – with the severity of such risks dependent on the length and level of exposure. Although data on exposure levels are limited, it has been estimated that *exposure to pollutants is 60 times greater in indoor environments in the rural areas of the South than in urban areas in the North*. The principal adverse effects on health are respiratory but in poorly ventilated dwellings, especially when biomass fuels such as charcoal (and coal) are used to heat rooms in which people sleep, carbon monoxide poisoning is a serious hazard. Exposure to carcinogens in emissions from biomass fuel combustion has been confirmed in studies in which exposed subjects wore personal monitoring equipment. For example, women who spend two to four hours a day at the stove have been found to have high exposure levels to total suspended particulates and benzo-a-pyrene. This can be presumed to cause some risk of respiratory cancer. Children are often kept close to the fire or stove, both for warmth and to allow their mother to supervise them. They can also, therefore, be exposed to similar risks.

Chronic effects of indoor air pollution include inflammation of the respiratory tract caused by continued exposure to irritant gases and fumes, which reduces resistance to acute respiratory infections; and infection in turn enhances susceptibility to inflammatory effects of smoke and fumes, establishing a vicious circle of pathological changes. These processes may lead to emphysema and chronic obstructive pulmonary disease, which can progress to the stage where impaired lung function reduces the circulation of blood through the lungs, causing heart failure (cor pulmonale). Cor pulmonale is a crippling killing disease, characterized by a prolonged period of distressing breathlessness preceding death.

In many countries in Africa, Asia and Latin America, girls and women tend the fires and do the cooking, inhaling larger concentrations of pollutants over longer periods of time than men. The prevalence of chronic bronchitis has been found to be doubled in those chronically exposed to biomass fuels. This may also result in reduced lung function and at a later stage, up to six times greater prevalence of cor pulmonale, particularly in hilly cold regions. Tobacco smoking may be an added factor. Women are the main victims of this form of chronic obstructive lung disease, a fact confirmed by observational and epidemiological studies in India and in several Southeast Asian countries, parts of Africa and Central and South America. Another cluster of effects arises when the cook crouches close to the fire and sustains heat damage to the conjunctiva and cornea. These become chronically inflamed. Prolonged exposure can lead to keratitis, causing impaired vision and probably also increasing the risk of recurrent infection, cataract and ultimately blindness.

Source: WHO Commission on Health and the Environment,
Our Planet, Our Health, *WHO, Geneva, 1992.*

CHEMICAL POLLUTANTS

Box 2.2 lists some of the chemical pollutants which impact on human health – or about which there is concern, even if the precise health impact remains unknown. Among these, lead remains a particular concern, especially for children since there is increasing evidence to show that relatively low concentrations of lead in the blood may have a damaging effect on their mental development – and this is an effect which persists into adulthood.[32] The three major sources of lead are: exhausts from petrol-engined motor vehicles (except for vehicles which use lead-free petrol), lead water piping (especially where water supplies are acidic), and lead in paint (although there is also a long-established move towards lead-free paints).

Fumes from coal, wood and other biomass fuels indoors are also thought to be sources of major health problems; hundreds of millions of people (most of them relatively poor households in Africa, Asia and Latin America) are regularly exposed to potentially harmful emissions from open fires or poorly designed stoves with inadequate attention to venting the flue gases. Box 2.3 outlines their health impacts and why it is generally girls and women who are most affected.

In regard to air pollution outdoors, WHO has noted that in many cities, the mix and concentration of pollutants are already high enough to cause illness in more susceptible individuals and premature death among the elderly, especially those with respiratory problems.[35] Current air pollution levels may also be impairing the health of far more people – especially infants, children and the elderly – but in many cities, the data on the most common air pollutants is very limited. In addition, it is often difficult to prove links between particular pollutants and health impairment.

An estimated 1.4 billion urban residents worldwide are exposed to annual averages for suspended particulate matter or sulphur dioxide (or both) which are higher than the minimum standards recommended by WHO.[36] Based on exposure to suspended particulate matter alone, an estimated 300,000 to 700,000 premature deaths a year might be avoided in the South if unhealthy levels of particulates were reduced to the average yearly level WHO considers safe.[37] The (limited) data available for cities in the South suggest the trend is towards increasing concentrations.[38] A study of air pollution in 20 of the world's largest cities found problems with sulphur dioxide and suspended particulate matter to be especially serious in Beijing, Mexico City and Seoul.[39]

Comparable estimates are not available for nitrogen oxides and carbon monoxide although there are studies in particular cities or city districts which suggest that current ambient air pollution levels of these gases can impair health. There are also concerns about the health impacts of secondary pollutants formed as a result of reactions between primary pollutants and the air – for instance acid sulphates and ozone (see Table 2.2).

Air pollution in urban areas is usually a mix of oxides of nitrogen and sulphur and suspended particulates – mostly from coal and oil fired power stations, certain heavy industries, motor vehicle exhausts and, where they are used, coal, wood and oil fired domestic stoves or furnaces. There are also often secondary pollutants – for instance photochemical smog formed by the reaction of primary pollutants with sunlight. Table 2.2 outlines the effects on health of some of the most common urban air pollutants.

In certain industrial centres, air pollution levels can be sufficiently high to show demonstrable health impairment, especially for children. Chapter 3 will describe examples of this from Brazil (Cubatao) and Poland (Katowice). Many cities or particular city districts in both the North and the South have air pollution levels comparable to or higher than these two cases.[40]

Links between health problems and air pollution levels have also been suggested by comparisons between the health of people in highly polluted areas within cities and those in less polluted areas; some of these have shown a strong association between the incidence of respiratory infections and pollution levels. However, the interpretation of such associations, has proved problematic, as high pollution levels are often directly associated with other risk factors for these diseases such as malnutrition and crowding. The links between air pollution and health can also be seen in cities where acute episodes of high concentrations of air pollution occur at

Table 2.2 *Main Urban Air Pollutants and their Effects on Health*

Pollutant	Action	Effect
1 Traditional (reducing) pollutants from coal/heavy oil combustion		
Smoke/suspended particulates (some contribution from diesel traffic too)	Can penetrate to lungs; some retained: possible long-term effects. May also irritate bronchi	**London smog complex** *Short term effects*: sudden increases in deaths in hospital admissions and in illness among bronchitic patients; temporary reductions in lung function (patients and some normal people)
Sulphur dioxide	Readily absorbed on inhalation: irritation of bronchi, with possibility of bronchospasm	*Long term effects*: increased frequency of respiratory infections (children) increased prevalence of respiratory symptoms (adults and children); higher death rates from bronchitis in polluted areas
Sulphuric acid (mainly a secondary pollutant formed from sulphur dioxide in air)	Hygroscopic; highly irritant if impacted in upper respiratory tract. Acid absorbed on other fine particles may penetrate further to promote bronchospasm	
Polycyclic aromatic hydrocarbons (small contribution from traffic also)	Mainly absorbed on to smoke; can penetrate with it to lungs	*Possible carcinogenic effects*: may take some part in the higher incidence of lung cancer in urban areas
2 Photochemical (oxidizing) pollutants from traffic or other hydrocarbon emissions		
Hydrocarbons (volatile: petrol etc)	Non-toxic at moderate concentrations	**Los Angeles smog complex** *Short term effects*: primarily eye irritation. Reduced athletic performance. Possibly small changes in deaths, hospital admissions
Nitric oxide	Capable of combining with haemoglobin in blood but no apparent effect in humans	

Nitrogen dioxide and ozone (mainly secondary pollutants formed in photochemical reactions)	Neither gas is very soluble: some irritation of bronchi but can penetrate to lungs to cause oedema at high concentrations. Urban concentrations too low for such effects, but evidence of reduced resistance to infections in animals	*Longer term effects*: increased onsets of respiratory illnesses (children), increased asthma attacks (adults). No clear indication of increased bronchitis
Aldehydes, other partial oxidation products, peroxyacetylnitrate	Eye irritation, odour	
3 Others from traffic Carbon monoxide (other sources contribute – smoking an important one)	Combines with haemoglobin in blood, reducing oxygen-carrying capacity	Possible effects on central nervous system (reversible unless concentrations are very high). Some evidence of effects on perception and performance of fine tasks at moderate concentrations
Lead (some industrial sources contribute to air lead; human intake often dominated by lead in food and drink)	Taken up in blood, distributed in soft tissues and some to bone	Possible effects on central nervous system (longer time scale than in case of CO and not necessarily reversible).Indications of neuropsychological effects on children within overall environmental exposure range, but specific role of traffic lead uncertain

Source: Waller, Robert E (1991), 'Field investigations of air' in Holland W W et al (Eds), Oxford Textbook of Public Health, Vol 2: Methods of Public Health, Oxford University Press, Oxford

particular times (for instance when high emissions coincide with particular meteorological conditions) and there is often an increased incidence of mortality among particular vulnerable groups.[41]

In Latin America, studies suggest that air pollution levels are sufficiently high in many of its largest cities and industrial centres (Sao Paulo, Rio de Janeiro and Belo Horizonte, Bogota, Santiago, Mexico City, Monterrey and Guadalajara, Caracas and Lima) that a high priority should be given to their control. One estimate suggests that over two million children suffer from chronic cough as a result of urban air pollution and that air pollution causes an excess of 24,300 deaths a year in Latin America.[42] This same source estimated that some 65 million person days of workers' activities are lost to respiratory-related problems caused by air pollution. While the authors emphasize that these are rough estimates, they give an idea of the order of magnitude of the problem. Local topographical and climate conditions can exacerbate problems, as in Mexico City where thermal inversions help trap pollutants within the valley in which the city is located.

Chemical wastes dumped into water bodies or onto land sites can also cause disease. In most cities in the South, toxic/hazardous industrial and commercial wastes are disposed of in water bodies or land sites without special provision to treat them prior to disposal (to render them less damaging to human health and the local environment) or without measures to ensure that disposal itself isolates them from the environment. Meanwhile, there is often little or no incentive for industry and commerce to cut down polluting emissions since few businesses are penalized and the penalties, when imposed, are so small as to be little deterrent. Reports from cities of severe health problems arising from human contact with toxic or hazardous wastes are increasingly common[43] although in most cities, they are unlikely to be a major cause of the disease burden compared to the biological pathogens described earlier.

There are also the health impacts of occupational exposures to chemical pollutants and of occupational injuries as a result of accidents. Estimates for 1993 suggest at least 220,000 deaths and 120 million injuries from accidents at work and 69 million new cases of occupational disease.[44] Environmental hazards are evident in workplaces from large factories and commercial institutions down to small 'backstreet' workshops and work done within the home. They include dangerous concentrations of toxic chemicals and dust, inadequate lighting, ventilation and space, and inadequate protection of workers from machinery and noise. Many case studies can be cited which show a high proportion of the female and/or male workers in particular industries or industrial plants whose health is affected by workplace exposures. For instance, a study of an Egyptian pesticide factory found that 'about 40 per cent of the workers had problems related to pesticide poisoning, ranging from asthma to enlarged livers',[45] while in Malaysia similar symptoms have been found among the largely female labour force in agricultural plantations.[46]

In most countries, the scale of occupational injuries and diseases is almost certainly greatly under-reported. For instance, the Mexican Social Security Institute reported an average of 2000 to 3000 cases of work-related illnesses across the country in 1988 but a study in just one large steel mill found 4000–5000 cases alone, with more than 80 per cent of the workers exposed to extreme heat, loud noise and toxic dust.[47] A paper on Bangkok's environmental problems noted that a remarkable number of Thai workers are exposed to poor working environments but that the number of workers suffering from occupational diseases is small: 'This may be a reflection of the difficulties of linking disease to working conditions rather than revealing a satisfactory condition'.[48] Other studies have shown serious health impacts for workers from exposure to toxic chemicals – for instance from benzene poisoning for leather workers in Turkey[49] and lead poisoning for people working in lead-acid battery repair shops in Kingston, Jamaica.[50]

Consideration must also be given to large scale accidents where chemicals had the central role in health impacts – for instance the accidental release of methyl iso-cyanate at Bhopal (over 3000 dead and perhaps 100,000 seriously injured)[51] or the natural gas explosions in Mexico City in 1984 (over 1000 dead) or the large loss of life, injury and damaged property resulting from explosions of gases which had accumulated in the sewers and drains in downtown Guadalajara in 1992.[52] There are also the various accidents that have happened in nuclear installations that have led to a release of radioactive materials – the fire in the Chernobyl nuclear power plant being the most serious such accident to date. Although dramatic and of very considerable local importance, these and other large scale accidents have a relatively minor health impact when compared to chronic problems, since they are local and acute in nature.

The attempts by European and North American industries to dispose of their toxic wastes in countries in Latin America, Asia and Africa have also received a lot of publicity. Although international action is seeking to control this – for instance through the Basel Convention[*] – the incentives to export such wastes or more general wastes contaminated with hazardous materials remain high as the production of such waste products continues to increase and as the costs of safely storing or disposing of them in the producing country are very high. However, in regard to the overall health impact of chemical pollutants, the scale of the impact arising from occupational exposures and from exposure to indoor and outdoor air pollution is likely to be larger and more widespread – but it remains poorly documented. The next 20–30 years may show that the health impact of pollutants in the South – in the air and water and through direct exposure in the home or workplace – has been considerably underestimated.

In regard to water quality, perhaps the two most worrying chemical pollutants are nitrates (mostly from chemical fertilizers washed by rain into water bodies) and pesticides. High levels of nitrates in drinking water may lead to serious or fatal consequences for infants under six months of age, as the nitrates are reduced to nitrites in the body which in turn impair the transport of oxygen from the lung to the tissues. In extreme cases, the result is severe methaemoglobinaemia (also known as blue baby syndrome).

Pesticides are the agricultural chemicals that cause most health concern.[53] Figure 2.1 illustrates the population groups at risk and gives estimates of the

---

[*] The Convention on the Control of Transboundary Movements of Hazardous Wastes and their Disposal that was adopted in 1989 and entered into force in 1992.

public health effect of pesticide use. Around three million people suffer from a single short-term exposure (including that linked to suicide attempts) with 220,000 deaths a year.[54] Over 700,000 people a year are thought to suffer from the chronic effects of long-term exposure.[55] Farmers and agricultural labourers working in farming operations which make intensive use of agricultural chemicals (pesticides included) are one group at particular risk.[56] For example, in Colombia, the 70,000 workers, mostly women, who do the cultivating, harvesting and sorting of flowers in the second largest flower industry in the world, have been found to suffer from a range of pesticide-induced symptoms.[57] The health impact is often much increased because of the extent to which toxic pesticides are used without adequate protective clothing or inappropriately used, especially where the labelling is poor (or in a foreign language) and where there is a high level of illiteracy.[58] Many highly hazardous pesticides which have been banned or whose use is very restricted in the North are still sold in the South.[59]

The scale and nature of pesticide poisoning is probably underestimated because the symptoms of the poisoning may be incorrectly ascribed to other causes.[60] It is also difficult for those affected or for medical personnel treating them to separate the effects of pesticide poisoning from the effects of other pathogens and of tiredness and overwork. The underestimation is also linked to the fact that a significant proportion of those exposed to pesticides have no health care system to which they can turn so their illnesses go unrecorded.

In regard to poisoning for infants and children, particular worries include:

- accidents, where toxic chemicals are not kept safely locked away from children's use;
- accidental contact through, for instance, spray drift when agricultural chemicals are being applied; and
- contact as a result of agricultural or horticultural work undertaken by children.

More details are given in Chapter 3 about the health risks to foetuses, infants and children, arising from pesticides.

THE AVAILABILITY, COST AND QUALITY OF NATURAL RESOURCES

The availability to any individual or household of such natural resources as food, fuel and fresh water is obviously central to their survival, health and development. The environmental dimension is prominent in that the ecosystem defines the limits for the availability of fresh water, fertile soils and trees. But social, economic and political factors tend to be dominant in influencing who has access to food, fresh water and fuel or to the land and water sources from which they can be drawn. For instance, worldwide and within most countries, there is no overall shortage of fertile land. Undernutrition is much more related to the undernourished people's lack

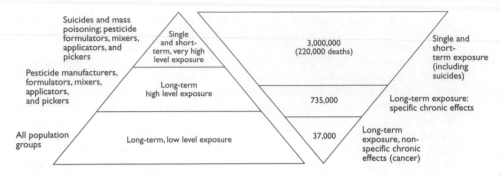

Source: WHO (1990) *Public Health Impact of Pesticides used in Agriculture*, World Health Organization, Geneva

Figure 2.1 *Population groups at risk from pesticides and the overall annual public health impact*

of economic and political power, rather than to an absolute shortage of the resource. This issue is explored in more detail in Chapter 4.

Similarly, only rarely does a shortage of freshwater resources explain why so many rural and urban households lack access to safe and sufficient water supplies. It is much more common for this to be the result of the low priority given to water supply (and sanitation) by governments and international agencies. In many urban areas, it is also linked to the refusal of public agencies or private utilities to provide services to illegal and informal settlements. Although there are cities and rural regions where overall shortages inhibit improved supplies, these are not the norm.

Water

As mentioned in Chapter 1, most households in the South lack safe, sufficient and convenient water supplies. Official UN statistics suggest that by the early 1990s, more than 80 per cent of the urban population and more than two thirds of the rural population in Africa, Asia and Latin America were 'adequately served' with piped water[61] – but these statistics considerably overstate the number. This is for two reasons. The first is the lack of an agreed definition of what is 'adequate' and the latitude given to governments in judging who is adequately served. The second is the tendency for governments to greatly exaggerate the proportion of people in their country with piped water supplies and UN agencies such as WHO, being inter-governmental organizations, are obliged to publish the water supply statistics supplied by their member governments.

People are considered adequately served with water if they have '...*access* to an *adequate amount* of *safe* drinking water located within a *convenient distance* from the user's dwelling.'[62] Each of the words in italics is defined within the respective countries, not by the international agencies responsible for monitoring and evaluating progress.[63] A considerable proportion of those who are said to have 'safe' water do not have drinking water at a convenient distance. Water is very heavy to carry any distance. A family of five or six persons needs around 300 litres of water a day to meet all its needs, the equivalent of 30 or more full buckets. Governments often claim that if a household is within 100 metres of a public standpipe, then it is adequately served. Even fetching and carrying water from a source 20–30 metres from a house is an onerous and time consuming task, if sufficient water is to be obtained for all basic domestic tasks. Eye and ear infections, skin diseases, scabies, lice and fleas are very difficult to control without sufficient supplies of water to permit regular washing and laundry.[64] The amount of water a family uses will be influenced greatly by the distance that water has to be carried to the home, so the convenience of a water source can be as important for health as its quality.[65]

Governments tend to include all those with public standpipes or boreholes with a handpump nearby as being adequately served. But there is often only one tap or pump for dozens or even hundreds of households. In low-income settlements in cities, especially the more peripheral illegal settlements, if there is piped water, there are usually hundreds of water users for each tap. Long queues at a public tap (especially if water is only available for a few hours a day, as is often the case) and time spent making repeated trips back to the house use up time that could be used in earning an income or completing other domestic tasks. In addition, many public water standpipes in urban areas are poorly maintained.

It is surprising to find how many countries claim that between 76 and 100 per cent of their urban and rural population have adequate water supplies when detailed studies from these same countries suggest much lower percentages. For instance, official statistics for India suggest that 87 per cent of its urban and its rural population had adequate provision for safe water in 1991, while those for Pakistan suggest a coverage of some 80 per cent for both rural and urban areas.[66] Burundi, Ethiopia and Ghana are among a number of African countries claiming that more than 90 per cent of their urban and rural population had access to safe water on this same date.[67] Even a cursory examination of conditions in low-income, urban settlements and in rural settlements in these countries suggest that these figures are greatly inflated. Thus, the proportion of the urban and rural population in Africa, Asia and Latin America that is said to have access to safe water supplies is certainly much larger than the actual proportion that has a regular, sufficient and convenient supply of good quality water at a cost they can afford.

One indication of this is the inadequacy in water supplies for much of the South's urban population living in squatter settlements. It is common for those in squatter settlements to pay private water vendors between 4 and 100 times as much per unit volume as middle and upper income groups pay for publicly provided piped water (see Table 2.3). Thus, it is generally neither an absolute lack of water nor indeed a lack of low-income households' willingness to pay which stops piped water supplies reaching poorer areas – but a refusal by government to extend the piped water supply to these areas.

Food

Certain forms of undernutrition are linked more clearly to environmental

Table 2.3 *Differentials in the Costs of Water between Poorer and Richer Groups*

Ratio of price charged by water vendors to the prices charged by the public utility (selected cities; mid 1970s–early 1980s).

City	Price ratio of water from private vendors:public utility
Abidjan	5:1
Dhaka	12:1 to 25:1
Istanbul	10:1
Kampala	4:1 to 9:1
Karachi	28:1 to 83:1
Lagos	4:1 to 10:1
Lima	17:1
Lome	7:1 to 10:1
Nairobi	7:1 to 11:1
Port-au-Prince	17:1 to 100:1
Surabaya	20:1 to 60:1
Tegucigalpa	16:1 to 34:1

Source: World Bank, World Development Report 1988, *Oxford University Press, p 146.*

Box 2.4 **Micronutrient Malnutrition**

Iodine: Goitre and cretinism are clinically obvious and easily recognizable forms of this deficiency, but the more pervasive but insidious effects of a milder deficiency on the survival and physical and mental development of children, intellectual ability and the work capacity of adults is not being recognized. About 1500 million people are affected in more than 118 countries; although iodine deficiency can be particularly prevalent in mountainous areas, the total global burden of this disease is probably greater in coastal areas and inland plains because of their greater population numbers. Excessive intakes of goitrogens (for example through eating cassava) interfere with the normal intake and metabolism of iodine and can amplify the effects of iodine deficiency.

Vitamin A: Vitamin A deficiency leading to xerophthalmia and sometimes blindness continues to be a widespread problem among children; this deficiency also decreases resistance to infections and thus increases mortality even at levels which do not cause clinical eye problems. A quarter of children under age five in the South are at risk of vitamin A deficiency. Analyses of food supplies from different regions show that the availability of vitamin A is limited and the problem exacerbated by any tendency to withhold foods with vitamin A (such as animal products, vegetables or fruits) from children for cultural or other reasons. The problem affects the greatest number of people in Asia because of its enormous population, and because maldistribution of foods high in vitamin A within populations can be very substantial. But very substantial numbers of people are also vitamin A deficient in many countries in Africa, the Pacific and probably, also, in parts of the ex-Soviet Union. Xerophthalmia continues to be a major problem in about 40 countries but sub-clinical vitamin A deficiency is much more widespread than this.

Iron: Anaemia, whose dominant cause is iron deficiency, remains a major problem; estimates made in 1980 suggest that it affected close to 200 million children between zero and four years of age and 217 million between 5 and 12. Over half the pregnant women in the South are anaemic (which also results in high rates of low birth weight). Most of the affected children and adults are in Southern Asia, although the proportion of the local population who are affected is also very high in Africa; in both these regions, half or more of all children in both age groups and close to half of all women are affected. More than three fifths of all pregnant women are affected in these two regions. Anaemia also affects significant proportions in each of the above groups in other regions. In many areas of the tropics or sub-tropics, existing dietary iron deficiency due to low intake of iron and/or its poor absorption may be complicated by hookworm infection which causes intestinal blood loss and may lead to profound iron deficiency anaemia. This, in turn, leads to lassitude, low work and educational output, and has particular risks both for the woman herself and for the foetus in pregnancy.

Others: Zinc has an essential role in many metabolic processes (and is especially needed in times of rapid growth) and there is a growing suspicion that zinc deficiency might be widespread among children in many countries in the South.[72] Fluoride deficiency increases the incidence of dental caries. (On the other hand, the much rarer excess consumption of fluoride leads to mottling of teeth and in severe cases to bone damage.) Rickets, which is still widespread in parts of Northern Africa and the Eastern Mediterranean and is reported to be increasing in Mexico, is attributable to insufficient exposure to sunlight and lack of vitamin D in the diet. Ascorbic acid deficiency is a problem in some drought-affected populations, especially in Africa. Vitamin B12 deficiency, which causes anaemia and, if severe, neurological disorders, may occur in those consuming exclusively vegetarian diets containing no foods of animal origin.

Source: Drawn mainly from WHO (1992), Our Planet, Our Health, *Report of the World Commission on Environment and Health, Geneva and WHO (1995),* The World Health Report 1995: Bridging the Gaps, *WHO, Geneva.*

factors, because of some specific deficiency in the diet being linked to a particular pathogen (for instance intestinal worms which often underlie or exacerbate anaemia) or to food supplies (for instance, the regions in which food with vitamin A or with iodine is limited). Certain kinds of food can also exacerbate particular deficiencies – as in the excessive intake of cassava which may amplify the effects of iodine deficiency (see Box 2.4). Yet most undernutrition linked to micronutrient malnutrition also has social and political dimensions in that the costs of remedying most such malnutrition is very small. As a result of severe iodine deficiencies in the mother during early pregnancy, there are some 60,000 miscarriages, stillbirths and neonatal deaths each year.[68] Iodine deficiency also causes a further 120,000 babies to be born mentally retarded, physically stunted, deaf-mute or paralysed and a million more to have such difficulties as poor eye–hand coordination, poor hearing or speech impediments.[69] Millions more will have their IQs significantly lowered. The cost of preventing this (for instance through iodizing salt supplies) is as little as $0.05 per person per year.[70] Vitamin A deficiency which lowers the resistance to disease of over 200 million children under five, as well as causing severe eye damage and blindness to half a million and being a major factor in the death of some 250,000 a year, can usually be solved with small, low-cost changes to diets or vitamin A capsules costing 2 US cents given three times a year to children over six months of age.[71]

PHYSICAL HAZARDS

The true extent of deaths and disabilities from accidents is often greatly underestimated, especially among low-income groups who lack access to the health care services on whose reporting public authorities rely for data about causes of mortality or morbidity. And for every accidental death, there are several hundred accidental injuries.[73] Most deaths and disabilities from accidents are those associated with motor vehicles, falls, drowning, burns and poisoning.[74] Estimates for 1993 suggested that there were 885,000 accidental deaths from motor and other road-vehicle accidents and another 1.8 million accidental deaths from falls, fires, drownings etc.[75]

Road accidents have long been a major source of premature death and serious injury in Europe and North America. In the USA, more than 40,000 people are killed each year through road accidents and over three million injured.[76] More than a million people have died from traffic accidents within the EU over the last 20 years, and more than 30 million have been injured and/or permanently handicapped.[77] However, road accidents can also become a common cause of accidental injuries or deaths even in relatively low-income countries with low levels of automobile ownership. For instance, in 1991, Kenya had a fatality rate for road deaths per person similar to that of the UK, Netherlands, Norway and Sweden, yet had less than a twenty-fifth as many motor vehicles per person. There were 580 deaths per 100,000 motor vehicles in Kenya in 1991[78] compared to between 18 and 21 in these four European nations.

Worldwide, domestic accidents represent about one third of all accidental deaths, with burns alone accounting for 15 per cent.[79] In the South, the incidence of domestic accidents and their impact on health is much greater than in the North. The incidence is much increased by overcrowding, poor quality building materials, and dangerous domestic appliances. For instance, burns, scalds and household fires are more common in over-crowded shelters, perhaps not surprising when five or more persons often live in one room and there is little chance of providing occupants (especially children) with protection from open fires, stoves or kerosene lamps and heaters. The risk of fires is further increased in most urban dwellings because of the use of flammable materials (wood, cardboard, plastic, canvas, straw) in their construction.

Overcrowded dwellings and limited amounts of indoor space make it difficult to create a home environment for parents to manage and supervise and for children to understand and avoid physical hazards. Physical limitations also make it difficult to keep medicines and dangerous household chemicals (such as bleach) safely stored. Here, as in many environmental problems, the level of risk is usually compounded by social factors, such as a lack of adult supervision if most or all adults have to work. The health impact of accidents is also compounded by the lack of a health service that can rapidly provide emergency treatment, followed by longer-term treatment and care.[80]

There are also physical hazards related to the land sites on which housing and settlements develop. This is evident in many rural and urban areas. In virtually all cities in Africa, Asia and Latin America, there are large clusters of illegal housing on dangerous sites (for instance steep hillsides, floodplains or desert land), or housing which has been built on polluted sites (for instance around solid waste dumps, beside open drains and sewers or in industrial areas with high levels of air pollution). Or they develop in sites subject to high noise levels – for instance close to major highways or airports. The issue is rarely a lack of land suitable for housing. Most major cities and metropolitan areas have large areas of centrally located land that is not prone to natural hazards which is left undeveloped or only partially developed, as the owners of such land benefit from the appreciation in its value as the city's economy grows. These owners also have the power to ensure that their land is not illegally occupied by those in need of housing. This, more than any overall shortage of space, is the main reason for the very high levels of overcrowding in the (mostly) illegal or informal settlements, where, in most cities, a high proportion of the population lives. For instance, in Nairobi, the informal and illegal settlements that house more than half the city's population occupy less than 6 per cent of the land area used for residential purposes.[81] Comparable estimates have been made for Metro Manila where more than two fifths of the population live in illegal or informal settlements that cover less than 6 per cent of the land area.[82] As with fresh water, in most instances it is not a shortage of the resource (unhazardous land sites within or close to the main centres of employment or income opportunity) that is the problem but the fact that poorer groups have no means to get access to them. In many rural areas, there are also large numbers of people living on lands at risk from floods, landslides, earthquakes or other natural disasters. Here too, the underlying cause is often not so much a shortage of land but a very inequitable land-owning structure.

ASPECTS OF THE BUILT ENVIRONMENT WITH NEGATIVE PSYCHOSOCIAL CONSEQUENCES

Psychosocial health problems such as depression, drug and alcohol abuse, suicide, and inter-personal violence (including child and spouse mistreatment and abuse and target violence such as teacher assault and rape) are now among the most serious health problems in many cities in Europe and North America.[83] Many psychosocial disorders are associated with poor quality housing and living environments through such stressors as noise, pollution, overcrowding, inappropriate design, and inadequate infrastructure and services.[84] For example, research done in the UK found high levels of depression among women living in high-rise public (municipal council) housing and the physical environment was found to be a contributing factor to this depression.[85] Many non-environmental factors are also important – for instance the stress associated with inadequate income and insecure and strenuous livelihoods and insecure tenure of the shelter (for tenants or squatters), especially for those living with a constant threat of eviction or displacement.

Psychosocial and chronic diseases are becoming a major cause of death and morbidity among adolescents and young adults in many urban areas in the South or in particular districts within urban areas. For instance, psychosocial and chronic diseases are among the most important causes of death in cities as diverse as Shenyang and Rio de Janeiro.[86] Homicides alone were responsible for 5 per cent of all deaths in Sao Paulo City in 1986[87] and are among the main causes of death in many major cities in North and South America.[88] Little is known about psychosocial disorders in rural areas, although they are more likely to be associated with stressors that are linked to low income, economic insecurity and civil conflict rather than to qualities of the environment. Poor quality and overcrowded housing and living environments contribute to the stress which underlies many such diseases. Coping with constant illness or injury among one's children is also stressful for parents, especially for the parent (usually the mother) who takes most or all responsibility for nursing and (where possible) ensuring treatment. Stress can contribute not only to psychosocial disorders but also to specific diseases and possibly to impairing the body's immune system.

Good quality housing and living environments can substantially reduce stress – through (among other things) providing sufficient space for indoor activities, adequate sound insulation, facilities for safe play for children and for recreation, and designs that minimize personal hazards.[89] Within the wider neighbourhood in which the house is located, it is clear that a sense of security, good quality physical infrastructure (roads, pavements, drains, street lights) and services (eg regular street cleaning and garbage collection) contribute to good mental health – along with other characteristics of 'good' housing such as the availability of emergency services and easy access to friends and family and to desired educational, health and social services as well as cultural and other amenities.[90]

Ekblad and others (1991) suggest the need to consider three aspects of the physical environment when considering its possible impact on people's psychosocial health:

- the subjective experience of the dweller, ie the level of satisfaction with the house and its neighbourhood and its location within the urban area (and also the degree of security of tenure);
- the dwelling's physical structure (eg the amount of space, state of repair, facilities – which may influence the level of privacy, the possibilities for meeting relatives and friends, and child-rearing practices); and
- the neighbourhood (including the quality of services and facilities, and the level of security).

Many characteristics of urban neighbourhoods which are not easily identified or defined may have important influences on an individual's level of satisfaction and on the incidence of crime, vandalism and inter-personal violence. These are aspects more fully explored in cities in Europe and North America – for instance the critique of urban planning by Jane Jacobs,[91] which is concerned about the characteristics of cities and city neighbourhoods and streets which make them pleasant, safe and valued and which avoid urban degradation. The work of Oscar Newman on what he termed 'defensible space' is another example; he showed how the particular form of open space within a neighbourhood, including the extent to which it was subject to informal supervision and the extent to which there was a clear visual definition as to who had the right to use it and who was responsible for its maintenance, could be linked to levels of crime and vandalism.[92] Perceptions of personal safety can be a powerful factor in women's and men's use of urban space. A survey undertaken in Greater London showed differences in the perceptions of personal safety on public transport on the basis of both gender and race.[93]

It is also clear that the extent to which any individual or household has the possibility of modifying or changing their housing environment and working with others in the locality to effect change in the wider neighbourhood is an important influence on psychosocial health. Many critiques of public housing and of urban planning in Third World cities (especially 'slum' and squatter clearance and redevelopment) have centred on the loss of individual, household and community control that they cause.[94] They often document the hardships caused to household members by eviction from their homes and neighbourhoods and on occasion the negative health consequences, although they do not examine the social pathologies which might be associated with such changes. Large scale resettlement programmes for rural people – for instance to remove them from the site of a reservoir or dam – have also created or contributed to serious psychosocial health problems. There is also a large and varied literature on the importance for the physical and mental health of individuals and communities of being able to command events which control their lives;[95] psychiatrists and other health workers are increasingly recognizing the importance of such a link.[96]

The precise linkages between different elements of the physical environment and each psychosocial disorder are difficult to ascertain – and to separate from other variables.[97] There are also interacting variables which can promote or prevent the process that might lead to disease.[98] There are buffers which can help people cope with stress – for instance a social support network which may mitigate the effect of inadequate physical environments on psychosocial health problems:

> *'strong social networks and a sense of community organization in many rundown inner city districts ... and squatter settlements ... might help explain the remarkably low level of psychosocial problems'.*[99]

The importance of such networks can also be seen in the increase in physical and mental ill health among populations relocated from inner city tenements or illegal settlements to 'better quality' housing, because such networks became disrupted.[100]

NATURAL RESOURCE DEGRADATION

The issue of natural resource degradation will be considered in detail in Chapter 4 – including soil erosion, deforestation and desertification. Any long term trend in natural resource degradation presents a profound threat to child health and survival since, for most of the world's children, the central natural resource issue is whether their parents have access to sufficient productive land and water for an adequate and sustainable livelihood and sufficient fresh water for drinking and household use. As in most other environmental issues, this is not simply an issue of the size and quality of the resource base since social, economic and political factors affect who obtains access to them.

NATIONAL/GLOBAL ENVIRONMENTAL DEGRADATION

The two major problems of global environmental degradation which have received most attention recently are the depletion of the stratospheric ozone layer and the increasing concentrations of what are termed 'greenhouse gases' in the earth's atmosphere and the possible, continued atmospheric warming. Both will have major health impacts for urban and rural populations. Some will be direct – for instance increased heat stress from higher temperatures and a growing incidence of skin cancer from stratospheric ozone depletion. But the indirect health impacts are likely to be much greater – for instance those arising from changes in agricultural production, sea-level rises (including flooding and damage to buildings, sewers and drains), disruption to freshwater resources and the expansion in the areas where some of the most serious tropical disease vectors can survive and breed (see Chapter 5 for more details). Other issues could also be raised under this heading – including the need to protect biodiversity worldwide. In this, the link to health is through its importance in guarding against the extinction of species because some may provide the basis for new foods or medicines or the biological control of pathogens or disease vectors.

ESTIMATING THE CONTRIBUTION OF ENVIRONMENTAL FACTORS TO THE GLOBAL DISEASE BURDEN*

New figures for the global disease burden and its main causes allow some estimate as to how much environmental factors contribute to ill health, injury and premature death worldwide. In 1993, WHO and the World Bank produced detailed estimates of the global burden of ill health or premature death for the year 1990 from a wide range of infectious and parasitic diseases and from injuries – as well as from other causes. These statistics allow comparisons to be made of the total disease burdens and the disease burdens per person between the world's main regions and the two most populous nations (China and India).

These statistics highlight the much larger disease burdens per person in the lowest income regions or the regions where governments and international agencies have not given a priority to supporting health care, promoting health and tackling the most life-threatening and health-threatening environmental hazards. They also emphasize the much greater toll that environmental factors take on ill health and premature death in the South when compared to the North. Some of the data are also disaggregated by age group, so the influence of environmental factors on ill health, injury and premature death among infants and children can also be considered.

Environmental factors account for a considerable proportion of the global disease burden, although for reasons already discussed in Chapter 1, it is difficult to estimate with precision their contribution, relative to non-environmental factors.[101] But it is also clear that there are enormous differences in the relative importance of environmental factors to disease, injury and premature death depending on where you live. Among the poorest nations, they may account for half or more of the disease burden, whereas among wealthy countries they may account for less than 10 per cent. There are differences between the relative importance of environmental factors within countries, especially between high-income and low-income groups. These differences are particularly large in most countries in the South where low-income groups living and working in the most life-threatening and health-threatening environments have much higher disease burdens attributable to environmental factors than wealthier groups.

The new statistics estimate the average disease burden for individuals which was acquired in 1990, as it affected them in 1990 and in future years. Diarrhoea and childhood diseases such as measles, respiratory infections, worm infections and malaria alone accounted for one quarter of the global disease burden in this year and a much higher proportion in most of the regions in the South. The burden of these largely preventable or inexpensively curable diseases was far larger in sub-Saharan Africa where they accounted for 43 per cent of the total disease burden but was also substantial in India (28 per cent) and the rest of Asia excluding China (29 per cent)

---

* Unless otherwise stated, the statistics in this section are drawn from World Bank (1993), *World Development Report 1993; Investing in Health,* published for the World Bank by Oxford University Press, Oxford, or derived from figures in its statistical tables.

and the Middle Eastern Crescent (29 per cent). The most important impli-cation of these figures is that a very substantial proportion of the ill health and premature death that occurs in the South has its origins in childhood and is easily cured or prevented at relatively low cost.

The disease burden was measured in terms of 'disability-adjusted life years' (DALYs). The measurement of the disease burden included not only life years lost from premature death but also the loss of healthy life years resulting from non-fatal illness or injury. However, not all years lost were counted equally – see Box 2.5. The figures suggest that premature deaths were responsible for two thirds of the global disease burden, with the rest attributed to disabilities from non-fatal illness or injury.

Box 2.5 **Notes on the Weighting used for Calculating DALYs**

The loss of disability-adjusted life years from premature death was not simply the difference in years between the age of death and the aver-age age of death in a healthy society. For instance, the death of a baby girl was assigned 32.5 life years lost, the death of a female at age 30 was assigned 29 life years lost and the death of a female at age 60 assigned 12 life years lost. This weighting is based on two factors. The first is because the periods of life when the individual is a net consumer, because they are dependent on others for their support (childhood and old age), were given less weight (value) than young adulthood or middle age, when the individual is a net producer within society. This is because the report from which the figures are drawn was making an economic argument for greater investment in health. The second is because years lost in the future were considered of lower value than years lost now, and an annual discounting of 3 per cent a year was applied to future years lost. This kind of weighting clearly reduces the global disease burden and the contribution of infant and child mortality to the global disease burden, compared to estimates that assume that all life years lost for whatever age group are of equal value. Reference should be made to World Bank (1993), *World Development Report 1993; Investing in Health*, Oxford University Press, Oxford, for more details of the weighting.

Figures 2.2, 2.3 and 2.4 show the total disease burden per person from all causes for the two most populous countries (China and India) and for the rest of the world, divided into six regions – for the total population, for 0–4 year olds and for 5–14 year olds. The disease burden in this and in the other figures in this section have been converted into the numbers of disability-adjusted life days lost per person, rather than disability-adjusted life years per 1000 inhabitants that was used in the original report. These figures show the enormous differences in the average disease burden per person between the regions.

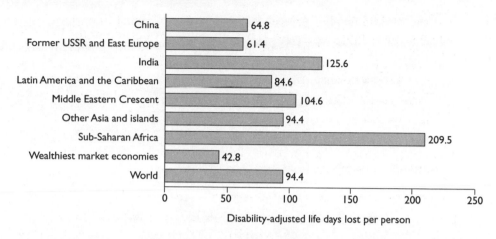

Figure 2.2 *The disease burden per person from all causes acquired in one year (1990)*

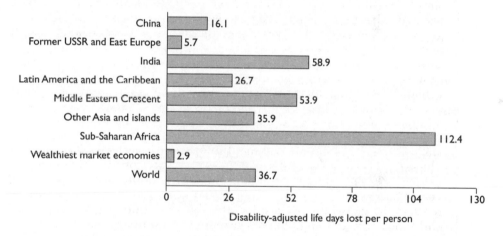

Figure 2.3 *The disease burden per person for 0–4 year olds from all causes acquired in one year (1990)*

Taking the disease burden for all ages (Figure 2.2), those living in the wealthiest market economies[*] had less than half the world average while those living in sub-Saharan Africa had more than twice the world average. The size of the differentials between regions becomes much larger when considering the disease burdens only for 0–4 year olds (Figure 2.3). Indeed, the figure shows the remarkably low disease burden for infants and young children in the wealthiest market economies (with less than a tenth of the world average) and the very high disease burdens in sub-Saharan Africa

---

[*] This group encompasses North America, Australasia, Japan and what used to be termed West Europe when the term East Europe included the countries that were formerly part of the Socialist Bloc. The World Bank termed this group the 'established market economies' – but they are termed in this book the 'wealthiest market economies' in that countries outside this group also have long-established market economies.

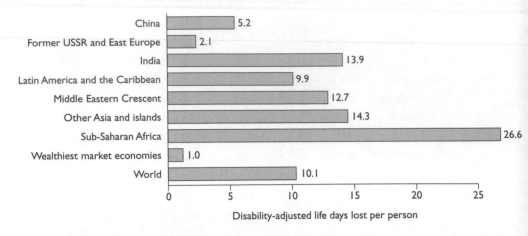

Figure 2.4 *The disease burden per person for 5–14 year olds from all causes acquired in one year (1990)**

(with each infant and young child having nearly 40 times the disease burden of infants and young children in the wealthiest market economies). The disease burden for infants and young children is also particularly high in India and in the Middle Eastern Crescent. Figure 2.4 also shows the remarkably low disease burden for 5–14 year olds in the wealthiest market economies, compared to the world average, and, again, the very high disease burden for children of this age group in sub-Saharan Africa and for India, the Middle Eastern Crescent and 'other Asia and islands'.

Comparing these figures also shows how the disease burden of infants and young children accounts for more than half the total disease burden in sub-Saharan Africa and the Middle Eastern Crescent and for nearly half the total disease burden in India – but less than a tenth of the disease burden in the wealthiest market economies and in the former USSR and East Europe.

Figure 2.5 shows the disease burden per person from infectious and parasitic diseases and highlights the enormous differences in the average disease burden per person between different regions. In sub-Saharan Africa, on average, for each person, 106 life days are lost to premature death or disability from new cases of infectious and parasitic diseases caught in 1990. By contrast, in the wealthy market economies and in the former USSR and East Europe, the average is less than two life days per person. The disease burdens per person from infectious and parasitic diseases in the other regions in the South are much lower than in sub-Saharan Africa but still much higher than in the wealthier countries. Most of the disease burden in this category of infectious and parasitic diseases comes from diseases which are substantially influenced by environmental factors (and highlighted in

---

* The figures for the disease burdens in Figures 2.2, 2.3 and 2.4 represent the average, current and future disease burden in disability-adjusted life days lost as a result of new cases of diseases or injuries acquired in 1990. Thus, they include the disability-adjusted life days lost in later years that arose from diseases caught or injuries sustained in 1990 but do not include the life days lost in 1990 from diseases or injuries sustained in years prior to 1990.

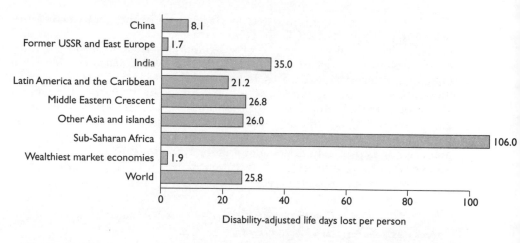

Figure 2.5 *The disease burden per person from new cases of infectious and parasitic diseases acquired in one year (1990)*

earlier sections of this chapter) – especially acute respiratory infections, diarrhoeal diseases, the vaccine-preventable childhood diseases, malaria, TB and intestinal worms.

Figure 2.6 shows the even larger relative regional differences in the disease burden per person for diarrhoeal diseases. The disease burden per person from new cases of diarrhoeal diseases caught in 1990 is around 200 times larger in sub-Saharan Africa than in the wealthiest market economies. It is also particularly high in India and the Middle Eastern Crescent – and still much higher in the other regions of the South, compared to what has been achieved in Europe, North America, Australasia, Japan, the former USSR and East Europe.

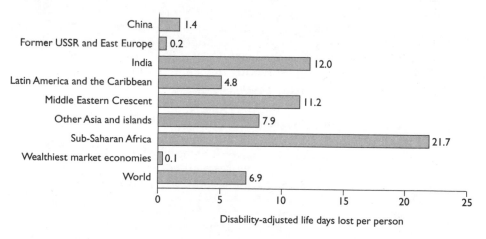

Figure 2.6 *The disease burden per person from new cases of diarrhoeal diseases acquired in one year (1990)*

There are also large inter-regional differences in the relative contribution of diarrhoeal diseases to the total disease burden from infectious and parasitic diseases in that region. For sub-Saharan Africa, for example, diarrhoeal diseases represent about a fifth of the total disease burden from infectious and parasitic diseases. In India and the Middle Eastern Crescent, they represent more than a third. In both regions in the North, they represent much smaller proportions of the total disease burden – for instance only some 5 per cent in the wealthiest market economies. This is despite the fact that they are still among the most common illnesses there.[102] The main reason is probably that a combination of better nutritional status and quicker and more effective access to treatment prevent most episodes of these illnesses becoming severe.

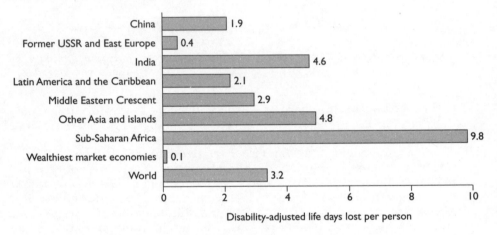

Figure 2.7 *The disease burden per person from new cases of tuberculosis acquired in one year (1990)*

Comparable relative differences between regions to those shown in Figure 2.6 also exist for tuberculosis – see Figure 2.7. Again, the disease burden in sub-Saharan Africa is particularly high – but also high in India and in 'Other Asia and islands' (ie excluding China and Japan).

The dataset on the global disease burden does have some disaggregation by age-group and region, but not with the same level of detail for particular disease categories. Figure 2.8 shows the disease burden per person for 0–4 year olds from new cases of communicable diseases and from perinatal causes in 1990 for the same eight regions. This category includes all the infectious and parasitic diseases. Again, the disease burden per person in sub-Saharan Africa is much higher than in any other region – and 27 times that in the wealthiest market economies. The absolute disease burden per person is also particularly high. In sub-Saharan Africa, in 1990, each young child, on average, lost almost one and a half disability-adjusted life years due to these diseases alone, and the equivalent figure exceeded

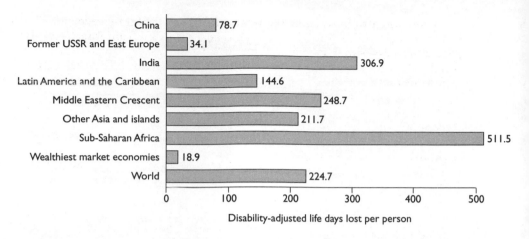

Figure 2.8 *The disease burden per person for 0–4 year olds from new cases of communicable diseases and perinatal causes acquired in one year (1990)*

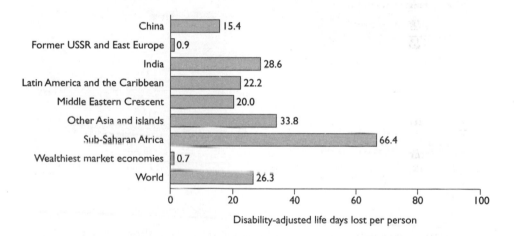

Figure 2.9 *The disease burden per person for 5–14 year olds from new cases of communicable diseases and maternal causes acquired in one year (1990)*

ten months for young Indian children (306.9 person days).* By contrast, it was less than one month in the wealthiest market economies.

The absolute disease burden for 5–14 year olds from communicable diseases and maternal causes is, not surprisingly, much lower than that for 0–4 year olds – see Figure 2.9. Chapter 3 will describe in more detail how the risk of premature death due to most of the infectious and parasitic

---

* The fact that each young child in sub-Saharan Africa suffered from more disability-adjusted life days from communicable diseases and perinatal causes acquired in 1990 than there were life days in 1990 is because of the high child mortality rate. As noted in Box 2.5, the death of one baby results in over 10,000 disability-adjusted life days of disease burden.

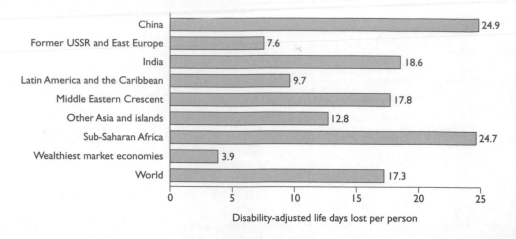

Figure 2.10 *The disease burden per person for 0–4 year olds from injuries sustained in one year (1990)*

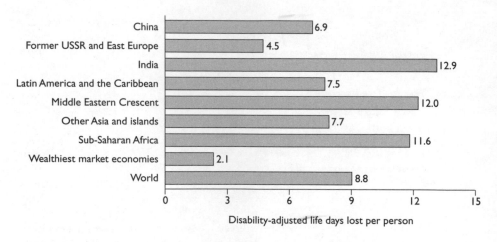

Figure 2.11 *The disease burden per person for 5–14 year olds from injuries sustained in one year (1990)*

diseases falls, as the child gets older. However, what is particularly notice-able is the scale of the differentials between regions which is actually even larger than those for 0–4 year olds. Thus, the disease burden per person for 5–14 year olds from communicable diseases and maternal causes in sub-Saharan Africa is nearly 100 times that in the wealthiest market economies. For all other regions in the South, it remains between 16 and 48 times that in the wealthiest market economies and the former USSR and East Europe. The main reason for this is probably that an even higher proportion of the infectious and communicable disease burden acquired in 5–14 year olds is preventable and/or easily treated – for instance schistosomiasis, intestinal parasites and tuberculosis – than in young children.

Figures 2.10 and 2.11 show the contrasts in the disease burden per person between the regions that arose from injuries in 1990 for different age groups. The relative disparities between regions are still large with the lower income regions having the highest disease burden per person, but smaller than those for communicable diseases. The relative importance of injuries compared to communicable diseases and maternal and perinatal causes tends to be higher in the wealthier regions, compared to the poorest regions.

In the wealthiest market economies, the former USSR and East Europe and China (which has a remarkably low disease burden from communicable diseases, relative to its per capita income), the disease burden per 0–4 year old from injuries sustained in 1990 was between a quarter and a fifth of that for communicable diseases and perinatal causes. By contrast, for the other regions, the equivalent ratio was between a tenth and a twentieth. This implies that while the disease burden from injuries for 0–4 year olds has been much reduced in the wealthier nations, in general, it has not been reduced as effectively as the disease burden from communicable diseases and perinatal causes.

For 5–14 year olds, the relative importance of injuries to total disease burdens is much greater. Figure 2.11 shows that the differences between regions are still large but less dramatic than in earlier age groups; the disease burden per person in the wealthiest market economies is only one sixth that in the worst-hit regions. But comparing Figures 2.9 and 2.11 show that in the wealthiest market economies and in the former USSR and East Europe, injuries are a much more serious disease burden for 5–14 year olds (2.1 and 4.5 disability-adjusted life days lost respectively) than communicable diseases (0.7 and 0.9 disability-adjusted life days lost respectively).

Thus, in concluding this section, note should be made of the large absolute and relative differences in the total burden of disease between regions of the world. Although this is true in all age groups, it is most marked in children (0–4 years and 5–14 years). The differences are even more extreme for the burden due to communicable diseases and injuries.

Environmental factors are important underlying causes of a high proportion of infectious and parasitic diseases, including most of the diseases that cause the greatest burden of disease in both young (0–4 years) and older (5–14 years) children and, as a result, they make up a very substantial part of the burden of disease in the poorest regions of the world that have the poorest environments. The same is true – to a lesser extent – in the poorest subgroups of the populations in richer regions. The same is true for injuries. The following chapter now turns to how and why children at different ages are particularly vulnerable to a great range of environmental hazards.

REFERENCES

1   WHO (1992), *Our Planet, Our Health*, Report of the Commission on Health and Environment, Geneva.

2   WHO 1992, op cit.

3   Rossi-Espagnet, A, G B Goldstein and I Tabibzadeh (1991), 'Urbanization and

health in developing countries; a challenge for health for all', *World Health Statistical Quarterly*, Vol 44, No 4, pp 186–244.

4   Official statistics exaggerate the proportion of the urban and rural population in the South with adequate sanitation. Many of the people judged to have 'access to sanitation' often have only a communal pit latrine that has to be shared by dozens of households. For more details, see Satterthwaite, David (1995), 'The underestimation of poverty and its health consequences', *Third World Planning Review* Vol 17, No 4, November, pp iii–xii.

5   WHO (1991), *Global Estimates for Health Situation Assessments and Projections 1990*, Division of Epidemiological Surveillance and Health Situation and Trend Analysis, WHO/HST/90.2, Geneva.

6   WHO (1986), *Intersectoral Action for Health - The Role of Intersectoral Cooperation in National Strategies for Health for All*, Background Document for the Technical Discussions, 39th World, Health Assembly, May, Geneva.

7   WHO 1991, op cit.

8   WHO (1995), *The World Health Report 1995: Bridging the Gaps*, WHO, Geneva.

9   World Bank (1993), *World Development Report 1993; Investing in Health*, Oxford University Press, Oxford.

10   WHO 1992, op cit; WHO (1984), *The Role of Food Safety in Health and Development*, WHO Technical Report Series, No 705; Report of a joint FAO/WHO Expert Committee on Food Safety, WHO, Geneva.

11   McGranahan, Gordon (1991), *Environmental Problems and the Urban Household in Third World Countries*, The Stockholm Environment Institute, Stockholm, pp 24–25.

12   Esrey, S A and R G Feachem (1989), 'Interventions for the Control of Diarrhoeal Disease: Promotion of Food Hygiene', WHO/CDD/89.30, WHO, Geneva, 1989, quoted in WHO 1992, op cit.

13   Rossi-Espagnet, Goldstein and Tabibzadeh 1991, op cit.

14   Surjadi, Charles (1993), 'Respiratory diseases of mothers and children and environmental factors among households in Jakarta', *Environment and Urbanization*, Vol 5, No 2, October pp 78–86; Songsore, Jacob and Gordon McGranahan (1993), 'Environment, wealth and health; towards an analysis of intra-urban differentials within Greater Accra Metropolitan Area, Ghana', *Environment and Urbanization*, Vol 5, No 2, October, pp 10–24.

15   WHO, 1992, op cit, p 204.

16   WHO 1992, op cit.

17   WHO 1995, op cit.

18   Ibid.

19   Cauthen, G M, A Pio and H G ten Dam (1988), *Annual Risk of Tuberculosis Infection*, WHO, Geneva; WHO (1990), *Environmental Health in Urban Development*, Report of a WHO Expert Committee, WHO, Geneva.

20   WHO (1996) *Creating Healthy Cities in the 21st Century*, background paper prepared for the Dialogue on Health in Human Settlements for Habitat II, World Health Organization, Geneva, 38 pages.

21   WHO 1992, op cit; Sapir, D (1990), *Infectious Disease Epidemics and Urbanization: a Critical Review of the Issues*, Paper prepared for the WHO Commission on Health and Environment, Division of Environmental Health, WHO, Geneva.

22   Sapir 1990, op cit.

23   WHO 1995, op cit.

24 WHO 1992, op cit.

25 Bradley, David, Carolyn Stephens, Sandy Cairncross and Trudy Harpham (1991), *A Review of Environmental Health Impacts in Developing Country Cities*, Urban Management Program Discussion Paper No 6, The World Bank, UNDP and UNCHS (Habitat) Washington DC.

26 Schofield, C J, R Briceno-Leon, N Kolstrup, D J T Webb and G B White (1990), 'The role of house design in limiting vector-borne disease' in Hardoy, Jorge E et al (Eds) *The Poor Die Young: Housing and Health in Third World Cities*, Earthscan, London.

27 Cairncross, Sandy and Richard G Feachem (1993), *Environmental Health Engineering in the Tropics – An Introductory Text*, John Wiley and Sons, Chichester.

28 Sapir 1990, op cit.

29 WHO 1995, op cit.

30 Briceno-Leon, Roberto (1990), *La Casa Enferma: Sociologia de la Enfermedad de Chagas*, Consorcio de Ediciones, Capriles C A Caracas.

31 WHO 1995, op cit.

32 Needleman, Herbert L, Alan Schell, David Bellinger, Alan Leviton and Elizabeth N Allred (1991), 'The long-term effects of exposure to low doses on lead in childhood: an eleven year follow up report' *The New England Journal of Medicine* Vol 322 No 2, pp 83-88.

33 Smith, K R (1988), 'Air pollution: assessing total exposure in developing countries', *Environment*, Vol 30, No 10, pp 28–35.

34 Ibid.

35 WHO 1992, op cit.

36 UNEP/WHO (1988), *Assessment of Urban Air Quality*, Global Environment Monitoring Service, UNEP and WHO.

37 World Bank (1992), *World Development Report 1992: Development and the Environment*, Oxford University Press, Oxford and New York.

38 UNEP (1991), *Environmental Data Report, 1991–2*, GEMS Monitoring and Assessment Research Centre, Blackwell, Oxford and Massachusetts.

39 UNEP/WHO (1992), *Urban Air Pollution in Megacities of the World*, Published on behalf of WHO and UNEP, Blackwell, Oxford.

40 See for instance European Environment Agency (1995), *Europe's Environment: the Dobris Assessment*, Copenhagen and Smil, Vaclav (1984), *The Bad Earth: Environmental Degradation in China*, M E Sharpe, New York and Zed Press, London.

41 WHO 1992, op cit.

42 Romieu, Isabelle et al (1990), 'Urban air pollution in Latin America and the Caribbean: Health perspectives', *World Health Statistics Quarterly* Vol 23, No 2, pp 153–167.

43 Hardoy, Jorge E, Diana Mitlin and David Satterthwaite (1992), *Environmental Problems in Third World Cities*, Earthscan, London.

44 WHO 1995, op cit.

45 Pepall, Jennifer (1992), 'Occupational poisoning' reporting on the work of Mohamad M Amr in *IDRC Reports* Vol 20, No 1, Ottawa, April, p 15.

46 Dinham, Barbara (Ed) (1993), *The Pesticide Hazard. Global Health and Environmental Audit*, Zed Books, London.

47 Castonguay, Gilles (1992) 'Steeling themselves with knowledge' report on the work of Cristina Laurell, *IDRC Reports* Vol 20, No 1, April, pp 10–12.

48 Phantumvanit, Dhira and Wanai Liengcharernsit (1989), 'Coming to terms with Bangkok's environmental problems', *Environment and Urbanization* Vol 1, No 1, April, pp 31–39.

49 Askoy, M et al (1976), 'Types of leukaemia in a chronic benzene poisoning', *Acta haematologica* Vol 55, pp 67–72.

50 Matte, T D, J P Figueroa, S Ostrowski, G Burr et al (1989), 'Lead poisoning among household members exposed to lead-acid battery repair shops in Kingston, Jamaica (West Indies)' *International Journal of Epidemiology* Vol 18, pp 874–881.

51 Centre for Science and Environment (1986), *The State of India's Environment 1984–5: The Second Citizens' Report*, New Delhi.

52 UNEP (1993), *Environmental Data Report 1993–94*, Prepared by GEMS Monitoring and Assessment Research Centre, Blackwell, Oxford.

53 WHO 1992, op cit.

54 Ibid.

55 WHO (1990), *Public Health Impact of Pesticides used in Agriculture*, WHO, Geneva.

56 Ibid.

57 Stewart, Sarah (1994), *Colombian Flowers: The Gift of Love and Poison*, Christian Aid.

58 Ibid; Conway, Gordon R and Jules N Pretty (1991), *Unwelcome Harvest*, Earthscan, London.

59 Ibid.

60 WHO 1992, op cit.

61 WHO/UNICEF (1994), *Water Supply and Sanitation Sector Monitoring Report 1994*, Water Supply and Sanitation Collaborative Council, WHO and UNICEF, Geneva.

62 WHO/UNICEF (1993), *Water Supply and Sanitation Sector Monitoring Report 1993*, WHO and UNICEF Joint Monitoring Programme, Geneva, p 13.

63 Ibid.

64 Cairncross, Sandy (1990), 'Water supply and the urban poor', in Jorge E Hardoy and others (Eds), *The Poor Die Young: Housing and Health in Third World Cities*, Earthscan, London, pp 109–126.

65 Ibid.

66 WHO/UNICEF 1993, op cit.

67 Ibid.

68 WHO, UNICEF and the International Council for the Control of Iodine Deficiency Disorders, (1993), *Global Prevalence of Iodine Deficiency Disorders*, quoted in UNICEF (1995), *The State of the World's Children 1995*, Oxford University Press, Oxford and New York.

69 Ibid.

70 WHO 1995, op cit.

71 UNICEF 1995, op cit.

72 Shrimpton, Roger (1993), 'Zinc deficiency - is it widespread but under-recognized?, *SCN News*, No 9, pp 24–27.

73 Manciaux, M and C J Romer (1986), 'Accidents in children, adolescents and young adults: a major public health problem' *World Health Statistical Quarterly* Vol 39, No 3, pp 227–231.

74 WHO 1991, op cit.

75 WHO 1995, op cit. These figures do not include suicides (779,000 deaths), 303,000 homicides and violence and 220,000 deaths from occupational accidents.

76 OECD, *OECD in Figures: Statistics on the Member Countries*, 1995 edition, Paris.

77 European Environment Agency 1995, op cit.

78 Odero, W, 'Road traffic accidents in Kenya', Paper presented at the Urban Health Conference, London School of Hygiene and Tropical Medicine, 6–8th December 1994.

79 WHO 1991, op cit.

80 Goldstein, Greg (1990), 'Access to life saving services in urban areas' in Hardoy, Jorge E et al (Eds) *The Poor Die Young: Housing and Health in Third World Cities*, Earthscan, London.

81 Alder, Graham (1995), 'Tackling poverty in Nairobi's informal settlements: developing an institutional strategy', *Environment and Urbanization*, Vol 7, No 2, October, pp 85–108.

82 ANAWIM (1990), published by the Share and Care Apostolate for Poor Settlers Vol IV, No 4.

83 WHO 1992, op cit; Cohen, Larry and Susan Swift (1993), 'A public health approach to the violence epidemic in the United States', *Environment and Urbanization*, Vol 5, No 2, October, pp 50–66.

84 WHO 1992, op cit.

85 Brown, George and Tirril Harris (1978), *Social Origins of Depression: a Study of Psychiatric Disorder in Women*, Tavistock, London.

86 Bradley and others 1991, op cit.

87 Leitmann, Josef (1991), 'Environmental profile of Sao Paulo' Urban Management and the Environment: Discussion Paper Series, UNDP/World Bank/UNCHS.

88 UNCHS (1996), *An Urbanizing World: The Global Report on Human Settlements 1996*, Oxford University Press, Oxford.

89 Ekblad, Solvig et al (1991), *Stressors, Chinese City Dwellings and Quality of Life*, D12, Swedish Council for Building Research, Stockholm; Schaeffer, B (1990), 'Home and health – on solid foundations?', World Health Forum Vol 11, pp 38–45.

90 Ibid.

91 Jacobs, Jane (1965), *The Death and Life of Great American Cities*, Pelican, London.

92 Newman, Oscar (1972), *Defensible Space: Crime Prevention through Urban Design*, MacMillan, New York.

93 GLC Women's Committee (1984), *GLC Survey on Women and Transport*, Vols 1–7, Greater London Council.

94 See for instance Turner, John F C and Robert Fichter (Eds) (1971), *Freedom to Build*, Macmillan, New York and London; and Turner, John F C (1976), *Housing By People - Towards Autonomy in Building Environments*, Ideas in Progress, Marion Boyars, London.

95 Duhl, Leonard J (1990), *The Social Entrepreneurship of Change*, Pace University

Press, New York.

96 Ibid; WHO 1992, op cit.

97 WHO 1992, op cit.

98 Kagan, A R and L Levi (1975), 'Health and environment: psycho-social stimuli – a review', in L Levi (Ed), *Society, Stress and Disease – Childhood and Adolescence*, Oxford University Press, pp 241–260, quoted in Ekblad and others, 1991, op cit; Ekblad, Solvig (1993), 'Stressful environments and their effects on quality of life in Third World cities', *Environment and Urbanization*, Vol 5, No 2, October, pp 125–134.

99 WHO 1992, op cit p 215.

100 See for instance Turner 1976, op cit.

101 An analysis of the causes of diseases usually points to a wide range of factors (environmental, social, economic, political, genetic…, also environmental factors often operate concurrently and are interrelated, and may contribute by very indirect paths – see Fox, John P, Carrie E Hall and Lila R Elveback (1970), 'Environmental factors in causation of disease', Chapter 6 in *Epidemiology, Man and Disease*, Macmillan, London, pp 94–110.

102 WHO 1992, op cit.

3

The Vulnerability of the Infant and Child to Environmental Hazards

INTRODUCTION

This chapter reviews why infants and children are particularly vulnerable to many of the most common environmental hazards. There is some overlap with Chapter 2 but the concern here is which environmental hazards pose particular risks for female and male infants and children, and how the relative importance of different hazards changes at different ages and at different points in children's development. Enormous gaps remain in basic data and in our knowledge – for instance about the dose-response relationships for toxic chemicals* and about the interaction of environmental factors with the many social, economic, political and demographic factors which also influence health.[1] In addition, data are often not disaggregated on the basis of gender, but in the small number of instances where data are available, the significance of gender as a variable in understanding environmental health is apparent.

The presence of an environmental hazard (eg a pathogen, pollutant, physical hazard or psychosocial stressor such as high noise level) does not necessarily imply that it will harm a child. For many environmental hazards, the level of risk is influenced by characteristics of the child (eg age, sex, genetic make-up and health and nutritional status) and of the household in which they live (eg the quality of the home and provision for water supply, sanitation and personal hygiene, family support systems and the possibility for the parents to obtain rapid treatment for their infant or child if they become seriously ill or injured). In any strategy to minimize environmental hazards for girl and boy children, consideration must be given to four aspects:

- preventive environmental measures (ie how to reduce or remove environmental hazards);
- preventive health measures (how to reduce health risks arising from

---

* The relationship between the administered dose or exposure and the biological change in one organism or part of an organism.

environmental hazards);

- how to limit the health impact of the illness or injury when it occurs; and
- how to help the child and its parents (or carers) cope with the illness or injury.

Children are particularly at risk from many environmental hazards, compared to most other age groups, from the time of their conception through their development in the womb, their birth, infancy, early and late childhood and adolescence through to adulthood. Age-related risk factors include weak body defences, susceptibility to particular chemicals and, for younger children in particular, inadequate or no understanding of how to avoid hazards. Other risk factors are determined or influenced by social and economic factors and relate to class, gender and in some societies, ethnicity/religion.

As children grow and develop, certain risks diminish: for instance, as the immune system of an infant or young child develops to protect them from various communicable diseases or as they are vaccinated to provide immunity from diseases such as measles, tetanus, tuberculosis and whooping cough (pertussis). Older children also learn to avoid certain environmental hazards; for instance, as children learn about the importance of handwashing after defecation and of personal hygiene in general, so may the risk of contracting various waterborne or water-washed diseases diminish. Although children can learn to avoid hazards from a relatively early age, their natural curiosity, increased mobility and learning through risk-taking exposes them to new hazards within the home and outside where they play. Where garbage is uncollected, sanitation inadequate (so sites around the house are contaminated with faecal matter) and drainage inadequate, their play with soil, water and waste materials in the areas around the house can be particularly hazardous.

As Chapter 1 stressed, a good home environment minimizes all the environmental hazards that can threaten the life or health of a child at all stages in their development. The same is true for other places where children spend significant parts of their day – for instance play groups, day-care centres and schools, the places where they play and in the paths, roads and forms of transport used to get to and from these places. In households and societies with sufficient resources and a commitment to children's health and development, only a very small proportion of infants and children suffer serious injury or die as a result of environmental hazards.

Within societies with sufficient resources and a commitment to child health, individual, household, community and state actions combine to ensure that environmental hazards for children are minimized, that their health impact is minimized if there is injury or illness, and that parents (or carers) can cope with the cost of their child's illness or injury. For instance, parents have the knowledge and resources to minimize hazards within the home and its surrounds. Local organizations and institutions also minimize hazards within the village, town or city neighbourhood (including the places where children play) and within the services used by children (day care, health centres, schools). Emergency services can ensure rapid and effective response when children become seriously ill or injured. In addition, parents can, if necessary, take time off work to look after a sick or injured child without a loss of income that threatens the health or survival of the household.

Another aspect of children's vulnerability to environmental hazards is their parents' vulnerability to these same hazards and the difficulties parents face in maintaining the household's income and in caring for the children, when one or more adults are sick or injured. The people who care for children (usually mothers or older female siblings) are often at risk from the infectious diseases that children catch and vice versa. And as Chapter 2 noted, a high proportion of the income-earning activities undertaken by household members in the South also expose them to many environmental hazards and cause or contribute to ill health or injury. Low-income households are generally not only at greatest risk from environmental hazards (as they cannot afford to live in homes and neighbourhoods with basic infrastructure and services) but they also have the least assets to draw on, to help meet household expenses when an income earner can no longer go to work and when payment has to be made for medical treatment. Here too, in wealthy societies and among middle and upper income groups in most other countries, there are provisions to provide families with sick or injured income earners with sufficient income to ensure this does not happen.[2]

For a large proportion of the world's infants, children and youth, their health (and life) and the health of their mothers and fathers is continuously threatened by environmental hazards. In addition, the burden of ill health and disablement and the likelihood of premature death is much increased, because of inadequate treatment and care from emergency and health services. Illness or injury for one adult in a household can bring health-threatening and even life-threatening declines in households' incomes. Box 3.1 provides an example from a settlement in Khulna (Bangladesh) where poorer households not only lost more paid work than richer households to illness and injury but also more income (and obviously a much higher proportion of total income). In addition, in households where income earners were severely incapacitated, both the children and other family members were likely to be undernourished.

THE CHILD IN THE WOMB

Human vulnerability to environmental factors precedes conception since both the mother's ova and the father's sperm may be damaged by radiation or by certain chemical pollutants. But the unborn child is most at risk during its nine month development within the mother's womb. Even in this relatively sheltered environment, the developing embryo/foetus is strongly influenced by external factors, including environmental factors. Perhaps the most important are those factors which influence the health and nutritional status of the mother since the embryo/foetus's nutrient supply is entirely dependent on the mother. One estimate suggested that around half of pregnant women in the world suffer from nutritional

Box 3.1 **The Impact of Adult Ill Health on Household Income and Nutrition in Khulna, Bangladesh**

A study of ill health and its impact on nutrition in an inner city *bustee* in Khulna, Bangladesh, found that it was the poorest households who lost most work days to illness or injury and also most income and much the highest proportion of income. Most such households were heavily in debt. Many of their incapacitated income earners had chronic illnesses that implied a continuous limitation on their capacity to work. Households with severely incapacitated earners were also much more likely to have severely undernourished children. In addition, among the households with severely undernourished children and incapacitated income earners, most family members were undernourished.

The *bustee* had a population of over 2200 within an area of some two hectares (five acres). The land and property there were claimed by 18 landlords all of whom lived within the settlement, mostly in good quality housing built with permanent materials. The rest of the population were tenants for whom environmental conditions were insanitary and overcrowded. Cross-sectional surveys undertaken in 1986 indicated that 7 per cent of children under five years old were severely undernourished and 43 per cent moderately undernourished using weight-for-age as an indicator. The top 10 per cent of households owned 70 per cent of all assets, while the bottom 10 per cent owned 0.07 per cent. Around 50 per cent of households were below a locally derived food poverty line.

Five relatively homogeneous livelihood groups were identified on the basis of a wide range of socio-economic and demographic variables:

- Group 1 households (2 per cent of all households) were the richest group. They were the largest and most politically powerful landlords. Labour participation was the lowest in the settlement overall, and women and children were not labour market participants. Incomes were four times the local poverty line, and households enjoyed a plentiful and diversified diet.
- Group 2 households (13.5 per cent of households) had incomes that were more than twice the local poverty line and assets were well above average. They had the lowest proportion of indebted households and loans incurred were mainly for business purposes. Household size and economic dependency ratio were well above the average. As in Group 1, labour participation was almost exclusively confined to men.
- Group 3 households (27 per cent of all households) were predominantly petty traders with an average income just above the local poverty line.
- Group 4 households (34 per cent of all households) were a relatively poor group with incomes below the local poverty line. This group owned few assets and were predominantly dependent upon male unskilled and semi-skilled casual labour for their

livelihood.

- Group 5 households (23.5 per cent of all households) had lower average values for assets, income and food supplies than any other group and a large average household size but, unlike the relatively richer groups, this was coupled with a low average dependency ratio. They had high levels of chronically ill adult men who were incapacitated from wage work. Female headed and supported households were also concentrated in this group. Group 5 households pursued a livelihood strategy based upon the unskilled labour of men, women and children. Consumption indebtedness from the informal credit market at usurious rates of interest, was also a characteristic feature.

Twenty four per cent of households lost labour days due to an illness or accident in the month prior to interview. In affected households, the average number of labour days lost was 10 days per month; 21 per cent lost more than 25 days per month. In the majority of cases (80 per cent) the incapacitated earner was the male household head. Total labour days lost due to illness in men as a percentage of total labour days worked by men in the settlement population was calculated at 8 per cent.

In general, the poorest households lost many more work days to illness than the wealthier households. In total, 51 per cent of Group 5 households lost labour days due to ill health as compared to only 7 per cent in Group 2 and none in Group 1. The average number of labour days lost for Group 5 as a whole was seven days per month, compared to only 0.4 days per month for Group 2. Most illnesses suffered by Group 5 incapacitated earners were either chronic in nature (70 per cent of cases including TB, chest and stomach pains, and asthma), or due to work related accidents (20 per cent of cases including cuts, burns and fractures). A broadly similar pattern was evident in Group 4, whereas in Groups 2 and 3 incapacitation from wage work was primarily caused by acute illnesses (65–70 per cent of cases including diarrhoea, colds and headache).

There was also a strong association between incapacitation from wage work at a household level and the prevalence of severe weight-for-age undernutrition in children under five years old. Thirteen point six per cent of children from households with incapacitated earners were severely undernourished compared to 5.3 per cent in non-incapacitated households. The relative risk of a severely undernourished child coming from a household with an incapacitated earner was thus two and a half times higher than from households without an incapacitated earner. It is striking that 40 per cent of all severely undernourished children came from households with incapacitated earners. These results indicate that the presence of an incapacitated principal earner in a household is a significant risk factor for severe undernutrition in young children in this community.

Source: Pryer, Jane (1993), 'The impact of adult ill-health on household income and nutrition in Khulna, Bangladesh', Environment and Urbanization *Vol 5, No 2, October.*

anaemia (low haemoglobin levels due to poor diet) which in turn may be linked to micronutrient dietary deficiencies (especially iron deficiency) and to diseases suffered by the mother (for instance diarrhoeal diseases and intestinal worm burdens). Pregnant mothers suffering from protein and calorie undernutrition face a greater risk of low birth-weight babies while such babies are more likely to die in infancy. Malaria contracted by pregnant mothers is also often associated with stillbirths or low birth weight and maternal mortality.

The mother may also be exposed to chemical pollutants which can have a marked influence on the development of her child. Anything that she eats or inhales may end up in the blood of the foetus, transferred from her blood to her child through the placenta. The placenta acts as a barrier against some toxic substances, but many diffuse through it and are found in foetal blood.[3] Some are found in equal concentrations in the mother and foetus while some have higher concentrations in foetal blood than in that of the mother; for instance, the mercury levels in the blood of mothers who ate contaminated fish was lower than that of their newborn babies.[4] Some types of exposure of the mother to chemicals may affect the foetus and not the mother.

Certain chemicals can cause cancer or birth defects in the foetus – or kill it. For instance, it has long been known that exposure to high concentrations of lead are associated with unusually high levels of infertility, spontaneous abortion, stillbirth, neonatal death and convulsions in children.[5] The sensitivity of the foetus or embryo to dangerous chemicals depends on its stage of development. For instance, it is highly susceptible to the toxic effects of various chemicals such as benzene, lead and methyl mercury for the first two weeks after conception, and since a pregnancy is normally detected only after the third week, an early death of an embryo is often undetected.[6] Exposure during the third to the ninth week of an embryo's development can cause severe malformation of the organs as this is the period of organ differentiation. Chemical exposures during the remaining period of prenatal development can cause less severe malformations or functional deficiencies.

A proportion of all birth defects may also be linked to the mother's exposure to certain toxic chemicals during pregnancy. Birth defects occur in between 2 and 3 per cent of all births; of these, an estimated 5–10 per cent result from the influence of environmental factors such as radiation, viruses, drugs and exposure to chemicals.[7] Examples of chemicals that are known to harm the foetus through being transferred through the placenta are lead, methyl mercury, certain pesticides, polychlorinated biphenyls (PCBs) and carbon monoxide, while there is concern that the exposure of pregnant mothers to some pesticides may result in miscarriage or birth defects (see Box 3.2).

Finally, mothers' exposure to ionizing radiation is a serious hazard for their unborn children – for instance, they are particularly vulnerable to brain damage if their mothers are irradiated between the eighth and fifteenth weeks of pregnancy.[8] This is the period during which the cortex of the brain is being formed and there is a high risk that radiation (for instance from X rays) will cause severe mental retardation.[9]

Box 3.2 **Toxic Chemicals which Pose Particular Threats to Embryos or Foetuses**

Methyl mercury: The exposure of pregnant mothers to methyl mercury (for instance through high consumption of contaminated fish) can lead to neurological disorders in offspring (WHO Industry Panel, 1992). For instance, many infants developed cerebral palsy after the epidemics of methyl mercury poisoning in Minamata (Japan) and in Iraq after the consumption of seed stock treated with a mercury-based fungicide.

Carbon monoxide: Carbon monoxide diffuses across the placenta and the haemoglobin in human blood which transports oxygen has about 200 times more affinity with carbon monoxide than with oxygen. Relatively small amounts of carbon monoxide can significantly reduce the blood's ability to carry oxygen to the tissues. When the mother is exposed to carbon monoxide, the concentration in a foetus is generally higher than that in the mother and the decreased oxygen level is associated with a redistribution of foetal blood to the brain, heart and adrenals. This may lead to a decrease in foetal weight, an increase in perinatal mortality and brain damage.

PCBs: Polychlorinated biphenyls (PCBs) can pass through the placenta and damage the foetus. Several pregnant Japanese women who ate rice oil contaminated with PCBs that had leaked from a heat exchanger gave birth to infants who suffered retarded growth later in life. So too did the children born to women in Taiwan who had eaten cooking oil contaminated with PCBs.[10]

Pesticides: Ten pesticides have been identified by the US General Accounting Office in 1991 as adversely affecting reproduction and development (including DDT) with a further 20 about which there is widespread concern about their possible reproductive and developmental consequences. Pesticides such as DDT can be transferred through the placenta. Some pesticides contain dioxin as a contaminant and there is laboratory evidence that dioxin is toxic to embryos, affects reproduction and causes birth defects and cancer in animals. There is some evidence to show that pregnant women's exposure to certain pesticides may result in miscarriage or birth defects, although little systematic research has been done in this area.[11]

Source: Drawn largely from UNEP and UNICEF (1990), Children and the Environment; the State of the Environment 1990, *UNEP and UNICEF, March and Braungart, Michael, Justus Engelfried, Katja Hansen and Joyce Rosenthal (1992),* Impact of Lead and Agrochemicals on Children, *Environmental Protection Encouragement Agency, Hamburg. Note also the effect of lead and of nitrates in drinking water on the foetus are described in the text.*

Pregnant mothers (like their foetuses) are particularly vulnerable to certain environmental hazards. As a WHO report noted:

> *'The reproductive system is particularly sensitive to adverse environmental conditions. Every stage of the multi-step process of reproduction can be disrupted by external environmental agents and this may lead to increased risk of abortion, birth defects, fetal growth retardation and perinatal death.'*[12]

Every year, an estimated half a million women die of causes related to pregnancy and childbirth and their deaths leave some one million children without mothers.[13] Virtually all are in Africa, Asia and Latin America. The risk for a mother of dying during pregnancy or childbirth in a poor village or urban settlement can be 1000 times or more that for a mother from a wealthy household living in a healthy environment with good quality health services and ante-natal and post-natal care. About three quarters of maternal deaths are from one of five causes: haemorrhage, infection, toxaemia, obstructed labour and abortion (especially unsafe abortion performed by untrained personnel in unhygienic conditions). In addition, a woman's health and nutritional status substantially affect her capacity to cope with difficulties during pregnancy, childbirth and the post-partum period, to produce a strong healthy baby and to nurse and care for it.[14] In some countries, gender-based discrimination in the quantity and quality of food available to women compared to men and thus in women's nutritional status from infancy to adulthood, put pregnant women at even higher risk.[15]

INFANCY AND EARLY CHILDHOOD

The quality of the environment into which an infant is born exerts a powerful influence on whether she or he will survive their first birthday and, if they do, their subsequent physical and mental development. In families and societies with the knowledge and resources to provide a safe environment, less than one infant in 100 dies before their first birthday and most such deaths are not linked to environmental factors but to conditions the infants had at birth – for instance a congenital deformity, a genetic disease, a birth injury or physical immaturity. By contrast, up to one infant in two may die before their first birthday in the poorest families living within villages or urban settlements with the least provision to protect the infant from communicable diseases and where health services are most inadequate or non-existent for both mothers and infants. Environmental hazards are the major factor in this – especially pathogens from human excreta ingested in food or water, airborne viral or bacterial pathogens or diseases such as malaria transmitted by disease vectors.

The increasing mobility of the infant and young child as they learn to crawl and then walk, and the natural curiosity of a healthy child, also means a much increased level of risk from environmental hazards in poor quality housing and living environments. From the time that an infant first learns to crawl, through childhood and adolescence, the size and quality of the home will exert a profound influence on the level of risk. For instance, a home with inadequate provision for sanitation and personal hygiene increases greatly the risk of the child ingesting faecal pathogens. Objects with faecal matter on them may be found on the floor or around the house and put by the child in its mouth. Or a young child's hands may be contaminated with faecal matter as it plays in the area around the house and also put in the mouth.

Infants and children are particularly at risk of serious injuries from falls down steps or slopes or from coming into contact with fires, stoves or hot water. Burns and scalds are particularly common in crowded, cramped conditions where families of five or more share one small room and where it is almost impossible to protect infants and children from open fires or stoves. Accidental poisonings are also common since in such circumstances; it is difficult to keep items such as household bleach, kerosene and other poisons away from children's reach. Here, as in so many environmental problems, the level of risk is usually compounded by social factors such as a lack of adult supervision if most adults have to work. The health impact of accidents is also compounded by the lack of a health service which can rapidly provide emergency treatment, followed by longer term treatment and care.[16]

Many factors lie beyond the ability of parents or their local communities to protect their infants' health. For instance, in urban areas, these usually include their access to safe, sufficient water supplies, provision for the hygienic removal of human excreta and affordable and acceptable health services (including preventive measures such as immunization and rapid treatment for diarrhoeal diseases and pneumonia).* Other factors depend on the extent to which parents and the wider society of which they are part can act to control the most common disease vectors. For infants living in unhygienic circumstances, it also depends to a large extent on whether the mother breastfeeds the infant, and introduces nutritious and safe complementary foods in addition to breastmilk after six months of age. Infants' health also depend on the level of education and knowledge of those who look after the infants (usually the mothers), including their awareness of the importance of hygiene, of the use of techniques such as oral rehydration therapy in managing diarrhoea and of the importance of infant and childhood immunization in providing protection against many of the most serious childhood diseases.

The transfer of infants and young children from exclusive reliance on breast milk to powdered milk and to semi-solid and solid foods is also hazardous, unless the food and bottled milk can be prepared and stored, free from pathogens. Housing where food and milk can be prepared hygienically (and where necessary with water that has been boiled) and stored in fridges and where childrens' bottles, bowls, mugs and feeding utensils can be easily washed and (where necessary) sterilized greatly reduces this risk. As a recent report on weaning foods noted:

---

* Examples are given in Chapter 6 of low-income communities that did manage to improve water supplies or provision for sanitation themselves and although there is great potential for such community-directed initiatives, these will usually need some external financial support and technical assistance, even if most or all costs can be recovered. There are also many examples of sophisticated political organization by the inhabitants of particular settlements to obtain publicly funded infrastructure and services. But in general, it is very difficult for predominantly low-income communities to solve these problems with no external support.

> *'Highly contaminated weaning foods are reported to be associated with severity of malnutrition in young children. Access to inadequate facilities – for both preparation and storage of foods – by many poor households contribute substantially to weaning food contamination. Under conditions such as lack of clean water, refrigerator, fuel, adequate sewage disposal, as well as enough time to prepare fresh food for every meal, it is hardly possible to provide young children with uncontaminated weaning foods. As a result of insufficient food intake and frequent diarrhoea, many young children, particularly between two months and two years of age, experience weight loss and impaired growth and development'.[17]*

In many societies, girls are more vulnerable to environmental hazards than boys, because their nutritional and health needs receive a lower priority within the household. For example in India gender differentials in nutritional status are established during infancy, with discriminatory breastfeeding and supplementation practices. Girl infants are breastfed less frequently, for shorter durations, and over shorter periods than boys. Weaned earlier, they may not receive adequate supplementary foods and are given lower quality foods than boys.[18]

Girls' health problems may also receive less attention than boys', with proportionately more male children being treated sooner in health services and with more financial resources allocated to their health.[19] These discriminatory practices have serious implications as to how girl infants and young children can cope with disease and the impact of environmental hazards. Some societies also practice female infanticide in order to save scarce resources for a desired future male child.[20]

Thus, for infants, as for all age groups, environmental hazards interact with other hazards, and it is often difficult to isolate the health impacts of one particular hazard from the others. For instance, interactions between malnutrition and infection produce the malnutrition-infection complex where the infection is usually due to a biological pathogen in the human environment and the malnutrition to non-environmental factors. Infection influences nutritional status through its effect on intake (for instance a child's loss of appetite), on efficiency of food and nutrient utilization and absorption, and, in some instances, on the body's requirement for them.[21] Thus, a child's rate of growth may be retarded by too little food and/or by too many infections or parasites. Malnutrition, perhaps especially vitamin A deficiency, lowers immunity, so the child may be more vulnerable to infection by pathogens in the immediate environment.[22]

The transmission of many of the infectious diseases associated with infancy and childhood is through airborne viruses (eg measles, chickenpox, mumps, influenza) or bacteria (eg pneumonia, tuberculosis). Chapter 2 noted the overall scale of their health impacts while Box 3.3 considers their health impacts for infants and children. In a recent survey of a representative cross section of households in Jakarta, interviews with women in 492 families who had children under six found a high prevalence of respiratory disease among the children. Of the 658 children under six in these households, 27 per cent had suffered from respiratory disease in the two weeks prior to the interview with 17 per cent having suffered from 'fever'.[23] A similar survey in Accra found that 12 per cent of children under six had suffered from acute respiratory infection in the two weeks prior to the interview.[24]

Box 3.3 **Airborne Diseases**

Many of the diseases that are major causes of infant and child death and illness are airborne viruses (eg measles, chickenpox, mumps, influenza) or bacteria (eg pneumonia, whooping cough/pertussis, diphtheria and tuberculosis). These can be divided into those that are preventable by immunization and those that are not.

Measles, whooping cough, polio, diphtheria and tuberculosis are among those that can be prevented by immunization. If combined also with tetanus immunization, such immunization could prevent over two million child deaths and protect even larger numbers from frequent illness and poor growth. Estimates for 1993 suggest that measles killed 1.16 million children in that year with tetanus killing more than half a million (and many hundreds of thousands of mothers). Here too, there is often a complex set of factors that contribute to ill health or death – for instance, measles often leads to nutritional losses, growth faltering, lowered resistance, more diarrhoeal and respiratory infections, and further nutritional losses which helps explain why many children die of malnutrition or illness in the few months following an attack of measles. However, note should also be made of the large decreases in the deaths of children under five from measles and of newborn infants from tetanus between 1983 and 1993, largely because of immunization of children under one against measles and tetanus immunization of pregnant women.

What are termed 'acute respiratory infections' such as influenza, pneumonia, bronchiolitis and bronchitis, cannot yet be prevented by immunization; they cause or contribute to the deaths of more than four million children a year and undermine the growth of many millions more.[25] Since children's lungs are not fully developed, they are more vulnerable to respiratory disease and a child who is weakened by frequent illness and poor nutritional health is more vulnerable still. A child who contracts bronchitis or pneumonia in the South is more than 50 times more likely to die than a child in Europe or North America.[26] For those who survive, growth is often set back; a severe case of bronchitis or pneumonia will weaken a child's body, making them more susceptible to further infection and further malnutrition. Meningitis and streptococcal infections are also among the airborne infections with major impacts on child health in poorer countries.

Source: Based on UNICEF (1986), State of the World's Children 1986, *Oxford University Press and UNICEF (1995),* The State of the World's Children 1995, *Oxford University Press. Oxford.*

As Chapter 2 described, diarrhoea remains one of the most pressing health problems for infants and children in the South and is usually caused by one of a number of food or waterborne pathogens. The average annual incidence of diarrhoea among children under five years of age in the South is 3.5 episodes; many children will have ten or more episodes each year.[27] Each episode lasts from 2–3 days up to two weeks or more and may result in severe dehydration.[28] The severity depends on the infectious organism, the intensity of the infection and such host factors as the age, nutritional status and immunity of the child. The weight loss which accompanies diarrhoea usually leads to acute malnutrition and repeated episodes lead to chronic malnutrition. The risk of dying from diarrhoea is greatly increased in malnourished children.[29] Box 3.4 presents an example of the scale of health impacts which can arise in the worst environments – in this instance in spontaneous settlements around Khartoum in the Sudan.

Box 3.4 **Health among Children in Spontaneous Settlements around Khartoum**

In 1990, over a million recently displaced persons lived in spontaneous settlements in or around Khartoum – most of them moving there as a result of the lack of security in their home area or a lack of food. Most built temporary housing and settlements on open spaces in and around the city – usually in small conical huts with up to 15 persons sharing each room. Some 80 per cent of the population had no latrine so most defecation was in the open; the 20 per cent that did have a latrine had simple pits. There were no public latrines and no service to remove garbage. Only a very small proportion of the population had regular employment.

Certain diseases emerged or their incidence much increased because of this large displaced population – for instance dermal and visceral leishmaniasis (transmitted by a bloodsucking sandfly) and malaria (transmitted by *Anopheline* mosquitoes) which is resistant to treatment with chloroquine. Meningococcal meningitis which had been controlled by vaccination programmes had appeared again with the disease focus traced to the displaced populations.

A four month survey in a settlement with some 67,500 persons found that 21 per cent of the population reported some illness in this period. More than two thirds of the illnesses were due to malaria, eye infections, diarrhoeal diseases and respiratory infections. Two thirds of the cases were children under 15. A survey of children found that 37 per cent of the population had at least one attack of diarrhoea within a two week period with an average of six attacks of diarrhoea per child. Diarrhoea was the main cause of death followed by measles, fevers (probably malaria) and respiratory infections.

Source: Omer, Mohamed I A (1990), 'Child health in the spontaneous settlements around Khartoum', Environment and Urbanization *Vol 2, No 2, Oct.*

It is common for a high proportion of all children in poor rural and urban settlements in Africa, Asia and Latin America to have intestinal worm infections. The intestinal roundworm (Ascaris) infects 1000 million people and 20 roundworms (not an unusual load) can eat up nearly 10 per cent of a child's total energy intake.[30] For instance, a study in one subdistrict in East Jakarta in 1985 showed that 69 per cent of the under five population were infected with *Ascaris* (roundworm) and 11 percent with *Trichuris* (whipworm) while 43 per cent were infected with both.[31] Many other studies in low-income settlements lacking basic services have found a high proportion of young children with intestinal worm infections and often with both roundworm and whipworm.[32]

Among the many insect vectors of disease, *Anopheline* mosquitoes deserve special mention in that malaria is one of the largest single causes of child death. Malaria kills more than one million children a year in the South;[33] in Africa alone, malaria is now estimated to be responsible for the deaths of over 800,000 children each year.[34]

Infants and young children are also exposed to a much higher risk of infection if they are put into contact with large numbers of other children (and adults) – for instance at a creche or day-care centre, infant or nursery school or though being in contact with a large number of people as they are taken to work by a parent (usually the mother). Infants whose immune systems are undeveloped are at particular risk. Box 3.5 gives more detail on the increasing proportion of children who are attending creches in many societies and the evidence of higher risks of infection there.

Chapter 2 outlined some of the health risks associated with indoor air pollution from the combustion of coal or biomass fuels on open fires or inadequately vented stoves. Infants and young children may be heavily exposed because they remain with their mothers – for instance strapped to their backs – while fires are tended and cooking done. The added exposure to pollutants combined with malnutrition may retard growth, lead to smaller lungs and greater prevalence of chronic bronchitis. When infants and children are exposed to these irritant fumes and develop respiratory tract inflammation, their reduced resistance can lead to repeated episodes of acute respiratory infections, paving the way for early onset of chronic obstructive lung disease.[43] Reducing indoor air pollution from very high to low levels could halve the incidence of children's pneumonia and also reduce acute respiratory infections.[44]

In regard to chemical pollutants, organochlorine pesticide residues in mothers' milk are a potential hazard for breast-fed children. Particularly high concentrations are found in mothers' milk in areas with high levels of use, either for agriculture or for the control of insect vectors (for instance malaria and tsetse fly control) or where food has high levels of pesticide residue. However, as yet, there is no proof of instances of infants suffering ill health from ingesting milk containing pesticide residues.[45]

Lead also presents a serious hazard for infants and children. Airborne lead remains a particular concern, especially for children, since there is increasing evidence that relatively low concentrations of lead in the blood may have a damaging effect on their mental development with an effect which persists into adulthood.[46] Children's exposure to lead comes not only

Box 3.5 **Creches and Communicable Diseases**

Over the past 20 years there has been a very rapid increase in the number of children attending child day-care centres (creches), both in the North and in urban areas of the South. For example, by the mid-1980s, it was estimated that about 30 per cent of all US children under six years of age were attending some form of out-of-home care,[35] with over one third of these children being cared for in formal child day-care centres.[36] A recent study in Brazil has shown that 13 per cent of children under six years of age in Campinas, a city in Sao Paulo State, were attending official, free day-care centres for between 40 and 50 hours per week, with an equivalent proportion of 5 per cent in Fortaleza, the capital of Ceara State in the poorer north east of the country.[37] It was planned to at least double the number of such day-care centre places in the two years from 1994–95 in both cities. Additional children attend either informal or fee-paying day-care centres, or ones run by companies for their employers' children. The reasons for so many young children attending day-care centres include the increasing number of single parent families, and the high proportion of poor women who work outside the home. They are an extremely important resource allowing single parents to gain an income without their children suffering from neglect, and giving other mothers the freedom to choose whether to work outside the home or not.

Studies in the North have shown that young children attending day-care centres experienced substantially more episodes of both upper and lower respiratory tract infections,[38] middle ear infections,[39] and diarrhoea.[40] The risks were usually found to be increased by 1.5–4-fold. Two recent studies in Brazil have shown even greater increased risks of pneumonia among young children attending day-care centres compared to their neighbours cared for at home; an almost 12-fold higher risk in Porto Alegre in southern Brazil,[41] and a five-fold higher risk in Fortaleza in north-east Brazil.[42]

The most likely explanation for these findings is that the environment in day-care centres, with relatively large numbers of young children mixing with each other in close proximity, and many children being attended by the same adult carers, is conducive to high levels of transmission of infectious diseases.

The need and demand for day-care centres in urban areas is substantial and increasing rapidly, but it is important that everything possible is done to ensure that the physical and social environment within these day-care centres is designed to minimize the risk of disease transmission (eg well-ventilated rooms, relatively small numbers of children per room, limited mixing of children and carers between rooms, and very high standards of hygiene, such as hand-washing and disposal of children's faeces).

from the exhausts of petrol-engined motor vehicles where lead additives are still used in the petrol but also from lead water piping, (especially where water supplies are acidic), lead in paint and some industrial emissions.[47] A study in Mexico City in 1988 found that over a quarter of the newborn infants in Mexico City had lead levels in their blood high enough to impair neurological and motor-physical development.[48]

Chapter 2 noted that high ambient levels of lead have been found around many industries in Central and Eastern Europe. One example is the Katowice district in Upper Silesia (Poland) where four non-ferrous metal industrial plants were responsible for a high output of lead and cadmium into the air and this showed up as elevated lead and cadmium concentrations in the blood of 20 per cent of children. Some of those tested were also found to exhibit the early detectable symptoms of toxic lead effects, especially among children.[49]

Another chemical hazard for infants is high nitrate concentrations in drinking water or diets that can be converted to nitrite which can give rise to methaemoglobinaemia (or blue baby syndrome). Infants are particularly susceptible for a variety of reasons including their large fluid consumption and their less acidic gastric juices (which encourages the bacterial conversion of nitrate to nitrite). Vitamin C and an absence of bacterial contamination in water reduces the risk of methaemoglobinaemia. But since in many countries in the South, nitrate and bacterial contamination of drinking water from domestic sources and from livestock are often high and diets often lacking in vitamin C, a high incidence of methaemoglobinaemia might be expected.[50]

Children are also more vulnerable than adults to pesticides in food. First, they are more susceptible to their toxic effects; many pesticides (like lead) can affect the brain and central nervous system which are still developing in a child. Young children also absorb chemicals more easily than adults and their kidneys are less capable of getting rid of poisonous substances. Finally, children may eat proportionately more pesticide residues – for instance because of much higher intakes of fresh fruit and vegetables relative to their bodyweight.[51]

There is some evidence of weak links between a variety of inorganic chemical pollutants and health impacts in children: exposure of children to nitrogen dioxide (especially in the home) or to ozone concentrations now common in heavily populated urban centres (linked mostly to emissions from motor vehicles which react in sunlight with other chemicals in the air to produce ozone) and some aspects of impaired lung function.[52] Box 3.6 gives an example of the links between air pollution and children's impaired lung function.

One of the most serious health impacts from chemicals is through the accidental poisoning from pesticides and other chemicals kept in the home. There are few detailed statistics – although those that do exist suggest that this is a serious problem. For instance, in California, most pesticide poisoning incidents are in the home and garden and some 12,000–17,000 people are poisoned at home each year, at least half of whom are children under six years of age.[53] Various factors would suggest that the scale and severity of accidental poisonings among children in the South is likely to be substantially higher: the greater availability of highly hazardous pesticides (some

Box 3.6 **Air Pollution and Health – the case of Cubatao**

Cubatao is a city in Southern Brazil which has a high concentration of industries and significant pollution problems. Three studies have been carried out which related air pollution to health. The first in 1983 took a sample of children from each school and measured their lung function. The tests were chosen because they are relatively easy to do. Comparisons of lung function against a standard (for age and height) found a very high proportion of children with abnormally low lung functions and a clear correlation between the children with the lowest lung functions and the school areas with the highest levels of industrial air pollution. In 1983, the state environmental body began to impose environmental controls, fining many industries and closing others down because they contravened the regulations.

In 1985, the lung functions tests were repeated. It was expected that there would be improvements since the levels of particulate matter, nitrogen dioxide and sulphur dioxide had gone down. This proved to be the case except in eight schools where there had been no improvement or lung functions had got worse. These were the schools near to the industries where air pollution levels had not improved.

A third study sought to measure lung function every day taking two cohorts of children – one already tested, another new. Children with bronchial problems or otherwise not in good health were excluded. The lung function of the children was normal but in each succeeding year the results, although still normal, were worse than those in the previous year. The conclusion was that if air pollution was not drastically reduced, then the children's lung function would reach abnormal levels.

Source: Hofmaier, V.A., Efeitos de poluicao do a sobre a funcao pulmonar: un estudo de cohorte em criancas de Cubatao, *(Doctoral thesis, Sao Paulo School of Public Health, 1991, quoted in WHO (1992),* Our Planet, Our Health, *Report of the World Commission on Health and Environment, Geneva.*

of which are banned or severely restricted in most countries in the North); the difficulties of keeping pesticides safely stored away from children in overcrowded conditions; and the fact that warning labels are rarely in a language that parents (or children) can understand. Pesticide misuse is widespread and often has serious health consequences.

Chapter 2 noted how domestic accidents are responsible for about a third of all accidental deaths. Even in homes in the wealthy nations of the North, injuries occuring within the home are among the major causes of hospital admissions for young children – and in some instances, the major cause (for instance in the USA). In the UK, over half of the fatal accidents to infants and children under five happen in the home.[54] In the South, injuries account for more than a fifth of deaths among boys and a seventh of deaths of girls.[55] Accidental deaths were the leading cause of death in the age group 1–24 years in more than half of a sample of 58 countries that included nations from the North and the South, in 1977–1981.[56]

An analysis of accidents in children in ten nations in the South in 1982 found they were the main cause of death for 5–9 year olds and 10–14 year olds.[57] Injuries from falls are common in sub-standard housing and in settlements with no all-weather paths or roads and on sites on steep slopes, and children are particularly at risk. A survey of 599 'slum' children of under five in Rio de Janeiro found that accidents accounted for 19 per cent of all health problems; most reported accidents were falls (66 per cent), cuts (17 per cent) and burns (10 per cent).[58] The age of the child was an important determinant of accidents; peaks in accidents were in the second and fifth year of life. The authors note that the hazardous physical environment is only one variable in this; another is the limited possibility for parental child care and supervision when all adult members work.

One final aspect of the relationship between the environment and the young child that needs stressing is the quality of the learning and play environment. Young (and older) children need a socially secure and physically safe environment in which to grow and play but they also need an environment that is stimulating, that allows them to take risks and test themselves, and that allows them to interact with other children and with adults. Poorer families are less able to afford the kind of housing that provides a safe and stimulating environment. Adults in low-income households are generally more constrained in the time that they can spend with their children – because all adult members have to work (often long hours) to maximize income. This may not pose problems where extended kinship networks (for instance grandparents), pre-school playgroups or child-care centres can provide the supervision and stimulation that infants and young children need. But many poor households lack such support. Certainly in many urban areas, and perhaps in many rural areas too, family support for and supervision of children is deteriorating as grandparents or extended family are no longer at hand to help with childcare and adult family members have to work.[59] Young children often remain for several hours each day with little or no adult supervision, or the supervision is entrusted to older siblings who are too young and inexperienced. They are less able to anticipate and prevent household injuries and have little capacity to act swiftly if the children become sick or injured. Without adult supervision, it is also much more difficult to teach them health-enhancing behaviours – for instance in regard to defecation and washing habits.[60] Mothers who have to return to work soon after the birth of a child are also less able to continue breastfeeding, except in the very rare instances where employers make special provision to help them do so.

THE OLDER CHILD

Most of the environmental risks associated with infancy and early childhood noted in the previous section continue to pose serious risks for older children – from age 5 to 14 – although the development of their body's immune system and immunization against many childhood diseases reduces some of the risks. The respiratory, enteric and vector borne diseases caused by biological pathogens described in previous sections are likely to remain the most serious environmental factors in the ill health or death of the older child in most countries in Africa, Asia and Latin America. Other environmental hazards also need to be noted – for instance accidents and, for child workers, occupational hazards.

The increasing mobility of children as they get older and their desire to explore the world around them and to take risks often means increasing exposure to serious environmental hazards, both indoors and outdoors. This can be seen in the incidence of certain communicable diseases. For instance, at least 100 million children of between 5 and 14 years of age are infected with schistosomiasis, a debilitating waterborne parasite. Infection takes place as the child washes or bathes in a canal or pond infested with the snail which serves as the intermediate host for the parasite. The peak prevalence and intensity of infection is among children of 10–14 years of age.[61] It is also evident in the toll taken by injuries, although the scale of the problem for older children is often not evident, as many statistics on accidental injuries are not broken down by age group.

The health impact of pesticides on younger children through their use, misuse or accidental ingestion was noted earlier, but older children are also affected. For instance, in rural Guatemala, the organophosphorus compound dichlorvus was widely used on the skin to treat botfly maggot infestation.[62] In many countries, paraquat is used on the skin or hair to control lice yet paraquat is extremely toxic to humans and one mouthful may be fatal.[63]

Another area where the environment exhibits a profound impact on child health and development is the quality of the older child's living environment – both in and out of the home and school. In most countries in the South, most schools are overcrowded and most have inadequate provision for defecation and personal hygiene and for food preparation. At their most extreme, hundreds of children have to share a few latrines which are themselves poorly maintained – and with little or no provision for handwashing. To give but one example, in research in seven districts in Tanzania, in one school there were four toilets for 379 pupils while in another, there was one for 234 pupils. To the health problems that this inevitably causes should be added a serious shortage of desks (children had to sit on the sand or grass because there was no proper floor or fight over broken bricks as chairs and perch precariously on them) and books and, in the less advantaged areas, many children coming to school hungry.[64]

The quality and accessibility of facilities where play and interaction with other children and with adults can take place are also critical for child development. There are obvious links between provision for play and physical health: adequate provision for children's play keep children away from roads, garbage tips and other hazards. Careful maintenance of the places where children play can ensure they remain free of faecal contamination and garbage and can minimize risks of infection from disease vectors.

One indicator of the importance of safe play environments comes from Chile, where injuries have superseded respiratory diseases as the most common cause of childhood deaths, after improved water supplies, childhood immunization and greater availability of oral rehydration had reduced risks from respiratory and enteric infections.[65] Where progress has been made in reducing the incidence or health impact of respiratory, enteric and vector borne diseases, accidents are often found to be a major cause of injury or death among children. For instance, motor accidents were found to be the leading cause of death for 5–14 year olds in the state capitals of Brazil.[66] In Sao Paulo city in 1992, deaths from accidents had become the most important cause of death among 5–14 year olds (and also 15–44 year olds) with traffic accidents and homicides the most common single causes.[67] In general, a much smaller proportion of women die from accidents and homicides. For boys, violence alone (mostly homicides) accounted for over half of all deaths in 5–14 year olds.[68]

But children need more than 'safe open play spaces' and school yards. They need places that are exciting and diverse, where they can direct their own play. This is also important for learning about social cooperation; children need time alone with their peers and with different age groups.[69] There are profound links between the quality of provision for play and children's development. The influence of play on child development includes the development of motor skills, communication, creativity, logical thinking, emotional development and social and socialized behaviour.[70] Much of children's play is a training ground for their later participation with adults in work; it is also a central part of learning about the properties of materials and developing physical skills.[71] It is also through play that a child develops an understanding of their relationship with the natural environment.

The need for special provision for children's play is particularly important in places where there is little open space – for instance densely populated urban areas. It becomes all the more urgent where there is also a need to keep children away from roads and other hazardous places. Play spaces need to remain attractive to older children, yet also be easily reached without crossing major roads. Box 3.7 describes an *adventure playground* – a concept of play provision whose importance has been acknowledged in Europe, especially in low-income urban communities. These allow play to be child directed. They are generally staffed by trained playleaders who can not only provide adult supervision (so parents can work) but also facilitate children 'play', but without taking over its direction. The importance of trained staff in such playgrounds and of the relationship between the children and the playleaders needs to be stressed since it is often assumed that the provision of the playground alone meets children's needs.

THE CHILD AT WORK

In most societies, older children make a contribution to work, especially to household chores and, in agricultural societies, to certain tasks linked to growing and harvesting food, fuel and fodder or to looking after livestock. In urban areas, children may also have an important role in urban agriculture. Their contribution may start at an early age. For instance, a study in a rural district of Nepal found that children as young as six helped to collect fodder, since by this age they could carry a basket, while by the age of ten

---

Box 3.7 **An Adventure Playground**

An adventure playground is an area of land, surrounded by a barrier such as a fence or stockade. The space within this boundary belongs to the children who frequent the playground. The space is normally staffed by several 'playworkers', adults trained in the operation of child-based play areas who are committed to the principles of free choice, personal direction and intrinsic motivation. Their function is to facilitate and enable the play process. This is achieved in three ways:

- By *environment modification* ie continually changing the nature of the space by landscaping and rebuilding in order to create areas which are perceived as secret, enchanting, interesting and exciting by the children.
- By *accessible ruralization* ie the provision of trees, wild flowers, grasses, streams, dirt banks, and allotments, all of which exist for the children's sole use and benefit. This encourages digging, building, cooking and growing. In addition, such spaces may include the keeping of livestock, which helps children understand their relationship with the wider environment. All these factors are particularly important in an alienating and 'non-organic' inner city environment.
- By *befriending* ie by the playworkers making time for children and by intervening only when judged to be appropriate and non-intrusive (playworkers are not play 'organizers' – they may play with children but their main function is to create and sustain a friendly, stimulating, interesting and exciting environment which motivates children to explore and experiment).

Source: Hughes, Bob (1990), 'Children's play – a forgotten right'
Environment and Urbanization *Vol 2, No 2, Oct, pp 58–64*

they could engage in wage labour.[72]

It is difficult to specify at what point children's work ceases to be a natural apprenticeship to the responsibilities of adulthood and, in farming or pastoral households, to natural resource management and becomes excessive and exploitative. Children's work is often still viewed and therefore disguised as socialization – and its extent and nature are influenced profoundly not only by age but also by gender relations.[73] But certainly, for millions of children, their work burden reaches the point where it impedes their development. An estimated 80 million children between the ages of 10 and 14 undertake work that is either so long or so onerous that it interferes with their normal physical and mental development.[74] Excessive work usually means not only exposure to physical hazards but also limited school attendance or early drop out from school. It also means a denial of all the learning and skills that come from play which were outlined above.

Although much of the work undertaken by older children is not remunerated, it is often crucial for the livelihood of poorer households. It is notable that among the households living in the low-income settlement in

Khulna described in Box 3.1, it was only among the poorest households that children had an important role in income generation with very few children working in other households.[75] Children's work can include food, fodder or fuel gathering, and household tasks such as collecting water and taking responsibility for supervising younger siblings to enable other children and adults to work outside the house (a task usually taken by girls). They may have important roles in production but with their role not only unpaid but also unrecognized.

For instance, in Kerala, although girls work in coir-making, their contribution is invisible because it is carried on among domestic tasks in the household, reinforced by customary attitudes and restrictions on girls' mobility: 'Small producers to this day still depend on the availability of this type of labour for remaining in the business.'[76] In the same area: '....boys, and to a lesser extent girls too, play an important role in fishing, in particular if we understand this activity as the totality of the offshore and onshore operations necessary to render a fishing expedition successful.'[77] A study of women waste pickers in Bangalore (India) showed how their children often helped to collect and/or sort the wastes before sale.[78] The scale of children's contributions to agricultural tasks is also often forgotten or underestimated.

With respect to work *outside* the home, some children are exploited in factories and sweatshops but the majority work in agriculture or in domestic service.[79] Below are outlined some of the environmental hazards to which children are exposed; Chapter 4 will return to the question of children's contribution to their households' livelihoods.

For children working in industry, there are many environmental hazards:

> '...children are more susceptible than adults to accident, injury and industrial disease. Small, weak and inexperienced workers are more at risk from dangerous machinery and materials, heavy weights and the heat of industrial processes; and more prone to chemical poisoning and respiratory complaints caused by the many air-borne hazards'.[80]

One example is the widespread employment of minors in the shoe industries in Novo Hamburgo, Brazil; with 30 major factories and 170 smaller ones, the industry employs over 35,000 people and at least 12,000 are minors.[81] Benzene-based solvents are widely used in the shoe factories, despite the known linkage with leukaemia.[82] There is normally inadequate ventilation so the vapour hangs around the work floor. It is also common for packed lunches to be brought, stored and eaten on the shop floor, which increases still further the exposure.[83] Box 3.8 gives examples of some of the environmental hazards to which working children are exposed.

Child labour is inextricably linked with poverty; it is not the product of particular cultures or 'stages' of development. Only 120 years ago, child labour (and the phenomenon of street children) were common in Europe and North America. They may have been as common there as they are today in many countries in the South, also with such unacceptable aspects as a high incidence of homeless street children and child prostitution.[84]

Box 3.8 **Examples of environmental hazards for children at work in India**

Brass moulding industry: A report on the workers who make brass instruments in Roorkee (Uttar Pradesh, India) mentions that 400 children are engaged in this industry, mainly in packing and moulding. In the moulding, gas escapes and is inhaled by the young workers; they also get burnt by sparks and accidental spillage from molten metal.

Carpet weaving: In Kashmir's carpet weaving industry, some 6500 children between the ages of eight and ten work in congested sheds in long rows behind giant looms; the air is thick with particles of fluff and wool and 60 per cent suffer from asthma and TB.

Agate processing: In the agate processing industry in Khambat, Gujarat, which employs some 30,000 workers including many children, – a study of 342 workers including 35 children found that half the children surveyed had lung diseases and five had pneumonoconiosis.

Match industries: Match factories in or around Sivakasi employ as many as 45,000 children between 4 and 15 years of age. Twelve hour days are common, working within cramped environments with hazardous chemicals and inadequate ventilation. A supervisor commented that 'we prefer child labour. Children work faster, work longer hours and are more dependable; they also do not form unions or take time off for tea and cigarettes.'

Glass industries: In and around Firozabad, there are some 200,000 people working in glass industries; roughly a quarter are children. Among the environmental hazards are exposure to silica and soda ash dust, excessive heat, accidental burns, accidents caused by defective machines or unprotected machinery, and cuts and lacerations caused by broken glass.

Sources: Kothari, Smithu (1983), 'There's blood on those matchsticks', Economic and Political Weekly Vol XVIII, 2 July, pp 1191; and Lee-Wright, Peter (1990), Child Slaves, Earthscan, London.

CHILDREN IN ESPECIALLY DIFFICULT CIRCUMSTANCES

UNICEF have a term 'children in especially difficult circumstances' to include working children, street children, abused, neglected and abandoned children, children caught in armed conflict and children affected by disasters.[85] They would also include children who become refugees because of disasters or armed conflict. Most of these face environmental hazards that are the result of the particular 'especially difficult' circumstances they are in. Some hazards have been considered already – for instance, the section above outlined some of the occupational health and safety problems facing children working in factories. A few examples are given below to illustrate some of the environmental problems these children face – but these deserve more detailed consideration as already mentioned in Chapter 1, particularly as the environmental hazards are rarely resolvable with environmental action.

A 1991 estimate suggested that seven million children were growing up in refugee camps (most of them in Africa), often deprived not only of adequate food, health care and education but also of identity and nationality.[86] Recent events in Rwanda, Burundi, Somalia, Angola and other countries means that the number has grown significantly. Those in refugee camps are often housed in substandard accommodation, depend on precarious supplies of food and water and suffer from poor sanitation and limited medical assistance.[87] In addition, when their number is large compared to the population of the host country or when they are highly concentrated in a small part of the country, their survival needs might have negative effects on the environment.[88]

Street children are particularly at risk from a number of environmental hazards. But the likely impact of the environment varies greatly depending on the extent of the street child's linkage with parents or with some other adult carer, the kind of work in which they engage and where they 'live'. Among the 100 million or so street children, most are 'children on the street', who have strong family connections, may attend school and in most cases return home at the end of the day. Here the environmental problems associated with being street children centre on the hazards to which they are exposed during their work (for instance traffic accidents, especially for those selling goods to passing motorists on roads or highways). For 'children of the street' (with family ties but who visit their families only infrequently) and 'abandoned children', who see the street as their home and seek shelter, food and a sense of community among their companions there, environmental hazards are much greater. For instance, the work they undertake may be particularly hazardous and they often have no adult to whom to turn when sick or injured. They generally have very poor quality accommodation (often sleeping in the open or in public places) and great difficulties in getting access to places to wash, obtain drinking water, latrines and health services. They are also exposed to child abuse – not least when child prostitution turns out to be one of the more dependable ways of ensuring sufficient income for survival. In addition, many children and youths imprisoned for crimes or vagrancy or simply placed in corrective institutions may not only have to live in a very poor quality environment but also be deprived of the child–adult relationships and stimulation which are so important for child development.[89]

There are also other children in especially difficult circumstances who face particular environmental risks. For instance, a study in Bombay identified children of pavement dwellers and construction workers and 'hotel boys' as particularly vulnerable, along with street children.[90] The children of construction workers who live on site lack access to schools, daycare, health facilities, water and sanitation, and life on construction sites also poses particular hazards for children.[91]

PARENTS AT PARTICULAR RISK FROM ENVIRONMENTAL HAZARDS

Since the health and development of infants and children are so dependent on the capacity of parents to earn incomes and to provide caring, stimulating supervision, children will be at risk where parents face injury, illness or premature death from environmental hazards. Just as a concern for the welfare of street children has led to a consideration of how to prevent children being expelled onto the street,[92] so a concern for a healthy environment for children must include a concern for limiting the health burden of environmental hazards for their parents and for addressing the social and economic factors which underlie their vulnerability to such hazards. The paper by Jane Pryer summarized in Box 3.1 illustrated the extent to which ill health among income earners in poor households can increase malnutrition for virtually all family members.

The quality of a child's environment is also affected by the mental health of parents. Again, poorer households often live in housing environments where both the children and the parents are subject to a higher level of stressors, such as higher and more continuous noise levels, overcrowding, air, soil or water pollution, inappropriate design, inadequate maintenance of the physical structure and inadequate services. Such housing environments tend to ensure a higher incidence of mental disorders and social pathologies.[93]

It is often assumed that such stressors are more evident in urban areas but a report on the links between health and environment noted that certain patterns of mental disorder associated with urban life may be more a function of poverty than of urban residence per se, especially when poverty implies social disorganization and social disintegration:

> 'Urban life may have more pernicious consequences for child behaviour because of the increased likelihood of family disintegration and negative peer and environmental influence.[94] The psychosocial development of children may become a major problem in areas characterized by poor-quality housing and basic services and low-income inhabitants. If cognitive, sensory/motor and social development is prevented or hindered, it may take a lifetime to reverse the consequences. The approach to these problems must be specific since there are inner city areas and declining urban centres which, although poor, are neither degrading nor destructive of human health. Social processes rather than geographic residence may be a critical factor.'[95]

There is growing evidence that the quality of the physical environment contributes greatly to the conditions which lead to the kinds of punitive parenting and abusive behaviour that has more often been associated with families in poverty.[96] Poor families often struggle with a most restrictive amount of indoor space and a lack of access to outdoor space. With children constantly underfoot, and a chaotic physical environment due to high density, small rooms, poor layout and inadequate storage, parents who already are under stress become even more so. Also, in such crowded situations, children's natural impulses to run, explore and play in the environment are often forbidden and their play sequences are unnaturally truncated because of competing demands for space. Recent evidence from a longitudinal study of low birth-weight premature children strongly indicates that a child's resilience is greatly affected by the quality of the physical environment. The availability of safe, secure and diverse play environments was found, alongside responsive parenting, to be the most important variables for healthy development.[97] Furthermore, there is some initial evidence that insufficient space, particularly outdoor space, may contribute to disturbances in a parent's attachment behaviour with their child.[98]

No review of the impact of environmental hazards on parents will be attempted here; Chapter 2 summarized the links between the environment and health while an earlier section in this chapter outlined the environmental hazards to which women during pregnancy and childbirth are particularly vulnerable. However, five examples follow of adult groups who often face particularly high health burdens from environmental hazards: particular occupational groups, low-income groups in general, women (especially women-headed households), migrants, and those living in poor quality housing. Obviously, these groups are not mutually exclusive.

Occupational Groups

Workers in many industries or occupational groups face particularly serious environmental hazards where there is no effective enforcement of occupational health and safety. The examples given in Chapter 2 of the Egyptian pesticide factory and the Mexico steel mill show the scale and severity of occupational health problems that can occur. There are also the millions of farmers and agricultural or horticultural workers exposed to high concentrations of toxic agricultural chemicals as noted in Chapter 2. For instance, the study by Loevinsohn detected a significant increase in non-traumatic mortality rates among adult males in an area in Luzon (Philippines) which coincided with an increase in pesticide use, at a time when such mortality rates were declining for women and children.[99]

Low-income Groups

Within most cities in Africa, Asia and Latin America, there is a strong association between the level of risk from environmental hazards and household income, with the lowest income women and men, girls and boys, usually facing the greatest risks and the largest environmentally-induced health burdens.[100] There is likely to be a similar association in many rural areas as poorer groups exploit more dangerous sites (for instance land subject to landslides or other disasters), live in poorer quality houses and rely most on smoky fuels for cooking and/or heating. Low-income rural households also have less money to spend on improved water supplies and sanitation, health care and measures to lessen the possibilities of infection or injury. A considerable proportion of poor rural households are also likely to live in particularly hazardous settlements.

In urban areas, the associations between income levels and environmental hazards are generally strongest in regard to the quality and quantity of water, the level of provision for sanitation, drainage and solid waste collection, and the risk from floods, landslides and other natural hazards. The reason for this is simply that poorer groups are priced out of safe, well-located, well-serviced housing and land sites. In many cities, there will be a strong correlation between indoor air quality and income because poorer groups use more polluting fuels and more inefficient stoves (or open fires) which ensure a much worse air quality indoors. The fact that poorer groups also live in more overcrowded conditions exacerbates this and the transmission of infectious diseases. A high proportion of poor groups live in shacks made of flammable material, with higher risks of accidental fires. Poorer groups will generally have the least access to playgrounds, parks and other open spaces managed for public use. The correlations between income level and level of air pollution may not be so precise. In certain 'hot spots', such as close to quarries, cement works and industries with high levels of air pollution in their immediate surroundings, the correlation is likely to be strong. But the correlations are less clear when an entire city suffers from air pollution.

The scale of the differentials in environmental risk between income groups can be greatly reduced where governments seek to ensure that all groups have access to basic environmental services and health care is available to all. But this is not the case in most nations in the South.

Women

Women are more vulnerable than men to many of the environmental hazards associated with poor housing and living conditions and inadequate service provision as women take sole (or primary) responsibility for child rearing, household management and subsistence production.[101]

The fact that women take most responsibility for child-care means that they also have to cope with most of the illnesses and injuries from which infants and children suffer to which environmental hazards contribute much. Caring for the sick and handling and laundering soiled clothes are particularly hazardous tasks when water supplies and sanitation and washing facilities are inadequate.[102] Those within a household who are responsible for water collection and its use for laundry, cooking and domestic hygiene suffer most if supplies are contaminated and difficult to obtain – and they are generally women.

Where smoky fuels are used for cooking and/or heating in indoor fires or poorly vented stoves, it is generally women (or girls) who take responsibility for tending the fire and doing the cooking who therefore inhale larger concentrations of pollutants over longer periods.[103] Usually women take responsibility for firewood gathering and subsistence crop and livestock production; in the millions of urban households where these are important components of households' livelihoods rarely, if ever, do urban housing schemes make allowances for these activities and urban land use and zoning regulations usually discriminate against such tasks.[104] Women and children are also most vulnerable to domestic violence, which may arise from or be much increased by poor quality and overcrowded housing and living environments.

As Crewe notes:

> 'The main reason why household energy management, indoor air pollution and other health consequences of unsafe kitchens are receiving so little attention is that the managers of energy resources in households are almost always women. In all cultures women's status tends to be lower than men's, which often means that neither women's household problems nor the technical expertise they can bring to bear on these problems are taken seriously enough. Moreover, household work everywhere is unpaid, invisible, low-status work which is not included in national economic statistics. Yet the enormous amount of time it takes a woman to do this work has significant implications for the health of her entire family.'[105]

Women's vulnerability to all the environmental hazards which are linked to the inadequate provision for water, sanitation, drainage and garbage collection is greatly increased because the practical needs of those responsible for child care and household management are rarely given the priority they should have in government-provided services or housing programmes. Even when they are, women are rarely consulted about the most appropriate designs and service provision.[106] For instance, provision for health clinics (and provision for ante- and post-natal care) rarely receives the priority it deserves in terms of its cost effectiveness in reducing health burdens. Health care services rarely provide the needed focus on women's reproductive health (including advice and support for fertility control) that can do so much to reduce maternal mortality and severe health problems.[107] Where there is some public provision for health services, rarely are the locations and opening hours well suited to women's needs.

Among low-income households, those headed by women usually face particular problems. In many low-income settlements, 30 or more per cent of households are headed by women either because a male partner is temporarily absent or because of separation or death.[108] The woman is often the only income earner in the household and has to combine income earning with child rearing and household management. Thus, she faces all the problems noted already concerning the inadequacies in provision for infrastructure and services and the discrimination that prohibits the kinds of income-earning activities in which women commonly engage or denies them access to government programmes.

Migrants

Migrants may move to an area where they lack immunity to an endemic disease. The susceptibility of recent migrants to an endemic disease can set off a serious epidemic;[109] migrants may be more at risk from diseases such as tuberculosis, leishmaniasis and malaria if these diseases are not common in their area of origin. Migrants arriving in a city might also be particularly at risk from being unable to find accommodation and a source of income, and thus having to live in very poor quality accommodation. However, except for migrants who suffer discrimination because of their migrant status (especially illegal immigrants) or who were forced into cities because of wars or other disasters, in most instances the scale of environmental hazards confronting any city dweller is much more likely to be related to their income level than to their status as a recent migrant, well-established migrant or city-born person.[110]

Those in Poor Quality Housing

It should be obvious from the evidence presented in Chapters 1 to 3 that it is parents (and children) in the poorest quality, most insecure and over-crowded housing with the least adequate provision for water supply, sanitation and drainage, and garbage collection that suffer most from environmental hazards. It is also obvious that it is overwhelmingly the lower-income groups who live in such housing as they can spend least on buying, building or renting housing. Also, many low-income households live in particularly dangerous housing and/or house sites as these have locations or other characteristics that are advantageous for their survival. The settlements with a predominance of low-income groups are also generally those with the least adequate provision for health care (including infant, child and maternal health) and for schools and day care. But if this is obvious, why have these problems not received a greater priority from governments and development assistance agencies?

Part of the explanation for this and for the lack of well-directed action on these problems is the lack of data about ill health, injury and premature death among those with low incomes and those living in poor quality housing. And even where some data exists, rarely are they disaggregated by age and by sex to allow a precise understanding of the main health problems faced by female and male infants, younger children, older children and parents. Part of the explanation is also the lack of attention given by housing specialists to environmental health problems associated with housing. But perhaps as important is the extent to which low-income parents who live in very poor quality housing and who struggle to keep their children healthy and safe have not been consulted about their needs and priorities. Within the low priority given by most governments and virtually all aid agencies and development banks to improving housing and living conditions and health care for low-income groups, what resources are made available are generally 'targetted' by specialists. There is little dialogue with the parents of the infants and children who are so often sick, injured or die prematurely. There is little understanding of the resources and actions that such parents can themselves contribute to improving housing and living conditions, with appropriate support. These are issues to which this book returns in Chapter 6.

REFERENCES

1   WHO (1992), *Our Planet, Our Health*, Report of the Commission on Health and Environment, Geneva.

2   There are examples of poorer groups who develop some community-based emergency/health insurance scheme themselves – see Patel, Sheela and Celine D'Cruz (1993), 'The Mahila Milan crisis credit scheme; from a seed to a tree', *Environment and Urbanization*, Vol 5, No 1, pp 9–17 – but most low income groups are not even protected by these.

3   Braungart, Michael, Justus Engelfried, Katja Hansen and Joyce Rosenthal (1992), *Impact of Lead and Agrochemicals on Children*, Environmental Protection Encouragement Agency, Hamburg.

4   Skerfvig, S (1988), 'Mercury in women exposed to methyl mercury through fish consumption, and in their new-born babies and breast milk', *Bulletin of Environmental Contamination Toxicology*, Vol 41.

5   Barlow, S and F M Sullivan (1982), *Reproductive Hazards of Industrial Chemicals*, Academic Press, London.

6   Braungart and others 1992, op cit.

7   Kalter, H and J Warkary (1983), 'Congenital malformations', *New England Medical Journal*, Vol 308; UNEP and UNICEF (1990), *Children and the Environment, The State of the Environment 1990*; UNEP and UNICEF, Geneva.

8   UNEP (1985), *Radiation: Doses, Effects, Risks*, UNEP, Nairobi.

9   Ibid.

10   Rogan, W J, et al (1988), 'Congenital poisoning by polychlorinated biphenyls and their contaminants in Taiwan', *Science*, Vol 241, p 334.

11   Dinham, Barbara, (Ed) (1993), *The Pesticide Hazard: Global Health and Environmental Audit*, Zed Books, London.

12   WHO (1992), *Reproductive Health: a Key to a Brighter Future*, WHO Special Programme of Research Development and Research Training in Human Reproduction, Geneva, p 21.

13   UNICEF (1991), *The State of the World's Children 1991*, Oxford University Press, Oxford.

14   World Bank (1990), *World Development Report – 1990; Poverty*, Oxford University Press, Oxford.

15   Mason, John B and S R Gillespie (1990), 'Policies to improve nutrition: what was done in the 1980s', *SCN News*, No 6, UN ACC/SCN, Geneva, pp 7–20.

16   Goldstein, Greg (1990), 'Access to life saving services in urban areas' in Hardoy, Jorge E et al (Eds) *The Poor Die Young: Housing and Health in Third World Cities*, Earthscan, London.

17   Lofti, Mahshid (1990), 'Weaning foods – new uses of traditional methods', SCN News, No 6, UN ACC/SCN, Geneva, p 21.

18   India, Government of (1990), *The Lesser Child*, Department of Women and Child Development, Ministry of Human Resource Development, with assistance from UNICEF.

19   Ibid.

20   Ennew, Judith and Brian Milne (1989), *The Next Generation; Lives of Third World Children*, Zed Books, London, page 16; see also Allsebrook, Annie and Anthony Swift (1989), *Broken Promise: The World of Endangered Children*, Hodder & Stoughton.

21   Mason and Gillespie 1990, op cit.

22   Ross, A C (1992), 'Vitamin A status: relationship to immunity and the antibody response', *Proceedings of the Society of Experimental Biology and Medicine*, Vol 200, pp 303–320; also K P West Jnr, G R Howard and A Sommer (1989),

'Vitamin A and infection: public health implications', *Annual Review of Nutrition*, Vol 9, pp 63–86.

23 Surjadi, Charles (1993), 'Respiratory diseases of mothers and children and environmental factors among households in Jakarta', *Environment and Urbanization*, Vol 5, No 2, October, pp 78–86.

24 Songsore, Jacob and Gordon McGranahan (1993), 'Environment, wealth and health; towards an analysis of intra-urban differentials within Greater Accra Metropolitan Area, Ghana', *Environment and Urbanization*, Vol 5, No 2, October, pp 10–24.

25 WHO (1989), *Programme Report 1988*, Programme for the Control of Acute Respiratory Infections, WHO Document WHO/ARI/89 3, Geneva; WHO 1992, op cit.

26 Pio, A (1986), 'Acute respiratory infections in children in developing countries: an international point of view', *Pediatric Infectious Disease Journal* Vol 5, No 2, 1986, pp 179–183.

27 WHO (1992), *Our Planet, Our Health*, Report of the Commission on Health and Environment, Geneva.

28 Ibid.

29 Ibid.

30 UNICEF (1986), *State of the World's Children 1986*, Oxford University Press, Oxford and New York.

31 Budiman, Gani and others (1988), 'The nutritional and health status of children under five in the subdistrict of West Padmangan, Metropolitan Jakarta', Paper presented at a workshop on 'Population Health Systems' Interaction in Selected Urban Depressed Communities', March.

32 See for instance such studies in Manila [Auer, C (1989), *Health Problems (especially intestinal parasitoses) of Children Living in Smokey Mountain, a Squatter Area of Manila, Philippines*, Msc Thesis, Swiss Tropical Institute, Department of Public Health and Epidemiology, Basel], Kuala Lumpur [Bundey, D A P, S O P Kan and R Rose (1988) 'Age related prevalence, intensity and frequency distribution of gastrointestinal helminth infection in urban slum children from Kuala Lumpur, Malaysia' *Transactions of the Royal Society of Tropical Medicine and Hygiene* Vol 82, pp 289–294], Lagos [Fashuyi, S A (1988), 'An observation of the dynamics of intestinal helminth infections in two isolated communities in south-western Nigeria', *Tropical Geographical Medicine*, Vol 40, pp 226–232], Mexico City [Forrester, M E, M E Scott, D A P Bundey and M H N Golder (1988), 'Clustering of Ascaris lumbricoides and Trichuris trichuria infections within households', *Transactions of the Royal Society of Tropical Medicine and Hygiene*, Vol 82, pp 282–288], Galle [Hettiarchi, S P, D G H de Silva and P Fonseka (1989), 'Geohelminth infection in an urban slum community in Galle', *Ceylon Medical Journal*, Vol 34, No 1, pp 38–39] and Dhaka [Stanton, B, D R Silimperi, K Khatun and others (1989), 'Parasitic, bacterial and viral pathogens isolated from diarrhoeal and routine stool specimens of urban Bangladeshi children', *Journal of Tropical Medicine and Hygiene*, Vol 92, pp 46–55]. The findings of these and other studies on mortality and morbidity of children are summarized in Bradley, David, Carolyn Stephens, Sandy Cairncross and Trudy Harpham (1991), *A Review of Environmental Health Impacts in Developing Country Cities*, Urban Management Program Discussion Paper No 6, The World Bank, UNDP and UNCHS (Habitat) Washington, DC.

33 The estimate for 1993 was for 1.16 million deaths of children under age five from malaria – WHO (1995), *The World Health Report 1995: Bridging the Gaps*,

WHO, Geneva. This includes deaths through malaria in association with acute respiratory infections and anaemia.

34 WHO (1991), *Global Estimates for Health Situation Assessments and Projections 1990*, Division of Epidemiological Surveillance and Health Situation and Trend Analysis, WHO, WHO/HST/90.2, Geneva.

35 Haskins R and J Kotch (1986), 'Day care and illness: evidence, cost, and public policy', *Pediatrics* Vol 77, pp 951–982.

36 Anderson L J, R A Parker, R A Strikas et al (1988), 'Day-care center attendance and hospitalization for lower respiratory tract illness', *Pediatrics* Vol 82, pp 300–308.

37 Barros A J D, L Correia L, and D A Ross, personal communication.

38 Anderson et al 1988, op cit; Gardner G, A L Frank and L H Taber (1984), 'Effects of social and family factors on viral respiratory infection and illness in the first year of life', *Journal of Epidemiol Community Health* Vol 38, pp 42–48; Hurwitz, E S, W J Gunn, P F Pinsky et al (1991), 'Risk of respiratory illness associated with day-care attendance: a nationwide study', *Pediatrics* Vol 87, pp 62–69; Wald, E R, N Guerra and C Byers (1991), 'Frequency and severity of infections in day care: three year follow-up', *Journal of Pediatrics* Vol 118, pp 509–514; and Woodward A, R M Douglas, N M H Graham and H Miles (1991), 'Acute respiratory illness in Adelaide children – the influence of child care', *Medical Journal of Aust*, Vol 154, pp 805–808 .

39 Henderson, F W and G S Giebink (1986), 'Otitis media among children in day care: epidemiology and pathogenesis' *Review of Infectious Diseases* Vol 8, pp 533–538; and Wald, E R, N Guerra and C Byers (1991), 'Upper respiratory tract infections in young children: duration of and frequency of complications', *Pediatrics* Vol 87, pp 129–133.

40 Alexander, C S, E M Zinzeleta, E J Mackenzie, A Vernon and R K Markowitz (1990), 'Acute gastrointestinal illness and child care arrangements', *American Journal of Epidemiology* Vol 131, pp 124–131.

41 Victora C G, S C Fuchs, J A C Flores, W Fonseca and B Kirkwood (1994), 'Risk factors for pneumonia among children in a Brazilian metropolitan area', *Pediatrics* Vol 93, pp 977–985.

42 Fonseca W, B R Kirkwood, C J Victora, S R Fuchs, J A Flores and C Misago (in press), 'Risk factors for childhood pneumonia among the urban poor in Fortaleza, Brazil: a case-control study', *WHO Bulletin*.

43 WHO (1992), *Our Planet, Our Health*, Report of the Commission on Health and Environment, Geneva.

44 World Bank (1993), *World Development Report 1993; Investing in Health*, Published for the World Bank by Oxford University Press, Oxford.

45 Conway, Gordon R and Jules N Pretty (1991), *Unwelcome Harvest*, Earthscan, London.

46 Needleman, Herbert L, Alan Schell, David Bellinger, Alan Leviton and Elizabeth N Allred (1991), 'The long-term effects of exposure to low doses on lead in childhood: an eleven year follow up report' *The New England Journal of Medicine* Vol 322 No 2, pp 83–88.

47 WHO 1992, op cit.

48 Rothenburg, Stephen J, Lourdes Schnaas-Arrieta, Irving A Perez-Guerrero et al (1989), 'Evaluacion del riesgo potencial de la exposition perinatal al plombo en el Valle de Mexico', *Perinatologia y Reproduccion Humana*, Vol 3, No 1, pp 49–56.

49 Jarzebski, L S (1992), 'Case Study of the Environmental Impact of the

Non-Ferrous Metals Industry in the Upper Silesian Area', in WHO, *Report of the Panel on Industry*, WHO Commission on Health and Environment, WHO/EHE/92.4, WHO, Geneva.

50 Conway and Pretty, 1991, op cit.

51 Timberlake, Lloyd and Laura Thomas (1990), *When the Bough Breaks : Our Children, Our Environment*, Earthscan, London.

52 WHO, 1992, op cit.

53 CFDA; California Department of Food and Agriculture (1990), *Summary of Illnesses and Injuries Reported by California Physicians as Potentially Related to Pesticides, 1990* (and reports in previous years), Sacramento, California, quoted in Conway and Pretty 1991, op cit.

54 Woodroffe, Caroline, Myer Glickman, Maggie Barker and Chris Power (1993), *Children, Teenagers and Health: The Key Data*, Open University Press, Buckingham.

55 WHO 1995, op cit.

56 WHO 1991, op cit.

57 Manciaux, M and C J Romer (1986), 'Accidents in children, adolescents and young adults: a major public health problem' *World Health Statistical Quarterly* Vol 39, No 3, pp 227–231.

58 Reichenheim, M and T Harpham (1989), 'Child accidents and associated risk factors in a Brazilian squatter settlement' *Health Policy and Planning* Vol 4, No 2, pp 162–167.

59 Sapir, D (1990), *Infectious Disease Epidemics and Urbanization: a Critical Review of the Issues*, Paper prepared for the WHO Commission on Health and Environment, Division of Environmental Health, WHO, Geneva.

60 Ibid.

61 UNEP and UNICEF 1990, op cit.

62 Hunter, John M (1990), 'Bot-fly maggot infestation in Latin America', *Geographical Review*, Vol 80, No 4, October, pp 382–398.

63 WHO (1992), *Our Planet, Our Health*, Report of the Commission on Health and Environment, Geneva.

64 Mabala, Richard (1995), *The Girl Child*, manuscript developed for UNICEF (Tanzania), Dar es Salaam.

65 See for instance Toucher, L (1981), 'Mortalidad de la 4 anos de edad: tendencias y causas; notas de poblacion', *Revista Latinoamericana de Demografia*, Vol 26, No 9, pp 27–54 quoted in Walsh, Julia A (1988), *Establishing Health Priorities in the Developing World*, UNEP, Adams Publishing Group.

66 PAHO (1988), 'Research on Health Profiles: Brazil 1984', *Epidemiological Bulletin of the Pan American Health Organization*, Vol 9, No 2, pp 6–13, quoted in Bradley and others 1991, op cit.

67 Stephens, Carolyn, Ian Timaeus, Marco Akerman, Sebastian Avle, Paulo Borlina Maia, Paulo Campanerio, Ben Doe, Luisiana Lush, Doris Tetteh and Trudy Harpham (1994), *Environment and Health in Development Countries: an Analysis of Intra-urban Differentials Using Existing Data*, London School of Hygiene and Tropical Medicine, London.

68 Violence (mostly homicides) also accounts for 86 per cent of all deaths in boys of 15–19; Stephens et al 1994 op cit.

69 Hart, Roger A (1992), *Children's Participation; from Tokenism to Citizenship*, Innocenti Essays No 4, UNICEF International Child Development Centre,

Florence.

70　Hughes, Bob (1990), 'Children's play – a forgotten right' *Environment and Urbanization* Vol 2, No, 2, October, pp 58–64.

71　Hart 1992, op cit.

72　Johnson, Victoria, Joanna Hill and Edda Ivan-Smith (1995), *Listening to Smaller Voices: Children in an Environment of Change*, ActionAid, London.

73　Nieuwenhuys, O (1994), *Children's Lifeworlds: Gender, Welfare and Labour in the Developing World*, Routledge.

74　UNICEF 1991, op cit.

75　Pryer, Jane (1993), 'The impact of adult ill-health on household income and nutrition in Khulna, Bangladesh', *Environment and Urbanization*, Vol 5, No 2, October, pp 35–49.

76　Nieuwenhuys 1994, op cit p 142.

77　Ibid, p 86.

78　See for instance Huysman, Marijk (1994), 'Waste picking as a survival strategy for women in Indian cities', *Environment and Urbanization*, Vol 6, No 2, October, pp 155–174.

79　UNICEF 1991, op cit.

80　Lee-Wright, Peter (1990), *Child Slaves*, Earthscan, London, p 10.

81　Ibid.

82　WHO (1992), *Our Planet, Our Health*, Report of the Commission on Health and Environment, Geneva; Askoy, M et al (1976), 'Types of leukaemia in a chronic benzene poisoning', *Acta haematologica* Vol 55, pp 67–72.

83　Lee-Wright, 1990, op cit.

84　See for instance Hibbert, Christopher (1980), *London: a Biography of a City*, Penguin Books, London, 1986, on homeless children and child prostitution in 19th century London.

85　UNICEF (1986), 'Children in especially difficult circumstances', Document based on the Executive Board Resolutions E/ICEF/1986/CRP 33, and 37 and distributed as CF/PD/PRO-1986-004, New York.

86　UNICEF 1991, op cit.

87　WHO (1992), *Our Planet, Our Health*, Report of the Commission on Health and Environment, Geneva.

88　Ibid.

89　UNICEF (1992), *Environment, Development and the Child*, Environment Section, Programme Division, UNICEF, New York.

90　Patel, Sheela (1990), 'Street children, hotels boys and children of pavement dwellers and construction workers in Bombay: how they meet their daily needs', *Environment and Urbanization*, Vol 2, No 2, October, pp 9–26.

91　Ibid.

92　Korten, David C (1990), 'Observations and Recommendations on the UNICEF Urban Child Programme', *Environment and Urbanization*, Vol 2, No, 2, October, pp 46–57.

93　WHO 1992, op cit.

94　Cederblad, M (1988), 'Behavioural disorders in children from different cultures', *Acta Psychiatria Scandinavica*, Vol 78 (Supplement 344), pp 85–92.

95　WHO 1992, op cit, p 217.

96 Sharp, C (1984), 'Environmental design and child maltreatment', in D Durke and D Campbell (Eds), *The Challenge of Diversity*, Proceedings of the 15th Annual Conference of the Environmental Design Research Association, EDRA, Washington DC; and Peterman, P (1981), 'Parenting and environmental considerations', *American Journal of Autopsychiatry*, Vol 5, No 2, pp 351–355.

97 Bradley, R H, L Whiteside, D J Mundfrom, P H Casey, K J Kellerher and S K Pope (1994), 'Early indications of resilience and their relation to experiences in the home environments of low birth weight, premature children in poverty', *Child Development*, Vol 65, pp 346–360.

98 Bartlett, S, forthcoming, *The Physical Environment of the Home as a Factor in Socialization*, Children's Environments Research Group, City University of New York, New York.

99 Loevinsohn, M E (1987), 'Insecticide use and increased mortality in rural central Luzon, Philippines', *The Lancet*, I, pp 1359–62, quoted in Conway and Pretty 1991, op cit.

100 Hardoy, Jorge E, Diana Mitlin and David Satterthwaite (1992), *Environmental Problems in Third World Cities*, Earthscan, London.

101 Moser, Caroline O N and Linda Peake (Eds) (1987), *Women, Human Settlements and Housing*, Tavistock Publications, New York and London; Lee-Smith, Diana and Catalina Hinchey Trujillo (1992), 'The struggle to legitimize subsistence: Women and sustainable development' *Environment and Urbanization* Vol 4, No 1, April, pp 77–84.

102 Sapir 1990, op cit; Jordan, Sara and Fritz Wagner (1993), 'Meeting women's needs and priorities for water and sanitation in cities', *Environment and Urbanization*, Vol 5, No 2, October, pp 135–145.

103 WHO (1992), *Our Planet, Our Health*, Report of the Commission on Health and Environment, Geneva.

104 Lee-Smith and Trujillo 1992, op cit.

105 Crewe, Emma (1995), 'Indoor air pollution, household health and appropriate technology; women and the indoor environment in Sri Lanka', in Bonnie Bradford and Margaret A Gwynne (editors), *Down to Earth: Community Perspectives on Health, Development and the Environment*, Kumarian Press, West Hartford, pp 94–95.

106 Moser, Caroline O N (1987), 'Women, human settlements and housing: a conceptual framework for analysis and policy-making', in Caroline O N Moser and Linda Peake (Eds), *Women, Housing and Human Settlements*, Tavistock Publications, London and New York, pp 12–32.

107 Germain, Adrienne and Jane Ordway (1989), *Population Control and Women's Health: Balancing the Scale*, International Women's Health Coalition in cooperation with the Overseas Development Council, New York.

108 Moser 1987, op cit.

109 Sapir 1990, op cit.

110 The reasons for this are discussed in more detail in Satterthwaite, David (1993), 'The social and environmental impacts associated with rapid urbanization', Paper presented to the Expert Group Meeting on Population, Distribution and Migration, UN Population Division, Santa Cruz, January. There is a tendency among commentators on urban problems in Africa, Asia and Latin America to assume that it is predominantly migrants to cities who live in squatter settlements and face the highest levels of unemployment, despite the many detailed empirical studies which have shown these generalizations to be inaccurate.

4

Children and Renewable Resources

INTRODUCTION

This chapter's main concern is how and under what conditions households obtain those natural resources on which their children's survival or development depend. Consideration is given to soil, forests and fresh water with a special interest in:

- the role of the resource in underpinning household livelihoods and the health of its members;
- current trends in terms of women's and men's access to the resource and how the quality of the stock is changing;
- the extent to which environmental factors underlie poverty; and
- the implications of current conditions and trends for girl and boy children.

Thus, this chapter is not so much on the relationship between children and renewable resources but on the issue of guaranteeing households and poor communities access to renewable resources. Guaranteeing poorer households access to those resources essential for adequate livelihood and health would probably do more to improve child health and development than any other factor. Although it is also important to consider the situation of children within households and communities that rely on renewable resources, the main environment/ development issue remains that of guaranteeing adequate livelihoods for individuals and households while also ensuring sustainable land-use and management practices.

With appropriate cultivation or management practices, most land and water ecosystems can sustain production and be considered as a renewable resource. Soil is usually classified as a renewable resource. Yet much fertile soil is being degraded through overexploitation or poor management and some is being destroyed. As the WHO Commission on Health and Environment noted:

> '... a growing proportion of land-based productive and protective ecosystems are being irreversibly degraded and lost as a result of

human activities. Many countries are facing an expanding demand for food, fuel and other primary commodities and at the same time a growing loss of farmland and diminishing water resources and biological diversity. For example, fertile soils developed by natural processes over millennia are being subjected to destruction or degradation by overuse or misuse in a few decades or, on occasion, a few years. Soil degradation from erosion, salinization, waterlogging and pollution are among the menaces that undermine soil fertility and the agricultural productivity of farmlands and rangelands'.[1]

For a large proportion of the world's children, the most important natural resource issue is whether their mothers and fathers have access to sufficient productive land and water for an adequate and sustainable livelihood and sufficient fresh water for drinking and household use. As in most other environmental issues, this is not simply an issue of the size and quality of the resource base since social, economic and political factors largely define who obtains access to these resources. Poor people's lack of access to fertile land and fresh water, or the high costs they have to pay to obtain access, are more often the result of highly unequal income and asset distributions within their society than a physical scarcity of these resources.

ACCESS TO RENEWABLE RESOURCES AND POVERTY

An estimate for 1988 suggested that there were some 940 million people living in rural areas who are living in poverty.[2] Two thirds were in Asia with just over a fifth in sub-Saharan Africa.[3] Most of them were in households with land holdings too small to provide them with an adequate income. Most of the rest were landless; the proportion of poor rural dwellers who were landless was particularly high in Latin America and the Caribbean and in Asia.

A high proportion of the world's undernourished people (including undernourished infants and children) are within these 940 million. A considerable proportion of the 1.6 billion or so urban dwellers that lived in Africa, Asia and Latin America in 1995 were also undernourished but this is only considered in this chapter where this is linked to their lack of access to renewable resources.

Most rural inhabitants in Africa, Asia and Latin America depend on access to soil, trees and fresh or marine water resources for their livelihoods. Where livelihoods are based on farming, livestock rearing, fishing or hunter gathering, all household members are dependent on the natural environment for many aspects of their food, health, shelter and development. For most rural households, it is from this natural environment that they obtain water and food, goods for sale, materials for shelter and, very often, raw materials for artifacts manufactured for the household's use or for sale. The natural environment is also a major influence on children's early development and provides the setting in which they learn and first begin to contribute to their household's livelihood. In many cultures, children begin quite early to help collect water and fuel and to help with some agricultural tasks. It is common for girls and boys to have different tasks and responsibilities.

Rural households and communities have usually evolved complex livelihood strategies that often involve a mix of agriculture, pastoralism, forestry and fishing. Any degradation in the natural resource base or decreasing access to such resources (for instance as forests or water sources that were previously common property resources become privatized or degraded) will usually mean less food or income. This implies a greater risk of malnutrition and ill health for all family members, including impaired physical and mental development for infants and children. It often means that adults have to spend more time in resource collection or exploitation and perhaps less time for mothers and fathers to spend with and care for their children. It often leads to one of the parents having to spend increasing amounts of time away from the home, through temporary, seasonal or permanent migration to obtain a more secure livelihood for the household. Thus, the degradation of resources generally makes it increasingly difficult for parents to provide the supervisory, nurturing and caring role that children need from parents.* It often increases the pressure on children to begin work before completing their education or to increase their workload and increasingly to miss school. Various case studies have shown how girls are more likely to have tasks assigned to them so they miss more school than boys or leave school earlier.[4]

A significant proportion of urban inhabitants of Africa, Asia and Latin America also depend on access to soil, trees and fresh or marine water resources for part or all of their livelihood – and this is considered in more detail in a later section on 'access to renewable resources in urban areas.'

SOIL

The Stock of Fertile Soil

Fertile soil and the water supplies needed to ensure that crops can be grown (or trees or other vegetation supported) can be considered the two natural resources with the most immediate importance for human livelihoods. They remain the source of most food production worldwide. More than half the world's children live in households whose livelihoods depend directly on access to fertile soil and water.

Although soil is a 'renewable resource' in that good farming or pasture management practice maintains its fertility, the supply of fertile soil is finite and the world's stock is declining through soil erosion, salinization, deforestation/desertification, waterlogging and pollution. In addition, there is the spread of urban areas over agricultural land – often among a nation's best quality soil (since so many major cities were founded in areas with

---

* The term parent will be used throughout this chapter, although other adults (for instance grandparents or other adult family members) and older children (usually siblings) often have important formal or informal responsibilities for caring for infants or young children.

fertile soil), although it may be overstated in many instances. Only in relatively urbanized countries with high population densities and countries with unusually small proportions of their total area as cultivable land (as in Egypt) is this likely to be among the most important factors depleting the stock of fertile soil. There are also other factors linked to urbanization, including the use of fertile soil for landfill and brickmaking to meet urban demands and the degradation of soil or vegetation as a result of air, water and land pollution originating from urban-based activities.* 'Soil is not an inert mass but a very delicately balanced assemblage of mineral particles, organic matter and living organisms in dynamic equilibrium'.[5]

The relationship between soil management, food production and ecological sustainability has been changing in recent decades. For most of its history, and in most areas, agriculture has been environmentally benign (although with notable exceptions – some of the great early city-states and cities are thought or known to have lost importance as the ecological base on which they depend was eroded or destroyed):

> 'Even when industrial technology began to have an impact in the 18th and 19th centuries, agriculture continued to rely on natural ecological processes. Crop residues were incorporated into the soil or fed to livestock, and the manure returned to the land in amounts that could be absorbed and utilized. The traditional mixed farm was a closed, stable and sustainable ecological system, generating few external impacts.'[6]

From the point of view of ecological sustainability, there is much to admire in the Chinese farmer in the 1930s, feeding a family on a fifth of a hectare or less and making very intensive use of organic wastes (including human wastes) to retain soil fertility.[7] Such a farming system was among the most land and energy efficient in the world. It could produce around 50 calories of food for every calorie of energy input which is one or two orders of magnitude more energy efficient than most modern farming.[8] From a development point of view, it had little to recommend it since it provided a very inadequate livelihood for the family and, very often, such farmers were tenants and paid very high rents to landowners.[9] Poverty in this context was much less the result of land shortages and more the result of inequitable land-owning structures and exploitative landowner-tenant relationships.

There are also many historic and contemporary examples of intensive agriculture or horticulture on relatively small plots of land that were or are ecologically sustainable without large chemical inputs and which provide households with adequate livelihoods. These provide examples of what can be achieved when there is relatively little land in relation to population. But supporting households with relatively small landholdings to improve

---

* Urbanization also has positive factors: the food grown and livestock raised within urban boundaries (which in many countries represents an important part of total food production); the extent to which urban demand for rural produce provides rural producers with the income to permit capital investment in soil and water conservation; and the goods and services provided to rural producers and consumers by urban enterprises which help sustain their production.

their incomes through more intensive cultivation and higher value crops and to do so in ways that are ecologically sustainable has not been the priority of governments or international agencies in their support for agricultural and rural development.

The objectives of agricultural research in the 1960s and 1970s focused on a technological solution to the problems of feeding the world. It essentially produced technical innovations which could be implemented in the most favourable agroclimatic regions and for those farmers with the best means for realizing the potential yield increases.[10] The last 30 years have brought impressive gains in terms of the growth in the world's total food production. Worldwide, the supply of calories per person increased by 14 per cent between the early 1960s and early 1980s; the increase in the South averaged 21 per cent in this same period.[11] But despite impressive yield increases in staple crops, Conway and Barbier identify two central problems.

The first problem is that: 'the new technologies are less suitable for resource-poor environments; farmers with small and marginal holdings have, on the whole, benefited less than farmers on large holdings.'[12] This is particularly so in Africa where large scale irrigation schemes were perceived as providing the means to protect harvests against hazards of drought but have run into serious problems of maintenance, high costs, low yields and poor incentives to farmers.[13] Meanwhile, the needs and priorities of women farmers in general, and poorer women and men in less productive areas have been largely ignored and, when some support was provided, it was often ill suited to local conditions. An estimated 1.4 billion people depend on what are termed low external input systems which are located in drylands, wetlands, uplands, near-deserts, mountains and hills[14] and their needs and priorities in regard to increasing production and conserving their soil base have received little support.

The second problem is that the increase in production may not be sustainable:

> 'intensive monocropping has also made production more susceptible to environmental stresses and shocks ... and ... there is growing evidence of diminishing returns from intensive production with high-yielding varieties... Moreover, it has become clear that these are not simple second or third generation problems capable of being solved by further technological adjustments.'[15]

Traditional pastoral societies also developed skills to manage large herds in spite of short grazing seasons, limited supplies of drinking water, irregular rainfall and periodic drought conditions. However, many traditional pastoral systems have now become destabilized and unsustainable due to increasing pressure on land resources (mainly from farmers) and unfavourable environmental conditions. Rangelands have been degraded in many parts of the world as a result of mismanagement and overgrazing.[16]

Soil Degradation and Desertification

A global assessment of human-induced soil degradation[17] suggested that some two billion hectares of soils worldwide were degraded (ie they had lost some of their natural productivity); this represents some 17 per cent of all vegetated land; 40 per cent of this land was lightly degraded while most of the rest suffered from 'moderate' degradation, ie its agricultural productivity was greatly reduced but it can still be used for agriculture. Some 300 million hectares have suffered from severe degradation which implies the need for major investments if its original biotic functions are to be reclaimed; nine million hectares were defined as unreclaimable and beyond restoration.*

The term 'desertification' is given to the degradation of soil and vegetation within the arid, semi-arid and sub-humid zones caused largely by harmful human activities. Drylands make up a third of the world's surface and provide a home for some 900 million people.[18] Estimates for 1991 suggest that around one fifth of the world's drylands is subject to human-induced soil degradation. Although Asia and North America have the

---

Box 4.1 **Africa's Drylands**

Excluding the hyper-arid deserts, dryland areas cover an estimated 43 per cent of the surface area of Africa and are home to 66 per cent of Africa's human population. Subject to low and uncertain rainfall within a short rainy season, dryland peoples have always had to cope with drought. However, the past few decades have witnessed growing problems of environmental degradation, food shortages, impoverishment and conflict through much of the drylands. In their acute form, rainfall failure and crop failure combined with political conflict, have produced refugees in their millions and a heavy human cost. Less clearly in evidence but of increasing importance has been the rising pressure of demand on all resources within the dryland region and increasing conflicts between different users for control over farmland, water, forests and pastures.

While low and unreliable rainfall is a key part of the vulnerability of dryland Africa to food shortage and famine, there are other very important contributory factors – institutional issues such as land tenure, economic policy such as food prices, questions related to international trade and debt, the low priority given to marginal regions by national governments, and military conflict. Together these factors help explain why tens of millions of people in Africa are at risk of serious food shortage while many millions more are chronically under nourished.

Source: Toulmin, Camilla, Ian Scoones and Josh Bishop (1992), 'Drylands' in Johan Holmberg (Ed), Policies for a Small Planet, Earthscan, London.

---

* Worldwide, agricultural activities accounted for 28 per cent of this with overgrazing accounting for about 35 per cent and deforestation for 28 per cent. Overexploitation for fuelwood accounted for 7 per cent. The relative importance of these varies greatly by region. For instance, in Africa, half of all soil degradation arises from overgrazing while overexploitation for fuelwood accounts for 13 per cent and agriculture for 24 per cent. In Central America, which has the highest percentage of vegetated land with moderate to extreme soil degradation, agricultural activities are the main cause (45 per cent) followed by deforestation (22 per cent). For Asia and South America, deforestation is the major cause, accounting for around 40 per cent, with most of the rest divided equally between agricultural activities and overgrazing.

highest percentage of drylands subject to desertification, it is in Africa where the human impact is most dramatic (see Box 4.1).

Many rural communities living in mountain areas are also particularly vulnerable to soil degradation.[19] While most such communities developed intricate adaptive mechanisms for managing soils and other natural resources to limit environmental degradation, a combination of internal and external forces have often resulted in serious environmental degradation.[20] For instance, this can be seen in the mountain areas of Central and South America, the hills of Indonesia, Nepal, the Philippines, Thailand and East Africa.[21]

Causes of Soil Degradation

In any particular location where soil degradation is taking place, there is usually a complex mix of immediate and underlying causes. There is also such variety between different locations in the range of causes or contributory factors and their relative importance that generalizations are difficult. But the immediate causes of soil degradation from agricultural activities include: shortening of fallow periods in shifting cultivation, or cultivating hillsides with inadequate protection against water erosion, or leaving soil exposed during fallow periods to wind erosion. Many soils cultivated by shifting cultivators and subsistence farmers in the tropics and sub tropics are subject to fertility depletion through a decline in soil organic matter, reduction in nutrient reserves by crop removal, leaching and acidification.[22] Waterlogging and soil salinization are major causes of declining yields on irrigated land, usually the result of poor water management (and drainage). Salt-affected soils are widely distributed throughout the arid and semi-arid regions. The problems are particularly severe in China (where 7 million hectares are affected), India (20 million hectares), Pakistan (3.2 million hectares) and the Near East.[23]

The underlying causes of soil degradation are usually complex and often interlinked.[24] For instance, one of the causes of over grazing in semi-arid regions is population pressure which is forcing farmers to cultivate marginal lands, often traditional grazing lands.[25] Poorer quality land formerly farmed extensively or left uncultivated has been brought into cultivation or fallow periods have been diminished. In many instances, this has meant serious damage to the soil with cultivation often abandoned after a few years; this has also led to the destruction of valuable sources of wild resources. However, the increasingly large agricultural and pastoral population who depend on land that is being degraded is often not the result of a shortage of good quality land. Three other factors are often important: land tenure and land-owning structures, commercial pressures, and inappropriate government policies and incentives.

Land Tenure and Land-owning Structures

In many instances, it is highly inequitable land owning structures that prevent poorer groups obtaining access to and control over sufficient land on which a livelihood can be sustained. Women often face more difficulties than men in obtaining land or rights to use land, even in societies where they are responsible for most farming and food production. Analyses as to the causes of soil degradation on the small land holdings of poorer households may stress population pressure as the underlying cause but this is often within a broader context of no overall shortage of good quality land. The northeast of Brazil provides one of the most dramatic examples. This has long been considered an area of extreme rural poverty, despite being located within one of the South's most wealthy and economically powerful nations. Poverty and malnutrition there are also associated with periodic droughts. The high proportion of rural dwellers with little or no land in this region has been the main cause of large migration flows out of the region or to the major northeastern cities. However, a reallocation of agricultural land in this region to small farms using only land which is currently unused or under-utilized by large landowners would provide an adequate livelihood for a million households and promote employment for many more (see Box 4.2).

Box 4.2 **Links between Poverty and Land-ownership**

A World Bank study shows that the main cause of poverty and out-migration from the northeast of Brazil is not a lack of land but a land-owning structure that keeps large amounts of high quality land unused or under-utilized. The study states that there are nearly one million farms or sharecropped plots in the northeast which provide an acceptable standard of living for farmers. There are also 'nearly 30 million hectares of under-utilized land of similar if not superior quality on the estates' on which 'nearly another million families could achieve comparable living standards'. Most of this land is unused or under-utilized and is the property of large land-owners; just 4 per cent of landowners own more than half the agricultural land and only one in four households in the region who are dependent on agriculture own the land they work.

If this land was transferred to those with no land or too little land, this could provide adequate incomes for perhaps another million families. The smallest farmers in the region:

> 'employ 25 times more labour per hectare on their land than do the largest farms and obtain vastly higher productivity levels. The smaller farms (less than 50 hectares) cover only 10 per cent of the agricultural land, produce over 25 per cent of the region's sugar, cotton and rice and 40 per cent of the beans, corn and manioc. Yet two million agriculturally dependent families own no land at all while an area of land the size of France is un- or under-utilized'

Such a land transfer would also bring a major stimulus to agricultural production (which would help feed city populations) and also to small urban centres there.

Source: Kutcher, Gary P and Pasquale L Scandizzo (1981), The Agricultural Economy of Northeast Brazil, *Johns Hopkins University Press, Baltimore.*

In their wide-ranging discussion of the factors which underlie rural poverty, Jazairy, Alamgir and Panuccio[26] included three related to social structures which inhibit large sections of national populations obtaining sufficient land:

- dualism in land-owning structures in ex-colonial societies where colonial production patterns persist and small and marginal farmers are hurt because resources, starting with the best land, are pre-empted by large, primarily export-oriented commercial farms;
- exploitative intermediation where landowners exploit share croppers and moneylenders exploit farmers and agricultural workers; and
- cultural or ethnic biases that limit or exclude large sections of the population from access to land and/or services – including the Amerindian populations of South and Central America, the nomadic pastoralists of the Near East and North and Southern Africa and the tribal and minority populations of Bangladesh, India, the Philippines, Thailand and elsewhere.

Commercial Pressures

Another key reason for increasing population pressure on soils by those with relatively little land is through commercial pressures that take over (legally or illegally) land that had previously been used by these people – as open access or common property resources. As commercial interests take over this land, poorer groups who have long drawn on forests and fresh-water sources and collected firewood or wild foods from unused land (or grazed their livestock there) are denied access to it. Or a conflictual relationship develops between these people and those who have appropriated the resource or growing conflicts within the community destroy the basis for community management. *The State of World Rural Poverty*[27] notes that poverty, commercially-induced encroachments and the extension of state jurisdiction seem to have broken the harmonious relationship between communities and the pastures and forested lands that they managed. Many examples of this destruction of or damage to effective community-based resource management systems are also presented in *Whose Common Future?*[28] The extension of state jurisdiction over natural resources during the colonial period is also noted by many authors as a key factor in undermining traditional community-based systems of common property resource management.[29]

A lack of secure land tenure for any farmer or pastoralist, particularly for smallholders, will discourage investment in better management and use. Insecure tenants are rarely willing or able to undertake longer-term investments in land improvement, irrigation, soil and water conservation and are also less likely to plant tree crops.[30]

In many instances, it is commercial farming or forestry operations that are the key cause of soil degradation – with population pressures having little or no role. For instance, the large mechanized farming schemes in eastern Sudan produced substantial returns for the large farmers but with high social and environmental costs. Large-scale wheat farms in northeast

Tanzania provide more than half the country's wheat requirements but have displaced thousands of herders.[31] In the case where large companies or corporations cleared forests in Amazonia for cattle ranges, the payback was sufficiently rapid (and the benefits arising from government incentives sufficiently high) for soil degradation not be a major concern.

Inappropriate Policies and Incentives

Good crop prices may be one of the most fundamental underpinnings for soil conservation. Low prices for crops (whether a result of market forces, government policies or other factors) limit the returns to farmers that can then be invested in soil and water conserving techniques. Governments' pricing policies may be favouring the cultivation of resource-depleting crops in marginal areas or providing subsidies to companies to expand soil-damaging operations (eg tropical forest clearance for cattle as in Brazilian Amazonia). In studies in 58 countries, domestic policy biases against agriculture and poor rural inhabitants were ranked as having a greater influence on rural poverty than population pressures.[32]

One reason for the inappropriate policies of so many governments is the difficulties in designing policies that mesh with the immense heterogeneity of different areas.[33] For instance, within dryland Africa, there are particular parts that have a high agricultural or grazing potential and it is important to understand these key micro-environments within dryland ecosystems.[34] In mountain areas, governments have failed to address the environmental degradation and impoverishment of the population with sufficient sensitivity to the diversity, fragility and inaccessibility that characterize these areas.[35] Moreover, government policies and agricultural extension systems are rarely aware of the different tasks within agriculture and natural resource management taken on by men and women; this lack of gender awareness about who is doing what also contributes to inappropriate and ineffective extension services.[36]

An increasing number of governments and external agencies are beginning to acknowledge and respect communal arrangements for common property management. However, the failure of the state to manage the resources that became its responsibility and to protect the rights of poor communities against encroachments by commercial pressures are underlying factors in much soil degradation. For instance, China's experience with the Contractual Responsibility System has brought personal enrichment for many rural households but also increasing inequity and the destruction of forests, pastures and irrigation channels:

> 'This is typical of a situation where the State, which is authorized to look after the common property, does not have adequate resources to do so and the people, who are using these common-pool resources, are not allowed to organize and manage them in the best way possible.'[37]

Population Pressure and Soil's Carrying Capacity

The agricultural or pastoral population that any region can support depends not only on the productivity of the soil but also on the crops grown and the technologies used. Rising population densities in areas where fertile soil and/or water is limited often pose serious problems for resource management, where people do not adapt their methods of farming and land use to take account of the reduced availability of the land.[38] However, increasing population pressure may produce improved soil fertility and less soil degradation as changing crop mixes and techniques permit increasing population densities to be supported without undermining ecological sustainability – or even improving environmental management. Box 4.3 gives an example of an area in Kenya which was considered 'overpopulated' in relation to its resources in the 1930s and 1940s, yet it has accommodated a fivefold increase in population since 1930. During this period, there has been a tenfold increase in output per hectare and a threefold increase in output per person, as well as much improved soil and water conservation practices.[39] Thus, there is not necessarily a direct link between increasing numbers of children and decreases in food production or declines in soil fertility.

Health Risks Associated with Agricultural Change

Forest clearance in preparation for agriculture or the movement of people into new areas as part of land colonization processes often brings with it new health hazards or existing health hazards being much increased. Box 4.4 gives some examples of the increased risk of malaria and leishmaniasis in the Amazon and of malaria in South-East Asia and of the many environmental and non-environmental factors that underlie such increased risks to human populations.

Irrigation schemes have also had serious health impacts in many countries, especially in the tropics and especially linked to certain vector-borne and water-related diseases – for instance malaria and schistosomiasis. A study of schistosomiasis in the upper region of Ghana suggested that there was an explosive increase in infection in areas where small agricultural dams were constructed, virtually tripling the prevalence rates and the incidence of other diseases such as river blindness and bancroftian filariasis may also have increased.[40] Box 4.5 outlines some of the impacts of irrigation systems on health.

There are few detailed accounts of what these sudden expansions in the incidence of such diseases actually mean for children or for their households and communities. But a few case studies show that their impact can be devastating. Box 4.6 outlines the impact on agricultural production and family livelihoods of infection with river blindness. It shows the transition of a family that was relatively young and healthy and even able to contribute some of their harvest to help other households to increasing impoverishment and finally destitution. As the adult male becomes visually impaired by river blindness and unable to work, so the wife and the 12 year old son have to take more responsibility for food production and to

117

Box 4.3 **Combining Population Growth and Environmental Recovery – Machakos in Kenya**

A study of Machakos District in Kenya which examined population growth, agricultural production and environmental conditions over a fifty year period (1930–90) demonstrated that a fivefold increase in population was compatible with environmental recovery, provided that market developments make farming profitable. In this district, over this period, there has been a tenfold increase in output per hectare and a threefold increase in output per person.

Many observers in the 1930s and 1940s saw Machakos as suffering from severe soil erosion and degradation of both cultivated and grazing lands, such that it could not support its 1948 average population density of 67 persons per square kilometre. The district's recovery from the situation of 1930–60, when there was both acute degradation and constant need for famine relief, shows that the point of reducing marginal returns may be further along the production-population density curve than many experts had predicted earlier. Thus, population growth exceeding 3 per cent per annum has been absorbed since the 1950s by a combination of developing new farmland, capitalizing older farms, and diversifying income sources into the non-farm sector. The most acute environmental degradation occurred in the 1930s and 1940s at much lower population densities than at present but this degradation has been reversed by human endeavour and by investment and employment diversification stimulated and made possible by the market.

Behind the physical recovery of the land lies a story of increasing value of production and investment per hectare. It is also demonstrated by the increase in the value of land – although this has also been influenced by its increasing scarcity. The increase in the value of output per hectare took place by several routes:

- increased and more efficient use of the second, long rains - almost all cultivated land is now double cropped, rains permitting;
- more careful husbandry and water retention in both seasons;
- increase in the ratio of cropped to pasture land (which has a lower output per hectare) combined with greater integration of livestock, utilizing crop residues for feed and manure for crops;
- investment in fewer but higher quality and healthier livestock per household;
- a switch of some land into higher value crops such as coffee, fruit trees and vegetables; and
- planting and/or protection of trees in grazing lands, croplands and hedgerows to provide fuel, timber and fodder needs for own use or for sale.

The effects of less rain are no longer so drastic - as a result of intensive land capitalization through investment: in bench terracing and cut-offs which collect water and bring it to the top of the terracing system or which are themselves planted with bananas and other trees; in fruit trees which have to be provided with pits, compost, manure or mulching; and ploughing along the contour and planting in lines rather than broadcasting so the first weeding can be done by plough (reinforcing the water trapping ridges as well as overcoming a previous labour bottleneck in weeding).

Thus, continuing population growth, in association with market development, has generated new technologies which have supported both increased productivity and improved conservation of land and water resources – although there has been a reduction in natural vegetation and wildlife. Increased involvement in the market has not only produced higher incomes from farming but also many new non-farm jobs in a way that would have been impossible if all farming had been for own consumption. The supporting technologies came from many different sources within and beyond local society. Society has changed in ways which have increased its access to information and its ability to organize, to obtain or to generate new sources of capital and labour. The family and the community have changed in ways which have enabled women as well as men to give leadership to the recovery and development of their district.

While Machakos is now showing some signs of decreasing returns to capital and labour applied to land, there is probably still scope for greater agricultural intensification and increased diversity of income sources, providing policies are followed which develop trade, transport, education and infrastructure. Policies that raise prices for farmers on their farm are probably the single most important action required from governments that want to encourage soil and water conservation, and the maintenance of the productivity of the agricultural resource base. Machakos would be assisted by the removal of restrictions on agricultural change in response to changing economic circumstances and by encouragement of regional specialization in products of comparative advantage rather than promotion of district self-sufficiency in food. Investments in roads should also help raise prices for farmers, as the costs of bringing in inputs and transporting crops to markets decreases. Electricity may also take pressure off land by supporting local industries and workshops.

Source: Tiffen, Mary and Michael Mortimore (1992), 'Environment, population growth and productivity in Kenya; a case study of Machakos District', Development Policy Review *Vol 10, pp 359–387*

Box 4.4 **Links between Land Clearance and Disease Vectors**

Environmental changes at the edge of forests often lead to new health hazards or existing health hazards being much increased. Such health hazards arise from many different factors such as new populations moving in and often lacking immunity to local diseases and environmental damage which increases human contact with new infections or vectors or provides new breeding sites for disease vectors. In Brazil, the Amazon forests have been invaded by road-builders and miners and settled by subsistence farmers. Major hazards are leishmaniasis and malaria. The parasites causing muco-cutaneous leishmaniasis and the cutaneous leishmaniases are usually transmitted by forest sandflies between the sloths, small rodents and other jungle mammals. The woodcutters entering the forest are bitten by the sandflies as well and suffer much more severe lesions from the parasites. The forest, especially where disturbed by human action, provides breeding sites for *Anopheles darlingi*, an efficient malaria vector so that malaria transmission is high near the forest edge and non-immune settlers are vulnerable to and suffer from malaria.

In South-East Asia, malaria is also related to environmental change at the forest fringe. The most efficient malaria vector there is a mosquito (*Anopheles dirus*) that breeds in the forest, closely followed by another (*Anopheles minimus*) that breeds in the pools along small streams, especially in areas of recently cleared forest. The forests are often close to national boundaries and inhabited by ethnic minority groups. They are often areas of political instability and the location for illegal logging, mining for gems and tin, and for smuggling. Mining produces many small craters which when filled with water provide a breeding ground for mosquitoes. Migrants to such areas may lack anti-malarial immunity.

Source: Bradley, David J (1993), 'Environmental aspects of public health in developing countries', Proceedings of a symposium 'Ambiente, Salute e Sviluppo', Accademia Nazionale dei Lincei, Rome, pp 85–95

take over the search for wages during the dry season. Crops are now changed to those that can be managed with less labour, but these are also less nutritious. The adult male is no longer able to migrate seasonally and this also depresses the family's income. He becomes blind while his wife becomes increasingly sick and finally dies and the family has become destitute.

Intensified land use often involves the overuse of fertilizers and biocides and sometimes with detrimental long term impacts on the productivity of agriculture. Pesticides may kill natural enemies of the pests as well as the pests themselves and groundwater needed for irrigation may become contaminated. Agricultural chemicals also have a serious health impact on human populations, as discussed in Chapter 2.

Box 4.5 **The Health Impacts of Irrigation**

Well designed and implemented irrigation systems will raise incomes and improve food security, increasing the potential for better nutrition and health. But irrigation development has often been associated with an increased incidence of disease. Irrigation schemes, especially in the tropics, carry a high risk of introducing or increasing the transmission of vector-borne and water-related diseases. More than 30 diseases have been linked to irrigation - the major vector-borne diseases being schistosomiasis, malaria, onchocerciasis and Japanese encephalitis. Vector-borne disease transmission is aggravated by human-induced environmental changes that favour the proliferation of the vector, by human behaviour which increases contact with the vector (for instance occupation, location of dwelling) and by economic expansion and migration.

The health problems associated with irrigation developments and the environmental changes they produce have been extensively reviewed over the past 15 years, although a lack of base line data prior to the construction of the irrigation system inhibits a better knowledge of the negative health and social aspects. For example:

- Hunter et al reviewed the negative effects on health of water resource development in 13 countries (including some from Africa, Asia and Latin America) and in all, there were indications that projects to develop water resources have resulted in a higher incidence of vector-borne diseases.[41]
- The implementation of a large irrigation scheme on the Cukurova plain of Turkey in the 1970s resulted in a resurgence of endemic malaria due to increasing breeding of the vector species in poorly drained ditches which received the run-off of surplus irrigation water. The absence of proper drainage systems in irrigation schemes is one of the most important factors contributing to the spread of vector-borne disease in irrigation developments. Gratz attributed the rise in malaria to:

> *'the sequence of construction ... with very inadequate or ... no provision for drainage, the increased agricultural activities requiring more and more irrigation and the vast increases in population densities of the main vector in the area, A. sacharovi, combined with an influx of migrants, inadequate surveillance activities and the failure to institute satisfactory control measures in good time.'*[42]

Different types of irrigation system (surface, subsurface, over-surface, continuous flow, demand flow and intermittent flow) and different cycles of water distribution have different effects on the transmission of vector-borne diseases.[43] The irrigation schemes which appear to present the greatest risk of increased transmission of vector-borne diseases are those located where:

- soils present drainage problems;
- rice is cultivated;
- reservoirs are constructed;
- canals are unlined;
- there is compacted settlement or resettlement.[44]

Source: This box is a shortened version of one which was published in WHO 1992 which drew on Chapter 3 of D E Cooper Weil, A P Alicbusan, J F Wilson, M R Reich and D J Bradley, The Impact of Development Policies on Health: a Review of the Literature, *WHO, Geneva, 1990.*

Box 4.6 A Household Coping with River Blindness

Areas of hyperendemic river blindness (onchocerciasis) are found in a belt of savanna across Africa roughly between 8° and 12° north of the equator. Villages in such areas are estimated to have 40 per cent of households 'sighted', 20 per cent visually impaired and 40 per cent blind or destitute. In endemic areas, the prevalence of blindness often exceeds 5 per cent of the population. The paragraphs below discuss a model of changes in agricultural production and family livelihoods for one family in this area.

In the first phase, the family is relatively young and healthy. Agricultural production is sufficient to feed the family for nine months of the year. In the remaining period (the dry season), the household head may migrate to earn money. Fishing, hunting, daily contract work, collection of wildfoods and market gardens are additional sources of food or income. The household is in a position to offer support to members of the extended family and contribute to the Muslim tradition known as *djaga* whereby 10 per cent of the harvest is put aside for elderly and disabled households.

In the second phase, the household head becomes visually impaired. At first, this is not particularly noticeable. The first change in livelihood activities is that hunting, one source of food during the season, is likely to be abandoned. There may be some additional expenditure on traditional medicines but this is not likely to be significant.

Three years later, the household head is likely to be severely visually impaired. In 70 per cent of cases, people with this condition cease to work but with very poor families this is not possible. The wife and 12 year old son are now responsible for food production. They change crops to those which are nutritionally inferior but which can more easily be managed with less labour. The reduced amount of labour available further reduces yields. The family unit can now only produce sufficient food for six months. The man can no longer migrate to find work in the dry season. The wife and son take whatever local work can be found. The family is now dependent on external assistance. The village may not help because of the young age of the household head; the extended family may be in a position to help.

The household head is blind in another two years. The wife is often sick due to the additional burdens. One daughter has left home through marriage, the remaining children are malnourished. The family in increasingly unable to maintain agricultural production. Wildfoods are gathered to supplement the grains. The eldest son continues to migrate in the dry season although his age (14) means that he is unlikely to earn sufficient money. His absence makes it harder to maintain the house.

In the final stage, the household is destitute. The wife has died and the blind household head is a widower (a marital status describing 17 per cent of blind people and only 3 per cent of sighted people). One daughter is also blind. The eldest son migrates permanently and the land is worked by the younger brother. In the dry season, the son undertakes contract work in order to earn money. The daughter also searches for local work in order to supplement the family's income.

Source: Evans, Timothy (1989) 'The impact of permanent disability on rural house-holds; river blindness in Guinea' in special issue of the IDS Bulletin on 'Vulnerability: How the Poor Cope', Vol 20, No 2, April.

WILDFOODS[*]

Although often ignored by those concerned with agricultural development, wildfoods are often important elements in diets and livelihood strategies. For example, in the apparently maize-dominated agricultural system of Bungoma in Kenya, people consume at least 100 different species of wild vegetables and fruits.[45] Within households, it is usually women and children who collect most of the wild produce and usually women who use or sell such produce. A wide range of foods is available from the forest including: wild plants, leaves, seeds and nuts, fruits, roots and tubers, mushrooms, and wild animals. Hunting and gathering these products is an important component of livelihood strategies, particularly for the poorest households. For example, wild foods may account for 20 per cent of the food supply among poorer groups in the dry season in parts of India.

In many societies, wildfoods are an important part of rural diets on a daily basis. They often have particular importance in times of famine. Famine foods include wild vegetables, berries, nuts, fruit, and insects. These are foods which may be eaten occasionally and more often by children and the poor but which are more widely consumed when more conventional food supplies are not available at a price which is affordable. It was noticeable in Box 4.6 that wildfoods were gathered to supplement the grains grown as the family's health deteriorated and limited their possibilities to grow food.

---

[*] This section draws on Ian Scoones, Mary Melnyk and Jules N Pretty (1992), *The Hidden Harvest; Wild Foods and Agricultural Systems – a Literature Review and Annotated Bibliography*, Sustainable Agricultural Programme, IIED London. The references quoted in this section are also drawn from this volume.

The commercial pressures that decrease or remove people's access to open access or common property land or forests obviously decreases their access to wildfood. As agrosystems change, so too does the availability of wild foods. For instance, as woodlands are cleared, non agricultural foods often disappear, although they may continue to be found on degraded sites and pathways, roadsides, home sites and field edges. In particular, the simplification of agroecosystems (eg. conversion of Brazilian forest areas to cattle) has the greatest impact on the poor through destruction of key food sources.[46]

IMPLICATIONS FOR CHILDREN

As noted already, for over half the world's children, the central natural resource issue is whether the household of which they are part has access to sufficient productive land and water for an adequate and sustainable livelihood and sufficient fresh water for drinking and household use. The welfare and development of each child also depend on gender relations and the pattern of decision making within the household about the distribution of resources in the household (including cash). For instance, there is the extent to which priority is given to children in regard to food – or, within this, to protein – and in this, boys may be favoured over girls. Another important issue is the extent to which the labour of girls and boys is needed within the livelihood or survival strategies of households who depend on natural resources and the implications this has for their health, education and development. Other environmental issues of relevance to children within farming or pastoralism include environmental hazards from biological pathogens and chemical pollutants (including biocides) and from physical hazards – as described in earlier chapters.

In poor rural households, it is very common for children to be assigned tasks in agriculture and/or the household to the point where this prevents or limits attendance at school. It is worth noting how children's economic contribution became increasingly important in the household described in Box 4.6, as the river blindness made it increasingly difficult for the household head to work. In a study of a Himalayan village (Box 4.7), children contributed more than a quarter of the total hours worked in the village. In a study of 'children's lifeworlds' in Poomkara, a village in Kerala, India, both poor girls and boys spend some 6–7 hours a day actively engaged in work with boys having more time to earn money and girls spending most time caring for younger children and undertaking such tasks as fetching water, gathering firewood, sweeping and scrubbing pots.[47]

Children's contribution can also begin relatively young. For instance, in a study of the role and priorities of children in a rural district in Nepal, children began to collect fodder from the age of six or seven, as this was the age by which they could carry a basket of fodder – and in the higher hill areas of this district, children spent many hours a day collecting fodder and fuelwood in the winter months.[48] Young children are also often left to look after infants and toddlers while the parents work.[49] Box 4.7 describes life in a Himalayan village in India and the extent to which children and adolescents (especially females) contribute to livelihood and household tasks and

Box 4.7 **Life in a Himalayan Village**

A study of female children in a Himalayan village showed that they generally began work well before boys and this greatly limited their possibility of educational advancement. The village has a population of 213 (37 households) who have access to 183 hectares in order to meet their biomass needs of fuel, food, fodder and manure. Agricultural land covers about 34 hectares. There are 92 main workers; 50 women and 42 men; approximately one third of men in the village and more than 50 per cent of the women are workers.

Women start work before they are 15 (two girls in the 10–15 age group are already putting in a full day's work in agriculture); men who wish to study generally start work when they are 20, otherwise they start between 16–18. Only 25 of Syuta's 42 men main workers are cultivators; the others work in the service sector in the village or as migrants in other parts of the country. All women main workers in the village are cultivators. Women break up the hard earth, and do all the heavy agricultural work. They generally start work within five days of giving birth and their diets remain meagre during pregnancy. Most women die between 35-55 when they are still active workers. One frequent cause of death is accidents while negotiating the narrow mountain path carrying heavy weights (70 kg is not uncommon). Nine of the men in the village are over 55, but only three women have reached this age.

Children undertake household activities such as collecting grass and firewood, grazing animals, fetching water, cooking and caring for the younger children. Babies are left to the care of siblings who take them to school - breast feeding is irregular and bottle feeding rare. There are 39 children in the village aged between 5–10. One boy and four girls were deemed important workers in their family. In primary school the number of boys and girls enrolled is equal but in high school all the girls drop out. Older girls work with their mothers assuming full responsibilities for grass and firewood collection, grazing cattle and assisting in farming tasks. Boys from 10–15 may also have an important role in many activities such as grazing animals and collecting firewood for domestic use and sale. Nine of the 11 children between 10–15 sell firewood for part of the year; they carry loads of about 20 kg on their heads - and spend more than eight hours a day collecting and selling. The children of between 10–15 years of age each work an average of 2885.5 hours a year. Over 700 hours are spent doing household chores and a similar amount of time looking after grazing animals. Women work between 9.5 and 14.5 hours a day. In April when firewood is scarce they may spend three hours a day on fuelwood collection, five hours in farm work and three hours in fodder collection. Women contribute 59 per cent of the total hours of work in the village, children 26 per cent and men 15 per cent.

Source: Agarwal, Anil (1992), 'Who will help her learn? To keep the girl at school, the environment must be improved', Down To Earth, Nov 15.

the ways in which this limits their possibilities of educational advancement. As this case study states, there are equal numbers of boys and girls at primary school but in high (secondary) school all the girls drop out.

It is also common in many rural areas for children to engage in wage labour – either seasonally (for instance during the slack period in farms or during the school holidays) or permanently. The study in the Sindhuli district of Nepal found that children as young as ten engaged in wage labour.[50] This study also found that both men and boys were migrating seasonally, with the boys involved in tempo (bicycle rickshaw) driving, portering, construction or carrying groceries or working in carpet factories. Girls generally remained with mothers, but with their work-loads much increased as both men and boys were away. Among certain families, boys and girls went to work permanently in carpet factories.

It is sometimes forgotten how widespread child labour was in Europe and North America a few generations ago. Here too, it was particularly important for low-income families in that while the child's income was relatively small, it still made an important contribution to total household income. In many countries in the South, children of 14 years or less represent a significant proportion of the workforce. Box 4.8 describes the use of child labour in agriculture in Brazil and highlights the high proportion of poor households who depend on working children. The children of families who work on estates are also often expected to work from an early age, and rarely are any educational or health services provided.[51]

Box 4.8 **Child Agricultural Labour in Brazil**

The Agricultural Census in Brazil recorded over 4.5 million children working – with 68 per cent working more than 40 hours a week. In 1987, an estimated 6.2 million children (between the ages of 10–17) were categorised as in the economically active population in rural areas. This is equivalent to 43 per cent of all children in this age category. A high proportion of them are in the 10–14 year old age category. Patterns vary from region to region but there are some common trends: the increasing polarization of rich and poor and the loss of land among the poor exacerbated by the presence of large families. Many small-holdings have been broken up so they all need to go to work as temporary wage labourers. In 1985, it was estimated that 37 per cent of families with working children are dependent exclusively on the wages of these children. Schooling obviously suffers as a result of the time spent working. As a consequence, many remain in employment sectors characterized by low wages and few prospects of advancement.

Source: Lee-Wright, Peter (1990), Child Slaves, Earthscan, London; and Marcondes Cupertino, Maria Amelia (1990), 'The employment of minors in Brazil', Environment and Urbanization Vol 2, No 2, October, pp 71–76.

However, care must be taken in making assumptions about when and where children begin to work early in their lives. It is perhaps surprising to find that children within hunter-gatherer societies do not necessarily have to make large contributions to household tasks and livelihood strategies – see Box 4.9. Children's labour generally becomes increasingly important as households experience economic stress. In addition, care must be taken not to consider children's involvement in agriculture or pastoralism as something to be stopped. Traditionally, in pastoral and agricultural societies, children's involvement in the household's livelihood is a combination of work and play and a central part of their education. Where school curricula are unrelated to the everyday reality of the children attending school and their future possibilities, children's learning as they work with other household members may be more important for their future than attending school. For instance, in Brazil, the standard school curriculum – teaching children in the Amazon about the Kings of Portugal – is hardly the best preparation for adult life.[52] The issue of how to integrate environmental concerns into education will be discussed in Chapter 7. For example, there is a community health project in the Brazilian Amazon called *Saude e Alegria* (health and hapiness) that fully involves children and that also has important environmental education aspects that relate to their local reality. Chapter 7 also includes examples of innovative ways in which children have been involved in environmental management.

FOREST RESOURCES

Forests and individual trees have importance to everyone: from their roles at the global level (which include maintaining biodiversity and their role within the carbon cycle) and the city level (providing a considerable range of goods and services of value to city dwellers and enterprises and protecting watersheds) to their many roles in rural areas (providing many resources important for the health and livelihoods of a wide range of households and communities).

Fuelwood is a critically important product obtained from logging, pollarding and lopping (removing branches from) trees. Many households in the poorest and driest African countries are dependent on wood for energy; in sub-Saharan Africa woodfuels are estimated to account for 60–95 per cent of total national energy use.[53] While forests are generally considered as sources of timber and fuel, in most rural areas, they have other important roles – for instance as sources of food or of food security to which people turn when harvests are poor or during certain parts of the year or as sources of fodder. Well managed forests can not only meet desired goals in terms of timber production but also contribute significantly to household security, providing food, fodder, fuelwood, trees to assist in arable crop production, and raw materials for forest enterprises.

Indirectly, trees and forests also supply a range of important environmental goods and services including:

- moderating temperature extremes within micro-climates (humidity,

Box 4.9 !Kung Childcare and Social Change

In hunting and gathering societies like the Baka and the !Kung, infants are carried by their mother most of the time and are nursed several times an hour. During their first year of life, !Kung babies are in physical contact with their mothers most of the time. The !Kung remain in close contact with their infants sleeping beside them and breast feeding until four years of age. The children are given almost no responsibility for chores and explore their environment at will. They play in naturally formed multi-age groups in which the older children watch over and teach the younger ones. By four and five, the children are wandering considerable distances from their mothers.

Between eleven and fifteen months, children become imitators and develop a capacity for pretend play. In a subsistence society such as the !Kung, they copy the activities of their mothers such as pounding roots, cracking nuts or digging in the sand with a stick. Toddlers are allowed to handle knives. Language development is similar to that in other cultures: babbling reaching a peak at eight months followed within three or four months by the beginning of a steep rise in the rate of meaningful vocalizations.

Birth spacing among hunters and gatherers like the !Kung average four years, mainly due to breast feeding; 92 per cent of fussing or crying episodes are responded to within 15 seconds. Fathers do not take a leading role in childcare but average more time with infants and young children than is the case in North America.

!Kung children during middle childhood are about as free of responsibility as are younger children. They have no formal education or work. Instead they watch adults and learn. Children spend their time playing and socializing. Girls do spend some time caring for babies and children of both sexes go on gathering expeditions. Boys learn to hunt through play and through dance with adults. Only as teenagers do they accompany their fathers on hunting expeditions.

Play is the children's main activity through their waking hours in the hunting and gathering societies, in contrast to the assignment of at least some chores and schooling after six years of age in most other societies. In herding and agricultural societies, obedient and responsible behaviour in middle childhood has to be encouraged. Children may look after younger siblings or herd fields of cattle. In !Kung households that have become settled, it has been observed that their attitudes to children have changed and they have begun to expect their children to undertake more household tasks.

Source: Myers, Robert (1991), The Twelve Who Survive: Strengthening Programmes of Early Child Development in the Third World, Routledge, London and New York.

temperature, shade, moisture availability);
- acting as windbreaks for crops and human settlements;
- preventing or limiting soil erosion, especially in watersheds;
- protecting critical or hazardous areas, including an important role in many systems of fallow land management, to permit soil regeneration for cultivation;
- maintaining hydrological cycles and regulating water supplies (helping moderate extremes of water flow, floods and droughts); and
- their role in global climate (including their influence on albedo and absorption of carbon dioxide) and as gene pools.

It is evident that the removal or degradation of forest resources can directly affect households (and their children) by reducing sources of household income and subsistence goods. These can indirectly affect them by reducing the productivity of agriculture and increasing the danger of flooding and other natural disasters. For example, deforestation often increases the rate of soil erosion which in turn reduces the productivity of the land and means increased sediment load which reduces water quality downstream.

Deforestation

Deforestation is not a new phenomenon. Since pre-agricultural times, the world's forests have declined from approximately five billion hectares to four billion hectares today.

> 'Temperate forests have lost the highest percentage of their area (32–35 per cent), followed by subtropical woody savannas and deciduous forests (24–25 per cent) and old-growth tropical forest (15–20 per cent). Tropical evergreen forests, now under most pressure, have lost the least area (4–6 per cent) because they were inaccessible and were sparsely populated'.[54]

An estimated 17 million hectares of tropical forests were being lost to deforestation every year in the late 1980s compared to 11 million hectares a year in the second half of the 1970s.[55]

Both the rate of deforestation and its underlying causes differ greatly from country to country. Current estimates suggest that the highest rates of deforestation are in South America, where average annual deforestation during the 1980s was estimated to be 1.3 per cent.[56] The UN Food and Agriculture Organization (FAO) estimates suggest that annual average deforestation equalled 0.5 per cent in Africa between 1981–5, with the highest rate, 2.2 per cent, being found in the region of West Africa; in Asia and Latin America the comparable figures were 0.7 per cent and 0.6 per cent respectively, with the highest rates being in Nepal (4 per cent), Haiti (3.7 per cent), and Costa Rica (3.6 per cent).[57] These figures offer only broad estimates and there remains many unanswered questions and much controversy as to the actual rate of forest depletion. For instance, national figures are subject to differing definitions of forest and forest resources. Such deforestation figures are difficult to interpret and may include diverse phenomena such as small scale (perhaps temporary) clearing for traditional slash and burn, large scale clearing for agriculture or pastoral development, and deforestation through logging. Deforestation also does not necessarily imply soil erosion; it depends on the use to which the land is put and the quality of the management.

In much of Latin America, a major reason for forest clearance is to create cattle ranches and small farms. In many instances, there has been a deliberate government policy to open up forest areas for colonization and development schemes although much of the colonization and land clearance takes place outside government schemes. In Brazil, one major reason for the drive to colonize Amazonia has been to reduce the pressures for land reform in the northeast and southeast. Hundreds of thousands of poor landless people, most of them from Brazil's northeast, have moved to Amazonia in search of a more adequate and stable livelihood.

In much of Africa, the main reason for deforestation is land clearance for agriculture, although the commercial exploitation of forests for timber and fuelwood is also important in many areas. In Asia, deforestation generally occurs because of commercial logging, fuelwood gathering, agricultural expansion and the establishment of plantations. The clearing of forests for large scale operations such as rubber and oil palm plantations may be encouraged by the need to generate income for debt repayment and this is also a factor driving governments to encourage the harvesting of valuable timber for export.[58] However, deforestation does not necessarily imply soil loss and reduced water retention – for instance if former forest land is converted to well managed permanent tree crops or agroforestry.

The unequal distribution of land ownership or tenure was highlighted by the United Nations Environment Programme (UNEP) as a major underlying cause of deforestation:

> 'People do not move into forests from choice, but from lack of it. Economic patterns in the (South), with grossly distorted distribution of wealth and inequitable land tenure systems mean that the forests are the only hope of subsistence for many people. In a number of tropical countries, governments have taken advantage of the peasant farmer's willingness to settle new lands. Schemes to promote resettlement have attracted massive numbers of people, but have often failed because the soils and other conditions were inappropriate.'[59]

Forest Degradation's Impact

Deforestation or forest depletion usually has an immediate impact on the livelihood of those who are directly or indirectly dependent on forest products. Perhaps the most serious impact of deforestation worldwide is the loss of employment, income and consumption goods for hundreds of thousands of rural settlements and small towns in areas where forest exploitation is a major part of the local economy. Many timber enterprises in tropical moist forests are itinerant, depleting their concession of the commercial wealth of the forest and then moving to another site, leaving the infrastructure they established to deteriorate. Only a tiny proportion of the world's natural forests are being managed in ways which allow current timber yields to be sustained. A study of natural forest management in six African nations, five Asian nations and six Latin American and Caribbean nations found that although many countries were aware of the need for sustainable management and have passed legislation accordingly:

> *'the extent of tropical moist forest which is being deliberately managed at an operational scale for the sustainable production of timber is, on a world scale, negligible..(and).. comprehensive and urgent measures are absolutely necessary if the tropical timber trade is to continue in the long term to handle material which even approaches the quantity and quality that it has become accustomed to.'*[60]

Likely consequences of deforestation and forest depletion include the migration of those who lose their livelihood as they go in search of work, loss of incomes due to lack of commercial opportunities and reduction in nutrition due to changes in diet. There is also the increasing difficulty experienced by those living in such settlements in obtaining fuel or other products collected from woods – which in many households is a task for women or for children. For example, in India, a woman may walk 1400 kilometres each year in the search for firewood – as all the most accessible areas have become deforested.[61] Similar changes can take place where commercial interests come to control forests which were formerly a common resource; it is this kind of appropriation that underlies the Chipko (tree-hugging) movement and many other citizen-led protests against logging companies.[62]

Many rural communities have also found that the forests that they have long used as a source of fuelwood and forest products become barred to them as fuelwood and charcoal traders from nearby cities take control of them; rural communities within a transportable range of cities have found it difficult to protect their rights to trees on their crop and pasture lands.[63] In addition, the viability of settlements belonging to indigenous peoples living in the forest areas may be destroyed by forest exploitation, for example through the introduction of disease and the loss of livelihood. Such people may require resettlement, possibly experiencing many problems in this process. Box 4.10 summarizes some of the social impacts of deforestation in Central America. It emphasizes the vulnerability of poorer groups and also notes that one of the impacts – the increasing price and growing scarcity of fuelwood – falls particularly on children.

Access and Tenure

In many rural areas, the inhabitants have been losing rights to use forests or particular forest products that have long been important in their livelihoods. Access to forests is often particularly important for low-income households who rely most heavily on off-farm subsistence food or fodder and off-farm income generating activities. The fact that many people drew products from forests rarely meant that the forests were degraded as effective management systems often developed to protect against this.

Box 4.10 **Social Impacts of Deforestation in Central America**

Throughout the 1960s and 1970s, Central America experienced one of the highest rates of deforestation in the world. The extent of forest cover has been reduced from 60 to 33 per cent of the total land area in about 25 years. The economic and social crisis that has affected much of the region throughout the 1980s is intimately related to this process of environmental destruction.

Four groups are particularly vulnerable to the process of deforestation in Central America:

- the peasantry and traditional peasant farming systems in the area being deforested;
- the peasant populations in the agrarian frontier areas where deforestation has occurred as a result of colonization processes;
- the Indian groups in forest areas affected by deforestation and encroachment by outsiders; and
- the groups living near or in urban centres located within densely populated rural areas who draw on forest products.

For centuries, the traditional peasant farming systems were based on the slash and burn system. This system is fragile and may break down as demand for land grows, and as the periods for which the land is left uncultivated are shortened. The peasant household often stops subsistence production and converts the land to cattle grazing in the belief that this will produce sufficient income. However, this generally results in increasing impoverishment of the peasants, environmental degradation and declining productivity, and increasing social differentiation in land holdings together with out-migration.

The indigenous Indian population in Central America is estimated to be 15 per cent of the region's 30 million inhabitants. Many of these people live in or near forest and agrarian frontier regions or in areas which have experienced extensive deforestation in recent decades. Two impacts need stressing. The first is a result of the extractive enterprises (timber and mining) as Indian communities become both wage labourers and consumers whereas previously they had participated in a subsistence economy. The second impact arises from settlement by farmers – and in many cases, the Indian population has been forced off their land.

Millions living in and around urban areas and those in densely populated rural areas have been affected by a lack of fuelwood and deforestation arising from previous fuelwood consumption. The cost of fuelwood in Central America has risen sharply in the last two decades and, reflecting similar trends, the time taken by poor families to gather fuelwood has also increased. Children are directly affected in communities where they are responsible for collecting wood (23 per cent of fuelwood gatherers in Nicaragua); and are indirectly affected as their carers have to spend more time collecting.

Source: Utting, Peter (1991), The Social Origins and Impact of Deforestation in Central America, UNRISD Discussion Paper No 24, Geneva.

There are also many examples of traditional agroforestry systems which combined intensive production with sustainable resource use.[64] Under the traditional system of land use, trees, shrubs, palms, bamboos etc are used in the same management unit as agricultural crops and/or animal feed. For example, traditional agroforestry is practised in Senegal over most of the groundnut basin, the area where agricultural output is highest in the country and where *Acacia albida* is a conspicuous feature of the farming landscape, together with its companion woody species such as *baobabs, roniers* and *tamarinds*. This applies especially to the central and south-western parts of the basin where over the centuries, the Serer people have developed a highly complex and stable agroforestry system alternating *Acacia albida*, cereals (millet and sorghum) fallowing and cattle raising. Other traditional agroforestry systems include the Chagga Homegarden in the Mount Kilimanjaro area of Tanzania which is characterized by an intensive integration of numerous multipurpose trees and shrubs with food crops and animals simultaneously on the same unit of land. There is also the *sheamba/taungya* system of east, central and west Africa under which landless people are allowed to grow various annual and perennial crops in rows between the trees in return for tending the trees.[65]

In the past, common property management systems have been a widespread and often effective means of managing forests and trees within non-forested areas. However, in many communities, traditional management systems have broken down, usually because of a mix of factors that include population growth, market forces, privatization, state interventions, and other socio-economic changes, ie very similar to those factors mentioned earlier in the chapter which have eroded or destroyed many common property regimes which were managing agricultural or pastoral land. In many instances, this disintegration of traditional systems of resource management may have begun many years or decades ago. For instance, in India:

> *'before the advent of the modern state, grazing lands, forest lands and water bodies were mostly common property and village communities played an important role in their use and management. The British were the first to nationalise these resources and bring them under the management of government bureaucracies. In other words, the British initiated the policy of converting common property resources into government property resources.'*[66]

In Pakistan, one important reason for deforestation is that:

> *'large tracts of forest traditionally used and owned by communities for subsistence level use were taken over by both the old colonial and newly independent state or powerful groups or individuals, and commercially exported to satisfy the demands of a growing urban and rural population.'*[67]

In spite of these pressures, many of these traditional management systems still have importance in the management of scarce natural resources,

133

complementing and combining with systems of private rights. For rural families without land, common property resources are often a particularly important resource.

The state is often reluctant to pass over (or return) control of forest resources to local inhabitants and their community organizations. But in many instances, the food security needs of the local people can be better served with flexible and more closely monitored forest management which responds to local needs and circumstances. These may involve the partial or complete transfer of forest land to local ownership, and the devolution of varying degrees of responsibility for control and use of forest resources to local communities. These issues are further discussed in Chapter 6.

Impacts on Children

The impacts of deforestation and of rural people's loss of the right to use or gather resources in forests has been documented in many instances – increased poverty, increasing undernutrition and additional work burdens, especially on women as the main collectors of fuel wood in most societies. However, it is rare for the documentation to include the specific impacts on children.

Two important impacts of declining availability of fuelwood are: the influences on what food is eaten and the use of inferior fuels. As Crewe points out, faced with a fuel shortage, a woman may turn to inferior, smokier fuels, particularly dung:

> 'She may cook food for less time, or boil less of the water her household uses. She may serve her family more leftovers from the meal before or the day before, or purchase more expensive, ready-made foods. She may prepare fewer meals ... or cook less food per meal. These coping strategies can have a disastrous impact on nutrition for all household members but especially for the woman herself since she is already likely to be malnourished and overworked.'[68]

If fuelwood scarcity reduces the number of cooked meals – for example once rather than twice a day – this may impact particularly on children if they are unable to digest sufficient calories in one meal alone.

The risk of foodborne diseases also rises, as fuelwood scarcity encourages shorter cooking periods for foods and greater use of uncooked or reheated food. This is particularly true of meats and for certain tubers and legumes that need to be adequately cooked to destroy toxic components. There may be a switch to foods that require less cooking but that are also less nutritious – for example, cereals replacing pulses. In addition, traditional means of preserving food that relied on fuelwood such as smoking and drying food, may not be used as much. The use of boiled water for drinking may also be reduced, resulting in additional risks of contaminated water – with this being particularly hazardous for infants and children.

Fuelwood scarcity usually means that more time has to be spent looking for fuel and those responsible for doing so (usually women) having less time for other activities such as agriculture, off-farm income generation and domestic tasks. The increasing demands on parents' time for fuelwood collection will limit the amount of time that they have to spend with their children. Such increasing demands on parents' (and usually women's) time and energy can also have serious health impacts. It is worth recalling that in Box 4.7, one frequent cause of death for women in the Himalayan village was accidents while negotiating narrow mountain paths with heavy loads. Fuelwood scarcity often means increasing reliance on children to help gather it – or other possible fuels. Box 4.7 pointed to the long hours spent by many children in gathering firewood. Box 4.10 also noted how increasing scarcity of fuelwood in Central America often meant increasing amounts of time spent by children in gathering firewood.

There are an increasing number of documented examples where rural inhabitants organize to protest against a loss of fuelwood or of their right to use forests. Box 4.11 describes the birth of the *Chipko* movement in India through which villagers sought to protect the forests they used from being cut down. It is worth noting that the *Chipko* movement's goal was not to save trees but to ensure the sustainable use of the forests with local inhabitants also being allowed an active part in managing the forests.[69]

Forests and trees are also important sources of medicines; for many rural dwellers, they are the sole source of medicines. Some are effective because they have high concentrations of particular chemicals; others because they have high concentrations of vitamins and minerals that can help counter illnesses caused by dietary deficiencies. Forests and trees are also important sources of building materials. Box 4.12 outlines the use of biomass in rural housing in India.

ACCESS TO RENEWABLE RESOURCES IN URBAN AREAS[70]

Although the conventional view of urban living and urban livelihoods is of one divorced from the growing of crops and the raising of livestock, a growing number of studies, most undertaken in the last 10–15 years, have revealed the importance of urban agriculture.[71] A significant proportion of the population of many urban areas grow crops and/or raise livestock which form an important part of their food intake and often an important part of their income as some produce is sold. The scale of urban agriculture is increased if it is taken to include food produced or collected by urban dwellers on land they own or to which they have use rights outside the urbanized area.[72]*

Urban agriculture's scale and importance is also much increased in many urban centres if it is taken to include the agricultural produce from what are often large areas of unbuilt-up land within or around the urbanized area that are officially part of the urban area. In many countries, the

---

* Although in many African countries, this inclusion within urban agriculture of urban residents who farm land outside urban areas is important, as it forms an important part of the livelihood and food intake of so many urban households, it can become misleading in countries or regions where a significant proportion of farmers live in urban areas or a significant proportion of farmland is owned by urban dwellers.

Box 4.11 **Community based Movements to Halt Deforestation: the *Chipko* Movement in India**

In the Himalayan areas of Uttar Pradesh in India, by 1970, forests had receded so far away from villages that women had to leave home as early as four o'clock in the morning to fetch wood and they returned late at night after long journeys, up and down hills, with a load of 25 to 30 kilograms. This problem was becoming increasingly acute and government agencies were not responding to this. The incidence and severity of floods was also increasing and this was linked to deforestation in the region. This led to the birth of *Chipko Andolan* (which literally means the 'movement to embrace'; should anyone try to fell a tree, the *Chipko* agitator threatens to hug it).

The *Chipko* movement began one morning in March 1973. A team of representatives and contractors from a sports factory reached Gopeshwar to cut ash trees which had been allotted to them by the State Forest Department. Not long before, the organization formed by local inhabitants to develop livelihood opportunities locally, the *Dasholi Gram Swarajya Mandal* (DGSM) had been refused permission to fell trees in a nearby forest for the manufacture of agricultural implements in its local workshop. The villagers provided the contractors with accommodation in their rest house, as there was no other in the village, but told them they should not try to cut the trees. The contractors ignored them. At the village meeting in the evening, one villager argued that 'a mother saves her child from the tiger by hugging the child to her breast, to take upon herself the wrath of the tiger.' The people at the meeting resolved to cling to the trees to prevent them from being cut.

Some weeks later, the contractors returned to Gopeshwar with a marked allotment from the Forest Department but they were again repulsed through local inhabitants hugging the trees earmarked for felling. The Forest Department tried to resolve the issue by offering the DGSM workers an allocation of trees but this was refused, since the workers were unwilling to allow the company its quota. The allocation of local trees to an outside company was seen as a symbol of an unjust forest policy that cared more about outside business than about the people who lived in the forest. Finally, the government gave in, the company's permit was cancelled and the trees assigned to the DGSM instead.

Later that month, the DGSM workers learnt that the same contractors had been offered trees in Phata forest, another part of the district. The villagers formed an action committee which organized a continuous watch over the approach to the forest. The contractors eventually retreated from the area. However, their permit was valid for six months and representatives from the company then visited the villagers, threatening them with the law if they tried to stop the tree felling and claiming that the *Chipko* leaders were only looking for bribes from the company. The *Chipko* leaders called a meeting and invited the contractors to present their viewpoint. The agents tried to intimidate the people with threats and insults but the villagers remained firm in their resolve to protect the trees.

As the meeting ended, word spread that the government was to show a movie in a nearby town. Many villagers and *Chipko* workers went to see it but, on arrival, found the film had been cancelled. The mountain buses had stopped running by that time and the people remained overnight in the town. The next day, on their return to the village, they heard that workers with axes and saws had gone into the forest. Immediately, the villagers organized a march. As they approached the area of the forest where the trees were being cut, the contractors' workers ran away leaving five fallen ash trees. The villagers then set up a permanent watch and prevented the contractors removing any trees - and then their permit expired.

The *Chipko* movement reached a climax when women in the village of Reni became involved. Months after a major river flood, the Forest Department announced the auction of almost 2500 trees in the Reni forest overlooking the Alakananda River. *Chipko* workers visited the villagers, explaining how the trees could be saved. The government auction took place in January 1974. The *Chipko* workers tried to warn the government and lumber companies both about the danger to the region from floods and landslides and about the resistance of the *Chipko* workers, but they were ignored. The trees were sold and the *Chipko* workers waited in Reni for the first timber workers to enter the area. The government tried to break the opposition by announcing that it would pay villagers for the land taken for military purposes after the war with China. The villagers had been waiting for this money for 14 years and immediately the village men rushed off to the nearby town of Chamoli to collect the money. The same day, *Chipko* workers and students were detained at Gopeshwar and Joshimath to meet officials of the forest departments bordering Reni. Later that morning, a bus with contractors and Forest Department officials was driven towards Reni forest.

However, the women of Reni barred their way to the forest, singing: 'This forest is our mother's home, we will protect it with all our might.' They told the lumberjacks: 'If the forest is cut, the soil will be washed away. Landslides and soil erosion will bring floods, which will destroy our fields and homes, our water sources will dry up, and all the other benefits we get from the forests will be finished.' Over the next month, rallies were held at this site and a constant watch was maintained over the forest. The campaign received widespread publicity and there was pressure from other parts of India for the protection of Reni forest. Eventually, the government responded by setting up a committee of experts to investigate the situation. Two years later, the committee made its report. It agreed with the *Chipko* movement that the forest was a sensitive area and that no trees should be cut in any part of a large section of the Alakananda watershed. The government responded to the report by banning the felling of trees in an area of over 450 square miles (1200 square kilometres) for ten years. Other villages have mounted similar forms of opposition to protect their forests.

Source: Chandi Prasad Bhatt (1990), 'The Chipko Andolan: *forest conservation based on people's power'*, Environment and Urbanization *Vol 2, No 1, April, pp 7–18.*

Box 4.12 **The Use of Biomass in Housing**

Various biomass materials are used in rural housing in India. The most common are: timber and wood, thatch from grasses, palmyra, agricultural residues (eg wheat and rice straw) and bamboo. These are used in four broad building systems: sub-structure for thatch, earth, tile and stone roofs; roof cladding material as bundled or laid thatch; wattle and timber framework for walls and as a binder in massive earth walls and plasters. In 1991, close to 10 per cent of the rural housing stock was built almost completely with biomass walls and roofs. This figure is falling very slowly. Many more houses are partially constructed using biomass; about 45 per cent of roofs and 13 per cent of walls.

The present shortage of materials is due to a rapid growth in rural demand combined with competing urban and industrial demand. In some areas, a shortage of timber has already resulted in the rural population being unable to afford to continue to build using timber.

There are four main constraints to increasing the amount of biomass materials available for rural housing. *Ecological constraints* limit what can be grown in each location. *Social constraints*, such as rural inequity, corruption and inadequate enforcement of what are usually inadequate laws, have failed to protect the existing stocks from unsustainable exploitation. The role of women in protecting livelihood resources has not been recognized. Tree growing to meet housing needs tends to be an activity of the poor; the returns from this activity are less than that of others and *economic constraints* limit the capacity of the poor to make such investments, ie the poor cannot afford to maintain adequate housing. *Policy constraints* remain significant; Indian forest policies developed to meet the needs for colonial exploitation and these policies cannot easily be changed to those that conserve forests while simultaneously meeting the needs of the rural poor.

Source: Drawn from Chapter 7, Aromar Revi et al (1992), BMTPC: Technology Action Plan for Rural Housing (1991–2001), *TARU: The Action Research Unit for Development*

boundaries of urban areas, municipalities or metropolitan areas are much larger than the built-up areas and they include large areas of intensively cultivated land and large livestock populations. In some instances, these boundaries encompass so much agricultural land that a significant proportion of the economically active population within these 'urban areas' are farmers.

That urban areas are often surrounded by intensively cultivated land is hardly surprising, given that many urban centres first grew within fertile areas to serve as market towns and the fact that urban areas provide markets for rural produce. Prior to the advances in transport that came with and after the industrial revolution, the size of cities was always constrained by the productive capacities of soils and fisheries nearby.[73] However, the potential for urban agriculture in terms of food production and of livelihoods for significant proportions of many urban populations is not utilized without a policy that encourages the use of agricultural or vacant land within or around built-up areas. With no such policy, agriculture in the land around cities with growing economies and populations is often in decline or even abandoned as speculative land markets develop in anticipation of profits to be secured from developing such land for urban use. In most cities in the South, a high proportion of all new dwellings are being developed in peri-urban areas, often on high quality agricultural land – and the urban authorities do little to control this. In most cities, a high proportion of the land developed for housing is on sites that are occupied or subdivided illegally. Such land often has considerable importance for low-income households as the only place in which they can afford to become home-owners (or to build their own home), even if this is done illegally. Although in theory, a well directed land policy could protect valuable agricultural land, promote urban agriculture and still ensure sufficient land to keep down the price of land for housing, in reality, very few urban authorities have shown the willingness or the capacity to use their planning and land development powers to do so.[74]

Scale of Urban Agriculture

Despite the lack of support for urban agriculture by most urban authorities, and the controls imposed on it by some, urban agriculture is an important part of the food intake and/or livelihoods for hundreds of millions of urban dwellers.[75] There is obviously great variation between cities in the proportion of households for whom some form of urban agriculture is important. Many case studies of urban centres in Africa have shown its importance – encouraged by relatively low density cities with open spaces suited to urban agriculture and a high proportion of households with low incomes for whom the returns from urban agriculture are attractive. A survey of over 1500 households in six Kenyan urban centres (including the largest city Nairobi) during 1984 and 1985 found that almost two thirds of respondents grew some of their own food or fuel and about half kept livestock – see Box 4.13.

Studies of urban centres in Tanzania have also shown that a significant proportion of the economically active population make a living from urban agriculture; for instance, in Dar es Salaam, much the largest city, 20 per cent of those employed work in urban agriculture.[76] A survey in Maseru (the capital of Lesotho) found that 55 per cent of all plots surveyed had some form of agricultural activity and where soils are decent, over 80 per cent of households in low-income and self-help housing areas have some form of agriculture/horticulture.[77] Other surveys of low-income households or of particular settlements with a high proportion of low-income households in Lusaka, Harare, Kisangani and Kampala showed that between 25 and 60 per cent of households engaged in urban agriculture – with even higher proportions in some instances.[78] The gathering of wild fruits and vegetables, fuelwood, fodder and other goods from plants and trees can also be important for low-income urban groups.

Box 4.13 **Urban Food Production in Kenya**

The importance of urban food production was shown by a study of six Kenyan towns completed between October 1984 and July 1985. In a survey of over 1500 urban households, almost two thirds of respondents grew some of their own food or fuel and about half kept livestock.

Nearly three quarters of urban households had access to land on which they could grow food (this proportion was highest in the smaller towns); 29 per cent of the urban population had access to local land and grew crops in the area in which they lived. Just under half of those with access to urban land farmed in their own backyards. Roadsides (used by 17 per cent of households with urban land) and riversides (13 per cent) were other sites which were farmed. The average farm was just 500 square metres in size. Maize and beans were the most popular crops, both grown by over 50 per cent of urban farmers; 95 per cent of these producers grew only for domestic consumption. Average household production for the season prior to the survey was 155 kilograms. Land productivity equalled 3200 kilograms/hectare and was highest in Nairobi (9000 kg/ha). Few urban farmers bought commercial fertilizer although 30 per cent used farmyard manure obtained from their own farms or those of friends and relatives. Women did most of the work growing crops in urban areas except where such work was paid.

Just over half of urban households kept livestock in urban or rural areas; 17 per cent kept livestock in the urban area in which they lived. The main reason why more families did not keep animals was lack of land. Of households with livestock, the largest number kept poultry (75 per cent) and/or goats (26 per cent). Just over half (52 per cent) kept livestock only for subsistence purposes; a further 39 per cent kept livestock for both subsistence and sale. In addition to the sale of livestock products, animals are an important form of saving. Prices are relatively low at the beginning of the year when many families sell in order to raise the money for school fees, and high at the end of the year when national and religious holidays increase the demand for meat. Small numbers of households kept more unusual livestock such as fish and bees.

The importance of urban subsistence farming is in part due to poverty; 57 per cent of the households interviewed were in the 'very low income' category. It was estimated that these households were unable to feed themselves on what they earned. Even among the poorest households, a majority were successful in obtaining access to urban land which could be used for farming. However, urban farming is not an activity confined to the poor; many richer households also undertake significant farming activities. Existing planning policies take no account of urban farming. According to most by-laws, the activity is illegal although it is tolerated in most towns. Government could do much more to support such activities. For example, low density residential areas favour farming practices as households can use backyard areas. Productivity might also be improved with a crop extension service designed to help the urban poor.

Source: Lee-Smith, Diana, Mutsembi Manundu, Davinder Lamba and P Kuria Gathuru (1987), Urban Food Production and the Cooking Fuel Situation in Urban Kenya, *Mazingira Institute, Kenya.*

Many middle and upper income households in African cities are also involved in urban agriculture and have better access to land, water, inputs, technology, security, credit and markets, which allows them to profit more from this. In many countries in Africa, there was a considerable expansion in urban agriculture during the 1980s as transport systems deteriorated, rural production atrophied and incomes fell in real terms for a large proportion of the urban population. Where government policy favoured urban agriculture, as in Nigeria, Zaire, Tanzania, Zambia and Malawi, it grew more rapidly.[79]

The proportion of households who engage in some form of urban agriculture may be higher in the many small and intermediate size urban centres in Africa. Most studies of urban agriculture have been made within the larger African cities. The study in Kenya whose findings are outlined in the box found that over half the households interviewed in the three smallest towns (Isiolo, Kagamega and Kitui) had access to urban land for agriculture; the proportion was much lower for the other urban centres that are the three largest cities in Kenya (Kisumu, Nairobi and Mombasa).[80] A 1990 masterplan in a relatively small urban centre in Tanzania, Songea, found that around 59 per cent of residents have farms with crops grown for food and for income generation – including maize, cassava, beans, rice, sweet potatoes, finger millet, peas and coffee. Goats, sheep, pigs, poultry and dairy cattle are also kept.[81]

The detailed case studies of urban agriculture in African cities are a reminder that this encompasses much more than the crops or livestock raised on private plots. For instance, urban agriculture in Africa often includes riverside farmers who use land on river flood plains, roadside farmers who grow crops or graze livestock alongside roads and 'squatter farmers' who plant crops or graze livestock on public land – for instance land owned by railway companies or in parks.[82]

Public authorities often greatly underestimate the diversity of food production within or around their boundaries and the fact that it often includes high value crops. A recent review of urban agriculture highlighted not only its importance but also the great variety of food and fuel items that it includes:

- aquaculture in tanks, ponds, rivers and coastal bays;
- livestock raised in backyards, along roadsides, within rights of way for railways or underneath electric pylons, in poultry sheds and piggeries;
- orchards, including vineyards, street trees and backyard trees; and
- vegetables and other crops grown on rooftops, in backyards, in vacant lots or industrial estates, alongside canals, on the grounds of institutions, on roadsides and in many suburban farms.[83]

This review also noted the extent to which rooftops, balconies and small backyards can be used and gave examples of medicinal herbs grown on rooftops in Santiago de Chile, silkworms on balconies in Delhi, pigeons in Cairo, rabbits in illegal settlements in Mexico City, orchids in houses in Bangkok and fruit and vegetables on rooftops and other spaces in a squatter area in Bogota.[84]

The particular form that urban agriculture takes and the scope for its development varies greatly, depending on the nature of the city and its surrounds, the formal and informal rules governing who can use open land or water (and on what terms), the natural resource base available for its support, the economic circumstances and the time constraints on potential farmers and fish-rearers and their knowledge of how to profitably engage in such activities. In some African and Asian cities, one influential factor is related to the colonial heritage;[85] the lack of planning and infrastructure provision in the 'indigenous quarters' of colonial cities (usually kept strictly segregated from the residential areas of the colonial elite and the non-indigenous population) permitted newly arrived rural settlers to develop urban settlements with house forms and plans similar to their rural settlements. Low incomes also encouraged indigenous food production.[86] However, the colonial heritage can also act to deter or ban urban agriculture as under colonial rule, urban agriculture had been strictly controlled or forbidden in the areas other than the indigenous quarters and these controls were extended to cover the whole urban area, by post-colonial authorities.

Although many recent case studies of urban agriculture have concentrated on urban centres in Africa, perhaps because urban agriculture is (or has become) so important for the nutritional status and livelihoods of so many of the urban population, it is in certain Asian countries where urban agriculture has been developed most and where it has long received government support. For instance, in China, the policies and attitudes of public authorities have greatly enhanced the role of urban agriculture. This builds on an ancient tradition of urban agriculture which has long used sophisticated methods of crop rotation, inter-planting, inter-sowing and use of human and animal wastes as organic fertilizer – and which has been developed and encouraged since 1949.[87] For instance, within the boundaries of Shanghai city region, there is some of China's most productive agriculture; this includes a belt of vegetable farms around the city which supply approximately 80 per cent of all vegetables shipped to Shanghai's core, while further out, cotton, food-crops and oilseeds are the major crops.[88]

China's largest cities are essentially self-sufficient in food except for grains because of support for and protection of intensive cultivation in their surrounding areas.[89] Agriculture practised within city or municipal boundaries feeds about one third of China's total population[90] although this might better be considered as peri-urban agriculture. A considerable part of the reason for the impressive statistics from China on urban agriculture is the result of boundaries being set for municipalities or cities which include large amounts of surrounding rural areas. Nonetheless, the public authorities have generally encouraged intensive agricultural production in these areas and protected such areas from urban sprawl, whereas its potential in other countries is often lost or diminished as agricultural land on city peripheries is purchased as speculative investments (and no longer farmed) or developed illegally for housing.

There are also many examples from China of spectacular yields and complex production systems within urbanized areas. Box 4.14 provides

---

Box 4.14 **Household and Courtyard Farming in Urban Areas in China**

Fish and livestock raising, vegetables and fruit can be grown together in small urban courtyards. One example comes from the courtyard of Yang Puzhong, located on the outskirts of Bozhou in Hebei Province. This courtyard is only 200 square metres in size. At the centre is a fish pool, 20 square metres in size and two metres deep where carp, black carp, grass carp, loach and turtle are raised. Around the pool is a grape trellis which produces more than 1000 kg of grapes a year. On one side of the pool is a pigeon house and a pigsty with about 40 pigeons and eight pigs. Above the pigsty is a chicken house with 20 chickens and on top of the chicken house, a solar water heater. Below the pigsty is a methane generating pit. On the other side of the pool is a small vegetable garden which supplies the family with vegetables all year round. Chicken droppings are used to feed pigs, nightsoil is used to generate methane for cooking and liquid from the methane pit is used to feed the fish - with the remainder used as manure for farmland or as a culture medium for mushrooms.

Intensive cultivation is also evident in many other cities. For instance, in Shanghai, China's most populous city, there are increasing numbers of backyards, roofs, balconies, walls and vacant spaces near houses being used to develop such agroforestry systems as orange tree/vegetable/leguminous plant, grapevine/gourd and melon/leguminous plant and Chinese tallow tree/vegetable/leguminous plant.

Source: Honghai, Deng 'Urban agriculture as urban food supply and environmental protection subsystems in China' Paper presented to the international workshop on 'Planning for Sustainable Urban Development', University of Wales, 1992 This drew from Li Ping, 'Eco-farming on Huaibei Plain', Beijing Review *Vol 34, No 28, 1991, pp 8–16.*

some examples of intensive household and 'backyard' farming in urban areas in China. However, there are factors in China that act against urban agriculture. For instance, the kind of housing with courtyards described in Box 4.14 are rapidly disappearing in the larger and more prosperous cities, being replaced by apartment blocks. The rapid growth of many major cities will mean new urban developments taking place over intensively farmed agricultural land on their periphery. And there are considerable worries about the lack of attention to pollution control from many new enterprises, including the very large expansion in enterprises in the townships that are not officially considered 'urban'.[91]

There are many examples of urban agriculture in other Asian countries – for instance small, intensively cultivated plots of vegetables can be seen on the periphery of nearly every major Southeast Asian city.[92] There are also many examples from Latin America, although the overall scale of urban agriculture is probably much less, especially in the countries which are most urbanized with urban land markets that have long been heavily commercialized and no tradition of support from governments for urban agriculture. However, in Fortaleza (Brazil), more backyards, vacant plots, roads and streamsides are being converted into food production in low income areas[93] while in El Alto, a large informal settlement in La Paz in Bolivia,* a household survey in 1984–5 found that between 31 and 55 per cent of households raised small livestock for self consumption (hens, rabbits, pigs, lambs and ducks) and these were often the main source of animal protein for households. Many households also grow food crops.[94] There are also examples of particular institutions supporting urban agriculture – for instance hospitals in Lima and the University of Manila which lease their land to people wanting to engage in urban agriculture.[95] There are also examples of intensive crop cultivation on balconies and rooftops in apartment blocks which by combining intensive production and high value crops still produce significant returns, despite small areas.[96]

Benefits of Urban Agriculture

The benefits from urban agriculture to the households involved in it are obvious in terms of the food or fuel produced either for household consumption or for sale. The high proportion of the total population in many African urban areas who engage in urban agriculture was noted earlier. In the study of urban food production in six Kenyan towns on which Box 4.13 was based, 40 per cent of urban farmers said that they would starve if they were not permitted to undertake urban agriculture.[97] One study in Kampala, Uganda's largest city, found that the children of low-income families who were involved in farming were generally larger and healthier than children from families with comparable incomes but not involved in farming.[98] But as the Kenyan study also noted, it is usually the very low-income households that most need to grow subsistence food but these are also generally the households with the least access to land for doing so. In this study, very low income earners were less represented among those owning the urban land they farmed and among those who could farm backyard spaces adjacent to their dwellings.[99]

The examples from China show the potential importance of urban (or peri-urban) agriculture in terms of total production and of the intensity of production that can be achieved. Urban agriculture within or around the urban settlement can also reduce environmental hazards.[100] For instance, solid and liquid wastes are reduced, as they are used as input into production, and what were generally derelict, waste-strewn land sites are converted into tidy, carefully managed fields or plots. There is usually less surface and ground water and, with careful management of the site, problems of disease vectors breeding there are lessened – although special attention may have to be paid to ensuring that the changes in crops, land cover and water management do not create or exacerbate problems with particular disease vectors. There are also many possibilities for involving children in urban agriculture and in including within land used for crops

---

* El Alto is part of La Paz in terms of an urban agglomeration although it has separate municipal status.

places where they can play and experiment with cultivation themselves.

There are also important city-wide benefits from urban agriculture in addition to the obvious benefits to those involved in terms of food, fuel or income. These include the relatively low energy intensity of the food produced compared to conventional commercial food production systems and (often) the intensive use of organic wastes from household garbage, which reduces waste volumes and reduces (or eliminates) the need for artificial fertilizers. For instance, in Calcutta, vegetable farms have developed on refuse dumps where the mixture of organic refuse, coal ash, street sweepings and animal dung allowed intensive production. These farms, combined with farms in adjacent villages which use garbage as fertilizer, provide some 150 tonnes of vegetables each day to the city.[101]

In many cities, peri-urban agriculture also serves as a cheap and effective means of providing primary treatment to sewage.[102] Again in Calcutta, fish-farms have long been functioning in the wetlands to the east of the city which are fed by the city's sewers and storm drains; the large, shallow ponds are fringed with water hyacinth (on which cows graze) and sustain several types of carp and tilapia.[103] Waterborne sewage from Mexico City is used to irrigate over 100,000 hectares for growing livestock feed.[104] The health risks to agricultural workers in fertilizing fields and crops with sewage and to consumers of the products can be minimized.[105] In addition, a combination of provision for urban agriculture and for parks, playgrounds and other areas of open space can have beneficial environmental impacts, providing shade and modifying the climate.[106]

Deforestation and Urban Areas

Deforestation will also have a major impact on urban settlements where consumers and producers rely on forest products. Many families are dependent on wood as a source of energy. Changes in either the availability or the price of this product may have important consequences on the well being and health of residents. For poorer and middle income urban households in the Sahel, fuelwood bills may represent as much as one third of the household's income, a sum similar to that paid in rent. The use of substitutes is mainly restricted to households with higher incomes who can afford the use of a kerosene, bottle gas or electric cooker. Deforestation around any urban centre generally implies increased costs for forest products.

The ecological effects of deforestation on urban areas, including changes in run-off and subsequent erosion, may add to the risk of small floods, reduce the capacity of hydro-electric stations and reduce the productivity of agriculture. Deforestation of river catchment areas and associated soil erosion may be a contributory factor in floods which devastate large areas downstream, including cities or city-districts built alongside rivers. When flooding does occur, the costs incurred through loss of life and the destruction of property may be large. For example, deforestation is held to be responsible for the flooding of the Alakananda river which swept away six bridges, 16 footbridges and 25 buses; hundreds of people and animals died and there was extensive destruction of houses and cropland.[107]

However, there may be considerable untapped potential in urban forestry.[108] Again, this might seem to be a contradiction but many major cities have millions of trees. Many urban dwellers rely on trees within the urban areas to provide various products for both subsistence and income generation needs. They can be a valuable source of food – particularly fruits, but also leaves, shoots and flowers. In many countries in the South, they are also used as fodder for livestock grazing in the urban areas. Trees can also be used as visual or acoustic screens and can provide pollution sinks for contaminants in land and air. Tree planting has a significant effect in cleansing the air of pollutants and trees have a role in energy conservation by providing shade in summer and, in colder climates or seasons, reducing the cooling effects of wind.

REFERENCES

1   WHO (1992), *Our Planet, Our Health*, Report of the Commission on Health and Environment, Geneva, p 62.

2   Jazairy, Idriss, Mohiuddin Alamgir and Theresa Panuccio (1992), *The State of World Rural Poverty: an Inquiry into its Causes and Consequences*, IT Publications, London.

3   Ibid.

4   For example see Johnson, Victoria, Joanna Hill and Edda Ivan-Smith (1995), *Listening to Smaller Voices: Children in an Environment of Change*, ActionAid, London.

5   Tolba, Mostafa K, Osama A El-Kholy, E El-Hinnawi, M W Holdgate, D F McMichael and R E Munn (1992), *The World Environment 1972–1992; Two Decades of Challenge*, Chapman and Hall on behalf of UNEP, London, p 289.

6   Conway, Gordon R and Jules N Pretty (1991), *Unwelcome Harvest*, Earthscan London, p 1.

7   Fei, H T and C Chang (1945), *Earthbound China*, University of Chicago Press, Chicago.

8   Leach, Gerald (1975), *Energy and Food Production*, International Institute for Environment and Development (IIED), London.

9   See for instance Thaxton, Ralph (1981), 'The peasants of Yaocun: memories of exploitation, injustice and liberation in a Chinese village', *Journal of Peasant Studies*, Vol 9, No 1, October, pp 3–46.

10   Conway, Gordon R and Edward B Barbier (1990), *After the Green Revolution: Sustainable Agriculture for Development*, Earthscan, London.

11   WHO 1992, op cit.

12   Conway and Barbier 1990, op cit

13   GRET (1991), *La Réhabilitation des Périmètres Irrigués*, Groupe de Recherche et d'Echanges Technologiques, Paris, quoted in Toulmin, Camilla, Ian Scoones and Josh Bishop (1992), 'Drylands', in Johan Holmberg (Ed), *Policies for a Small Planet*, Earthscan, London.

14   Pretty, J N, I Guijt, I Scoones and J Thompson (1992), 'Regenerating agriculture: the agroecology of low-external input and community based development' in Holmberg J (ed), op cit.

15   Conway and Barbier 1990, op cit, p 11.

16   Tolba and others 1992, op cit.

17 Estimates for soil degradation are drawn from a Global Assessment of Soil Degradation (GLASOD), as reported in Oldeman, L R, R T A Hakkeling and W G Sombroek (1991), *World Map of the Status of Human-Induced Soil Degradation*, International Soil Reference and Information Centre, Wageningen and in WRI (1992), *World Resources 1991–92: a Guide to the Global Environment: Toward Sustainable Development*, Oxford University Press, Oxford.

18 Toulmin, Camilla (1995), *The Desertification Convention: the Strategic Agenda for the EU*, EC Aid and Development Briefing Paper No 1, January, IIED, London.

19 Bajracharya, D (1992), 'Institutional imperatives for sustainable resource management in the mountains, in N S Jodha, M Banskota and Tej Partap, *Sustainable Mountain Agriculture: Perspectives and Issues* Vol 1, Oxford and IBH Publishing, New Delhi, pp 205–234.

20 Ibid.

21 Jazairy, Alamgir and Panuccio 1992, op cit.

22 Tolba and others 1992, op cit.

23 El-Hinnawi, E (1991), 'Sustainable agricultural and rural development in the Near East', Regional Document No 4, FAO/Netherlands Conference, on Agriculture and Environment, FAO, Rome.

24 Toulmin, Scoones and Bishop 1992, op cit.

25 Tolba and others 1992, op cit.

26 Jazairy, Alamgir and Panuccio 1992, op cit.

27 Ibid.

28 The Ecologist (1992), *Whose Common Future: Reclaiming the Commons*, Earthscan, London.

29 See for instance Agarwal, Anil and Sunita Narain (1989), *Towards Green Villages – a Strategy for Environmentally Sound and Participatory Rural Development*, Centre for Science and Environment, Delhi, India; and Hasan, Arif and Ameneh Azam Ali (1992), 'Environmental problems in Pakistan: their origins and development and the threats that they pose to sustainable development', *Environment and Urbanization*, Vol 4, No 1.

30 Arulpragasam, L C (1990), 'Land reform and rural poverty in Asia', *The State of World Rural Poverty Working Paper 21*, IFAD, Rome.

31 Lane, Charles and Jules Pretty (1990), 'Displaced pastoralists and transferred wheat technology in Tanzania', Sustainable Agriculture Programme *Gatekeeper Series no 20*, IIED, London.

32 Jazairy, Alamgir and Panuccio 1992, op cit.

33 Toulmin, Scoones and Bishop 1992 and Bajracharya 1992, op cit.

34 Ibid; Chambers, Robert (1990), 'Micro-environments unobserved', Sustainable Agriculture Programme *Gatekeeper Series no 22*, IIED, London.

35 Bajracharya 1992, op cit.

36 See for instance Brydon, Lynne and Sylvia Chant (1989), *Women in the Third World: Gender Issues in Rural and Urban Areas*, Edward Elgar; Whitehead, Ann (1992), 'Gender-Aware Planning in Agricultural Production', Module 7 of *Gender and Third World Development*, Institute of Development Studies, University of Sussex.

37 Bajracharya 1992, op cit.

38 Toulmin, Scoones and Bishop 1992, op cit.

39 Tiffen, Mary and Michael Mortimore (1992),'Environment, population growth

and productivity in Kenya; a case study of Machakos District', *Development Policy Review* Vol 10, pp 359–387.

40 Hunter, John M (1981), 'Past explosion and future threat – exacerbation of Red Water Disease (schistosomiasis haematobium) in the Upper Region of Ghana', *Geojournal*, Vol 5, No 4, pp 305–313; WHO 1992, op cit.

41 Hunter, John M, et al (1982), 'Man-made lakes and man-made diseases: towards a policy resolution', *Social Science and Medicine*, Vol 16, pp 1127–1145.

42 Grazt, N (1987), 'The effect of water development programmes on malaria and malaria vectors in Turkey', in FAO, *Effects of Agricultural Development on Vector-Borne Diseases*, Document AGL/MISC/87.12, FAO, Rome.

43 Goonasekere, K G A and F P Amerasinghe (1987), 'Planning, design and operation of rice irrigation schemes – the impact of mosquito-borne disease hazards', in *Vector-borne Disease Control in Humans through Rice Agro Eco-system Management*, International Rice Research Institute, Los Banos.

44 Tiffen, Mary (1989), *Guidelines for the Incorporation of Health Safeguards into Irrigation Projects through Intersectoral Cooperation with Special Reference to Vector-borne Diseases*, Unpublished WHO Document, WHO, Geneva.

45 Juma, C (1989), *Biological Diversity and Innovation: Conserving and Utilizing Genetic Resources in Africa*, African Centre for Technology Studies, Nairobi.

46 Hecht, S B (1982), 'Agroforestry in the Amazon basin: practice, theory and limits of a promising land use', in S B Hecht (ed), *Amazonia: Agriculture and Land Use Research*, CIAT, Cali, pp 331–371.

47 Nieuwenhuys, Olga (1994), *Children's Lifeworld: Gender, Welfare and Labour in the Developing World*, Routledge, London.

48 Johnson, Hill and Ivan-Smith 1995, op cit.

49 Examples of this are described in Nieuwenhuys, Olga (1994), op cit; and Agarwal, Anil (1992), 'Who will help her learn? To keep the girl at school, the environment must be improved', *Down To Earth*, November 15.

50 Johnson, Hill and Ivan-Smith 1995, op cit.

51 Lee-Wright, Peter (1990), *Child Slaves*, Earthscan, London.

52 Hart, Roger (1996), *Children's Participation in Sustainable Development: The Theory and Practice of Involving Young Citizens in Community Development and Environmental Care*, Earthscan, London, 1996.

53 Leach, Gerald and Robin Mearns (1989), *Beyond the Woodfuel Crisis – People, Land and Trees in Africa*, Earthscan, London.

54 WRI (1990), *World Resources 1990–91: a Guide to the Global Environment*, Oxford University Press, Oxford, p 107.

55 Tolba and others 1992, op cit.

56 WRI 1990, op cit.

57 FAO (1988), *An Interim Report on the State of the Forest Resources in the Developing Countries*, FAO, Rome.

58 Gradwohl, J and R Greenberg (1988), *Saving the Tropical Forests*, Earthscan, London.

59 Tolba and others 1992, op cit, p 63.

60 Poore, Duncan (1989), *No Timber without Trees*, Earthscan, London.

61 Agarwal, Anil (1987), 'Between need and greed – the wasting of India; the greening of India', in Anil Agarwal, Darryl d'Monte and Ujwala Samarth, *The Fight for Survival: People's Action for Environment*, Centre for Science and Environment, Delhi.

62   Bhatt, Chandi Prasad (1990), 'The Chipko Andolan: forest conservation based on people's power' *Environment and Urbanization* Vol 2, No 1, April, pp 7–18.

63   Toulmin, Camilla (1990), 'Drylands and Human Settlements', Internal paper, IIED.

64   This paragraph is drawn from Chapter 10 of Jazairy, Alamgir and Panuccio 1992, op cit.

65   Jazairy, Alamgir and Panuccio 1992, op cit.

66   Agarwal and Narain 1989, op cit, p 13.

67   Hasan and Azam Ali 1992, op cit, p 13.

68   Crewe, Emma (1995), 'Indoor air pollution, household health and appropriate technology; women and the indoor environment in Sri Lanka', in Bonnie Bradford and Margaret A Gwynne (eds), *Down to Earth: Community Perspectives on Health, Development and the Environment*, Kumarian Press, West Hartford, p 93.

69   Bhatt 1990, op cit.

70   This section draws largely on Smit, Jac and Joe Nasr (1992), 'Urban agriculture for sustainable cities: using wastes and idle land and water bodies as resources' *Environment and Urbanization* Vol 4, No 2, Oct.

71   See for instance Smit and Nasr 1992, op cit, Mougeot, Luc J M (1994), *Urban Food production: Evolution, Official Support and Significance*, Cities Feeding People Series, Report 8, IDRC, Ottawa, and Yeung, Yue-Man (1985), *Urban Agriculture in Asia*, Food-Energy Nexus Programme, UN University, Tokyo.

72   See for instance Lee-Smith, Diana, Mutsembi Manundu, Davinder Lamba and P Kuria Gathuru (1987), *Urban Food Production and the Cooking Fuel Situation in Urban Kenya*, Mazingira Institute, Kenya.

73   Mougeot 1994, op cit gives some examples of the intensive agriculture and horticulture associated with historic cities.

74   This chaotic and haphazard expansion of cities and its impact on land use is described in more detail in Hardoy, Jorge E and David Satterthwaite (1989), *Squatter Citizen: Life in the Urban Third World*, Earthscan, London.

75   Smit and Nasr 1992 and Mougeot 1994, op cit.

76   See Mougeot 1994, op cit, for a review of the studies in Kenya and Tanzania.

77   Greenhow, Timothy (1994), *Urban Agriculture: Can Planners Make a Difference?*, Cities Feeding People Series, Report 12, IDRC, Ottawa.

78   See Mougeot 1994, op cit.

79   Smit, Jac, personal communication.

80   Lee-Smith and others 1987, op cit.

81   Lamba, Davinder (1993), *Urban Agriculture Research in East Africa: Record, Capacities and Opportunities*, Cities Feeding People Series, Report 2, IDRC, Ottawa.

82   Lee-Smith and others 1987, op cit; Freeman, D B (1991), *A City of Farmers: Informal Urban Agriculture in the Open Spaces of Nairobi, Kenya*, McGill-Queens University Press, Montreal.

83   Smit and Nasr 1992, op cit.

84   Ibid.

85   Douglas, Ian (1983), *The Urban Environment*, Edward Arnold, London.

86   See for instance Mbiba, Beacon (1994), 'Institutional responses to uncontrolled urban cultivation in Harare; prohibitive or accomodative', *Environment and*

Urbanization, Vol 6, No 1, April, pp 188–201. A more detailed discussion is available in Mbiba, Beacon (1995), *Urban Agriculture in Zimbabwe*, Avebury, Aldershot.

87 Honghai, Deng (1992), 'Urban agriculture as urban food supply and environmental protection subsystems in China' Paper presented to the international workshop on 'Planning for Sustainable Urban Development', University of Wales.

88 Hawkins, J N (1982), 'Shanghai: an exploratory report on food for a city', *GeoJournal*, Supplementary issue; Zhongmin, Yan (1988), 'Shanghai: the growth and shifting emphasis of China's largest city' in Victor F S Sit (Ed), *Chinese Cities: the Growth of the Metropolis since 1949*, Oxford University Press, Hong Kong, pp 94–127.

89 Smit, Jac, personal communication.

90 Honghai 1992, op cit.

91 Kirkby, Richard (1994), 'Dilemmas of urbanization: review and prospects', in Denis Dwyer (Ed), *China: The Next Decades*, Longman Scientific and Technical, Harlow, pp 128–155.

92 Sommers, Paul and Jac Smit (1994), *Promoting Urban Agriculture: a Strategy Framework for Planners in North America, Europe and Asia*, Cities Feeding People Series, Report 9, IDRC, Ottawa.

93 Yves Cabannes, personal communication quoted in Mougeot 1994, op cit.

94 Prudencio, J (1994), *Institutional Assessment for Research Initiative on Urban Agriculture (Latin America and Caribbean)*, Draft consultancy report (mimeo), La Paz, quoted in Mougeot 1994, op cit.

95 Smit and Nasr 1992, op cit.

96 Smit and Nasr 1992, op cit.

97 Lee-Smith and others 1987, op cit.

98 Maxwell, D G and S Zziwa (1992), *Urban Farming in Africa: The Case of Kampala, Uganda*, ACTS Press, Nairobi; and Maxwell, D G and S Zziwa (1993), 'Urban agriculture in Kampala: indigenous adaptive response to the economic crisis', *Ecology of Food and Nutrition*, Vol 29, pp 91–109.

99 Lee-Smith and others 1987, op cit.

100 This point was made by Jac Smit, when reviewing an earlier draft of this manuscript.

101 Furedy, Christine (1990), 'Social aspects of solid waste recovery in Asian cities' *Environmental Sanitation Reviews* No 30, ENSIC, Asian Institute of Technology Bangkok, December, pp 2–52.

102 Ibid; Smit and Nasr 1992, op cit.

103 Furedy 1990, op cit.

104 Smit and Nasr 1992, op cit.

105 Mara, Duncan and Sandy Cairncross (1990), *Guidelines for the Safe Use of Wastewater and Excreta in Agriculture and Aquaculture*, WHO, Geneva.

106 Douglas 1983, op cit; Rabinovitch, Jonas (1992), 'Curitiba: towards sustainable urban development', *Environment and Urbanization*, Vol 4, No 2, Oct, pp 62–77.

107 Bhatt 1990, op cit.

108 This paragraph is based on a box in UNCHS (1996), *An Urbanizing World: Global Report on Human Settlements 1996*, Oxford University Press, Oxford and New York, which draws on Carter, J (1993), 'The Potential Of Urban Forestry In Developing Countries: A Concept Paper', FAO, Rome.

5

Sustaining Environment and Development[1]

BRINGING DEVELOPMENT INTO SUSTAINABLE DEVELOPMENT

The achievement of development goals ultimately depends on human capacities both to shape the living and working environment in ways that promote and safeguard health and to draw resources from natural systems in ways that do not threaten their integrity. Healthy and safe living environments for children and their parents and ready access to the resources on which their livelihoods and health depend have to be achieved without requiring levels of resource use (and waste generation) which are ecologically unsustainable. The term 'sustainable development' has become widely used to stress the need for the simultaneous achievement of development and environment goals.

For the agencies of governments and international institutions that are involved in different aspects of 'development', 'sustainable development' is most easily interpreted as adding onto existing development goals the requirement that their achievement does not contribute to the depletion of natural capital – for instance the degradation of renewable resources such as soil, the depletion of scarce non-renewable resources and/or the degradation of ecosystems. Although the origins of a concern for combining environmental and developmental goals go back several decades and were much discussed throughout the 1970s,* this concern was made more

---

* There is also an assumption that the concern for sustainable development is new when its key conceptual underpinnings were widely discussed and described in the early 1970s and possibly earlier. The term 'sustainable development' arose primarily to acknowledge the development needs of low-income groups and low-income countries within the growing interest in local, national and global environmental issues in the North and the understanding of the international dimensions of environmentalism. The need to reconcile these two aspects was widely discussed before, during and after the UN Conference on the Human Environment at Stockholm in 1972, even if this was not called sustainable development at that time. The Brundtland Commission's stress on 'meeting the needs of the present without compromising the ability of future generations to meet their own needs' had been a central theme in the writings of Barbara Ward throughout the 1970s - although this was usually phrased as meeting the 'inner limits' of human needs and rights without exceeding the 'outer limits' of the planet's ability to sustain life, now and in the future.[2]

explicit, and the use of the term 'sustainable development' promoted, by *Our Common Future,* the report of the World Commission on Environment and Development (WCED) (also known as the Brundtland Commission), published in 1987.[3] The statement that we must meet 'the needs of the present generation without compromising the ability of future generations to meet their own needs'[4] is drawn from this report and this has become one of the most widely used and quoted summaries of the goals of sustainable development.

The two key goals within this statement have obvious implications for children. *Meeting the needs of the present* requires actions on all the preventable illness, injury and premature death described in previous chapters and on providing children and their parents with the means to ensure this happens. The implications for children yet unborn of '...*without compromising the ability of future generations to meet their own needs*' is obvious as future generations have the right to come into a world whose ecosystems have not been degraded, whose natural resource base has not been depleted, and where human activities have not disrupted global climate to the point where many people's livelihood or health is at risk. On this second goal within sustainable development, such sayings as 'we hold the world in trust for our children and their children' and 'the world is on loan to us from our grandchildren' remain valid even if these may have been stated too often to get our attention.

It has often proved difficult to engage the interest of development practitioners in environmental issues, especially when they have so often found their concerns largely excluded from discussions about sustainable development. Much of the discussions on sustainable development are about what actions are needed to sustain the global resource base (soils, biodiversity, mineral resources, forests) and about limiting the disruption to global cycles as a result of human activities – especially greenhouse gas emissions and the depletion of the stratospheric ozone layer. Such global issues do pose serious threats to child health and survival, especially in the future. But global discussions about environment and development should not ignore the other environmental crises referred to in Chapter 1, which underlie the ill health or premature death of millions of infants and children each year and also contribute so much to the ill health and disablement of tens of millions of children and to the ill health, disablement and premature death of adults. To recall just two examples of this, the environmental modifications that could contribute so much to lessening the million or more children who die each year from malaria or the three million who die from diarrhoeal diseases should be at the centre of all international discussions about the environment. Discussions about 'sustainability' in regard to soil erosion and deforestation also must not be abstracted from the needs of the hundreds of millions of people whose livelihoods depend on access to soils and forest products.

THE DIFFERENT COMPONENTS OF SUSTAINABLE DEVELOPMENT

The focus of this book is on how to ensure the environment in which children live is safe and healthy and therefore meeting 'the needs of the present generation' can be taken as meeting the economic, social, health and political (or participatory) needs of children (and their parents). This can be considered as the *development* part of sustainable development and the key components are listed in the first part of Box 5.1. They include the environment-related needs discussed in earlier chapters such as living environments in which biological, chemical and physical hazards are minimized and where there is adequate provision for schools, health care, play and social interaction with their peers. They obviously include the need for parents to have an adequate livelihood that allows the needs of all household members to be met, without requiring from the children themselves an excessive work burden. Children also have needs and rights in regard to participation in environmental issues – and this is considered in Chapter 7.

The *sustainable* component of sustainable development can be taken as meeting these needs for all children and the households of which they are part but without a level of resource use and waste generation which threatens local, regional and global ecological sustainability. The sustainable component requires no depletion or degradation of four kinds of 'natural capital' (or 'environmental capital') listed in the lower part of Box 5.1. The first is the finite stock of *non-renewable resources* – for instance fossil fuels, metals and other mineral resources. Most of these resources (especially fossil fuels) are consumed when used, so finite stocks are depleted with use. Others are not consumed since the resource remains in the waste – for instance metals used in capital and consumer goods. But for most non-renewable resources, there are energy and cost constraints to recovering a high proportion of the total amount used from waste streams. These may be considered as partially 'renewable', with the extent defined by the proportion of materials in discarded goods which can be reclaimed and recycled. Biological diversity, one key part of environmental capital, might also be considered a non-renewable resource.

The second component of environmental capital is what might be termed the *non-renewable natural sink capacity* which is the finite capacity of local and global eco-systems to absorb or dilute non-biodegradable wastes without adverse effects. As Chapter 2 noted, one area of concern is the increasing concentration of persistent biocides. There are also large volumes of non-biodegradable wastes arising from human activities that have to be stored and kept entirely isolated from ecosystems because of the damage to ecosystems and to human health they would pose – for instance there are large volumes of hazardous wastes that are generated by many industrial processes. The wastes from nuclear power stations are also a particular concern; these include wastes which will remain with dangerously high levels of radioactivity for tens of thousands of years. Globally, one of the most pressing problems is the finite capacity of global systems to absorb greenhouse gases without changes in climate that can cause very serious direct and indirect impacts on health and on ecosystems.

Box 5.1 **The Multiple Goals of Sustainable Development as Applied to Children**

Meeting the needs of the present...

- *Economic needs* – parents having access to an adequate livelihood or productive assets and economic security when unemployed, ill, disabled or otherwise unable to secure a livelihood. No undue work burden for children, including pressure to skip school or leave school early because of parents' inadequate incomes.
- *Social, cultural and health needs* – includes a shelter for the household of which the children are part which is healthy, safe, affordable and secure, within a neighbourhood where environmental health hazards are minimized through the provision for piped water, sanitation, drainage etc. Ready and safe access to schools, health centres and places with adequate provision for safe, largely child-directed play. This should include access to the natural environment and their involvement in environmental issues within their schools. Full immunization against the vaccine-preventable diseases and good quality maternal health services for their mothers. Emergency first aid and health care available to rapidly treat accidental injuries. Good quality and stimulating day care provision for children when both parents have to work.
- *Political needs* – the right to express their views and to be involved in discussions and decisions that affect them. Their involvement in participatory learning about the environment.

...Without compromising the ability of future generations to meet their own needs

- Minimizing the use or waste of *the finite stock of non-renewable resources* – includes minimizing the consumption of fossil fuels in housing, commerce, industry and transport plus substituting renewable sources where feasible. Also, minimizing waste of scarce mineral resources (reduce use, re-use, recycle, reclaim). There are also cultural and natural assets that are irreplaceable and thus non-renewable – for instance, historic city districts and parks and natural landscapes which provide space for play, recreation and access to nature.
- *Non-renewable natural sink capacity* – minimizing the generation of non-biodegradable wastes, especially those that have harmful impacts on human health and natural systems or cycles, eg minimum generation of persistent chemicals and most greenhouse gases.

> • *Renewable resources* – human activities drawing on soils and fresh-water resources at levels that ecosystems can sustain without damage or degradation. This includes cities keeping to a sustainable ecological footprint in terms of land area on which producers and consumers in any city draw for agricultural crops, wood products and biomass fuels.
> • *Renewable sink capacity* – biodegradable wastes kept within the absorptive capacity of local and global sinks – eg capacity of river or lake to break down biodegradable wastes from local industries and urban centres.
>
> *Source: Adapted from a box on sustainable development and cities in Mitlin, Diana and David Satterthwaite,* Cities and Sustainable Development, *the background paper to Global Forum '94, Manchester City Council and IIED, 1994.*

The third is the finite capacity of ecosystems to provide sustainable levels of *renewable resources*. Human use of some renewable resources (eg the direct use of solar power or its indirect use through wind or wave power) does not deplete the resource. But many renewable resources (especially pasture, crops and trees) are renewable only within finite limits set by the ecosystem within which they grow. Freshwater resources are also finite; in the case of aquifers, human use often exceeds their natural rate of recharge and such levels of use are unsustainable.

The fourth component of environmental capital is the *renewable sink capacity*, the finite capacity of ecosystems to break down biodegradable wastes. Although most wastes arising from production and consumption are biodegradable, each eco-zone or water body has a finite capacity to break down such wastes without itself being degraded.

WHAT IS TO BE SUSTAINED?

One of the main sources of confusion in regard to sustainable development is what precisely is to be 'sustained'. Some consider that the *sustainable* component of sustainable development is in regard to natural or environmental capital; this is how it is understood in Box 5.1 and in this chapter. But for many people writing on sustainable development, it is used to refer to different aspects of development (ie sustaining economic growth or social or political sustainability). Thus, a discussion of sustainable development might be discussing how to sustain a development project, an institution, a business, a society or some subset of a society (eg a 'community'), culture or economic growth (in general or for some specific country). It may also be focusing on sustaining a nation, a city or a region.

In many such discussions, there is no *development* component in the sense of better meeting human needs.[5] It is also common to find the terms 'sustainable development' and 'sustainability' used interchangeably with no recognition that the two mean different things. A comment about this in a review of the literature on sustainable development published in 1992 still remains accurate for much that has been published on sustainable development since 1992:

> *'Much of the writing, and many discussions, in the North concentrate primarily on sustainability rather than sustainable development. These authors' main focus is how present environmental constraints might be overcome and the standard of living maintained. The need for development, of ensuring that all people in the world might obtain the resources they need for survival and development is ignored or given little attention.'*[6]

As a recent paper commented, 'the most serious problem with broad definitions of sustainability is that they tend to marginalize the primary environmental concerns of the poor, even as they claim to incorporate them.'[7] In addition, most of the literature on sustainable development does not question the current distribution of power and of the ownership of resources except where this is considered a factor in 'unsustainable practices'. Box 5.2 gives more details of the different meanings given to the sustainable part of sustainable development and explains why we suggest

---

Box 5.2 **The Meaning of Sustainability**

There is considerable confusion as to what is to be *sustained* by sustainable development. For instance, is it natural systems or human activities that are to be sustained and at what scale are they to be sustained (eg local projects, cities, nations, the sum of all activities globally).

The term 'sustainable' is most widely used in reference to ecological sustainability. But during preparations for the Earth Summit (held in 1992) and ever since, an increasing number of writers and international organizations began to include such concepts as social sustainability, economic sustainability, community sustainability and even cultural sustainability as part of sustainable development. Meanwhile, many aid/development assistance agencies were giving another meaning to the term sustainable development as this was the label given to ensuring that their development projects continued to operate and meet development objectives when these agencies' external support was cut off at the end of the project. In this sense, sustainability was far more about operation and maintenance (or *institutional and managerial sustainability*) than about any concept of ecological sustainability. A concern for project sustainability may give little or no consideration as to whether the sum of all the 'sustainable' projects would prove sustainable in an ecological sense.

Some of the literature about sustainable development discusses 'social sustainability' although there is no consensus as to what this means. For instance, some consider social sustainability as the social preconditions for sustainable development while others imply that it is the need to sustain specific social relations, customs or structures. But it is difficult to equate social sustainability with the goals of *Our Common Future*. When judged by the length of time for which they were sustained, some of the most 'successful' societies were also among the most exploitative, where the abuse of human rights was greatest. These are not societies we would want to 'sustain'. Development includes strong and explicit social objectives and achieving the development goals within sustainable development demands social change, not 'sustainability' in the sense of 'keeping them going continuously'. Indeed, the achievement of most of the social, economic and political goals which are part of sustainable development requires fundamental changes to social structures including changes to government institutions and, in many instances, to the distribution of assets and income. This can hardly be equated with 'social sustainability'.

Discussions on 'social sustainability' when defined as the social conditions necessary to support environmental sustainability are valuable in so far as they stress that natural resources are used within a social context and it is the rules and values associated with this context that determine both the distribution of resources within the present generation and between the future generations and the present. Discussions of 'social sustainability' that stress the value of social capital or the social conditions that allow or support the meeting of human needs are also valuable. Our avoidance of the term is both because it can invite confusion with the other interpretations and because it can imply that there is only one way to achieve ecological sustainability whereas there is generally a range of possible options.

There has also been some discussion of 'cultural sustainability' because of the need within human society to develop shared values, perceptions and attitudes which help to contribute to the achievement of sustainable development. It is clear that development should include as a critical component a respect for cultural patrimony. Culture implies knowledge and a vast wealth of traditional knowledge of relevance to sustainable natural resource use (and to development) is ignored or given scant attention in development plans. But the term 'cultural sustainability' seems rather imprecise for the need to recognize the importance of culture and respect it within development. Culture is never static; to argue that it should be sustained is to deny an important aspect - its changing and developing nature.

We choose to use the concept of *sustainability* only in regard to ecological sustainability, both because of the lack of consensus as to what sustainability might mean when applied to human activities and institutions and because we believe the term has been inappropriately applied. Meeting economic, social and political goals fall within the *development* component of sustainable development. Obviously their achievement has to be sustainable in an ecological sense since human life and wellbeing depend on this.

Source: Developed from Hardoy, Jorge E, Diana Mitlin and David Satterthwaite (1993), Environmental Problems in Third World Cities, *Earthscan, London.*

that the term 'sustainable' is best kept in reference to natural capital. It also outlines the confusions inherent in such concepts as social sustainability or cultural sustainability. Thus, desirable social, economic or political goals at community, city, regional or national level are best understood as being within the *development* part of sustainable development while the *sustainable* component includes goals relating to ecological sustainability – for instance no overall depletion of natural or environmental capital within nations or worldwide.

If the criterion of *sustainability* is used only in terms of environmental capital, there is a further distinction needed between particular projects/ activities and in reference to larger systems (sometimes city-wide or nation-wide or world-wide). It is useful to differentiate between the two applications of the term since both are important in considering sustainable development. Simple inter-relationships between specific development activities (for instance, expanding a piped water supply or developing an irrigation system) and environmental capital can be assessed and judged according to whether there is a decrease in any of the four kinds of environmental capital outlined above. Alternatively, the focus can be much broader, concerned with large aggregates and systems of activities. The first approach is concerned with making a single part of the system ecologically sustainable. The second approach recognises that it is difficult to make all activities sustainable and that what is important is that the sum (or net effect) of the activities within a specific area is ecologically sustainable.

Not all human activities can be supported only by the natural resources and ecosystems in which they are located. For instance, it is unrealistic to demand that major cities must be supported by the resources that are produced in their immediate surrounds although it is entirely appropriate to require that consumers and producers in high consumption, high waste cities reduce their level of resource use and waste, and reduce or halt the damaging ecological impacts of their demands for fresh water and other resources on their surrounds.

The successful achievement of sustainable development requires society to establish institutions which are capable of ensuring that individual projects sum to an acceptable aggregate outcome without demanding such stringent conditions on individual projects that they inhibit the achievement of development goals.

WHAT IS CURRENTLY UNSUSTAINABLE?

There is growing evidence that many current global trends in the use of resources or sinks for wastes are not sustainable – and this is something that is unique to the late 20th century.[8] Although there are many examples of human activities destroying or seriously damaging natural resources and systems throughout history, only relatively recently has the sum of all human resource consumption and waste generation reached the point where it can adversely affect the present and future state of the global environment and the availability of certain natural resources. This obviously alters the parameters of the environmental debate as the scale and scope of global environmental problems are recognized.[9]

Although much uncertainty remains about the current level of risk and how much the risk will increase in the future (and its ecological consequences), the costs are already apparent (as in the health effects of stratospheric ozone depletion) or likely to become apparent soon. In the South, the problems are largely the worrying trends in terms of unsustainable levels of use for some renewable resources (for instance through deforestation and soil degradation) that were described in Chapter 4. In the North, the problem centres on the scale of renewable and non-renewable resource use, waste, pollution and greenhouse gas emissions.

The link between what is unsustainable in terms of environmental capital and what needs to done to meet development goals does not appear to be problematic in the short term. However, while meeting the needs of poorer women and men of all ages and ethnic groups in both the North and the South need not imply an unsustainable level of resource use, it is clear that extending the levels of resource consumption and waste generation currently enjoyed by the rich minority to an increasing proportion of the world's population almost certainly does.[10]

If consideration is given to more sustainable patterns of use for the four different kinds of environmental capital noted earlier, some progress has been achieved in two of them. The first is in limiting wastes that were previously dumped into local ecosystems. For instance, in most countries, environmental legislation has limited the right of industries and utilities to use local sinks for wastes – for instance disposing of untreated wastes in rivers, lakes or other local water bodies or in high levels of air pollution. However, the extent to which the environmental legislation is enforced varies widely and in many countries in the South there is little enforcement. Rivers, lakes and estuaries in or close to major cities or industrial complexes in the South are usually heavily polluted and this has often led to a drastic reduction in fish production and the loss of livelihoods for those who formerly made their living from fishing.[11] In addition, most countries have also been less successful in controlling air pollution arising from motor vehicles, except for the reduction in lead emissions that has been achieved in many countries by the increasing proportion of vehicles that use lead-free petrol.

There has also been some progress in many nations towards more sustainable use of certain resources. For instance, the protection of renewable resources is being promoted in many countries where fertile soil and fresh water are in short supply, and forests are being rapidly depleted – especially in the wealthier nations. But one problem that has yet to be addressed is the extent to which the wealthier nations or regions can achieve this by appropriating the soils and water resources of distant ecosystems as the cheapest means of reducing pressure on their own ecosystems.[12] Wealthy nations now import many of the land- and water-intensive goods their consumers or producers need so the depletion of soil and the overexploitation of freshwater resources these cause are not environmental costs borne within their boundaries. William Rees coined the term 'ecological footprint' to highlight the large area of productive land on which city-based consumers and producers draw – with the size of this footprint obviously growing, as consumption levels for renewable resources rise. Wealthy nations can also import goods whose production has high environmental and health costs – for instance, the high use of pesticides which are applied without adequate protection for the workforce involved in the production – but with none of these health or environmental costs affecting their own inhabitants or ecosystems. Thus, the wealthiest nations can maintain the highest environmental standards within their own countries, even though the ecological and health costs of producing the goods they import are very high.

There is much less progress on achieving more sustainable patterns of resource use and waste generation in the two other types of environmental capital – the use of non-renewable resources and sinks for non-biodegradable wastes. This includes the 'global sink' as the reduction in the stratospheric ozone layer brings new environmental and health costs and as global warming appears likely to continue and to bring increasingly serious health and environmental costs. Progress on addressing environmental problems is easier where those creating or exacerbating the problem (for instance the polluters) and those affected by the problem are within the same locality or nation. Even if those whose livelihoods and health have been adversely affected by the environmental consequences of other people's or businesses' activities have often found it difficult to get these activities halted or their environmental impacts reduced, at least within most societies there are laws and institutions which allow such problems to be addressed.

Where environmental problems are caused or exacerbated by activities in other countries, it is much more difficult for those affected to stop this. For instance, how can those people who are adversely affected by floods or extreme weather conditions that are probably linked to global warming get redress from the past and current middle and upper income households with high consumption levels who have been a major cause of global warming?

The problem becomes even more complex when considered across generations – how can those who are likely to lose their livelihoods (and possibly their lives) from storms and floods and changes in rainfall patterns that are linked to global warming in the future get redress from the people whose high consumption and waste levels were the main underlying cause of their losses? It has proved possible to halt or modify investment decisions which imply serious social and environmental costs either in the immediate locality or at least within that nation's boundaries (although much more needs to be done) but it is very difficult to halt or modify investment decisions that imply serious social and environmental costs in distant (foreign) ecosystems or for future generations.

In addition, if governments and international agencies give such inadequate attention to the needs and priorities of so many children and their parents today, will they act to safeguard the needs and priorities of future children? The lack of a commitment to intra-generational equity, ie to lessening unequal access to natural resources and to safe and healthy living environments within the contemporary world, does not augur well for obtaining a real commitment to inter-generational equity. Achieving the inter-generational equity aspect of sustainable development is, in effect, a commitment by middle and upper income groups all round the world to change lifestyles and consumption patterns to safeguard the needs of children in future generations. Although the extent of the needed changes is strongly debated, the need for changes has become evident.

Achieving what can be termed the three major principles that underlie sustainable development[13] – more inter-generational equity, more intra-generational equity and transfrontier responsibility by resource users and waste generators – implies major political changes. It implies major changes in ownership rights for land and natural resources.[14] And as Graham Haughton and Colin Hunter point out, it implies changes in the configuration of the political system at local and global levels that had previously allowed or even encouraged undesirable environmental impacts.[15] Achieving this is made all the more difficult by incomplete knowledge about the scale and nature of the environmental costs that current production and consumption patterns are passing onto current and future generations.[16]

One of the most difficult issues to resolve is on what basis to value the different kinds of environmental assets widely used in production and consumption[17] and how to ensure that this valuation contributes to greater inter-generational and intra-generational equity. Another is the extent to which one form of natural capital is substitutable for another – and the extent to which other forms of capital are substitutable for natural capital.[18] Another is how to ensure that social capital (including social institutions that have great importance in ensuring human needs are met) and human capital (including people's knowledge and level of education and their health) are also not depleted.[19]

Earlier chapters looked in some detail at the environmental problems facing girl and boy children (and their parents) and at the link between development needs and renewable resource use and management. What has not been considered is the issue of non-renewable resource use and non-renewable natural sink capacity. These will be considered briefly in the sections below with most attention given to the possible ecological and health consequences of global warming, since in the long term, these pose the greatest threat to children and their parents.

NON-RENEWABLE RESOURCE USE

It was a concern about possible global shortages of key non-renewable resources (oil, natural gas and certain minerals) which provided a strong stimulus to the environmental movement in the early 1970s – as in, for instance, the Club of Rome report, *Limits to Growth* (1972). If the concerns about environment and development in the early 1990s are compared to those in the mid 1970s, this concern now receives less prominence. Two other concerns have grown in prominence. The first is the much increased concern about damage arising from human activities to global natural systems: the depletion of the stratospheric ozone layer and atmospheric warming are now perceived as far more serious threats to sustainability than was the case in the early 1970s. The second is the much increased concern about the finite nature of many renewable resources (especially fertile soil and freshwater resources). They are only renewable within particular limits.

However, because of the scale of the disparities between the wealthiest and the poorest nations, a concern for the use of non-renewable resources remains. Levels of resource use per person for non-renewable resources vary by a factor of between ten and 100 or more, when comparing per capita averages between wealthy and poor nations. The same is also true for levels of waste generation.[20] The disparities become even larger, when considering the contribution to date of non-renewable resource use and the contribution to currently existing persistent chemicals or greenhouse gases in the atmosphere. But, in one sense, comparisons of averages for resource use or waste (including greenhouse gas emissions) per person between nations is misleading in that it is essentially the middle and upper income groups who account for most resource use and most waste generation; this only becomes a North-South issue because most of the world's middle and upper income people with high consumption lifestyles live in Europe, North America, Japan and Australasia. High income households in Africa, Asia and Latin America may have levels of non-renewable resource use comparable to high income households in the richest nations; it is the fact that there are so many fewer of them that keeps national averages much lower.

However, levels of household wealth alone are insufficient to explain the disparities in terms of averages for resource use per person and other factors must be considered. For instance, figures for the use of gasoline per person in different cities are particularly interesting, since this represents both a draw on a finite non-renewable resource (oil) and a major contributor to greenhouse gases. In 1980, gasoline use per capita in cities such as Houston, Detroit and Los Angeles was five to seven times that of three of Europe's most prosperous and attractive cities: Amsterdam, Vienna and Copenhagen.[21] Averages for resource use per person are not only linked to incomes and prices but also to the incentive and regulatory framework provided by governments to encourage resource conservation or penalize high levels of resource use and waste.

Two points in regard to non-renewable resources need to be emphasized. The first is that the finite nature of the resource base is not in doubt, even if the predictions as to when resource shortages (or price rises associated with shortages) will begin have receded. The second is that high consumption levels for non-renewable resources are also associated with high levels of waste generation and greenhouse gas emissions. Reducing greenhouse gas emissions certainly implies lower levels of use and waste in non-renewable resources. There may be sufficient non-renewable resources to ensure that 9–10 billion people on earth, late in the next century, have their needs met. But it is unlikely that the world's resources and ecosystems could sustain a world population of 9 or 10 billion with a per capita consumption of non-renewable resources similar to those enjoyed by the richest households today or even the average figure for the world's high consumption cities such as Houston and Los Angeles.

NON-RENEWABLE SINKS

The disparities between rich and poor nations in terms of averages per person for the warming potential of total greenhouse gas emissions or, until recent moves to control them, emissions of stratospheric ozone depleting chemicals, are as striking as those noted above for non-renewable resource use and waste generation. For instance, cities such as Canberra, Chicago and Los Angeles have between six and nine times the per capita CO_2 emissions of the world's average and 25 or more times that of cities such as Dhaka.[22]

Stratospheric Ozone Depletion

The gas ozone, a form of oxygen that is a serious danger to health at ground-level (as described in Chapter 2), is at the same time a critical shield in the stratosphere, protecting human, animal and plant populations against biologically damaging components of sunlight.[23] There has been a severe depletion of stratospheric ozone since measurements began in the early 1960s, largely as a result of emissions of chlorofluorocarbons (CFCs) and other halocarbons that are used for refrigerants, aerosol propellants, solvents, foam blowing agents and fire retardants.[24] The problems are most serious over the South Pole where what is sometimes termed as a large ozone hole appears during the spring due to severe ozone depletion. A comparable, although less extensive, ozone hole also appears over the Arctic. The main direct effect on human populations is increased incidence of skin cancers and cataracts.[25] It has been suggested that a decrease in the stratospheric ozone layer of 10 per cent would result in a 26 per cent increase of more than 300,000 additional cases of non-melanoma skin cancer and 4500 cases of malignant melanoma.[26] But the importance of reducing the emission of gases currently responsible for depleting stratospheric ozone is much increased because they are also among the largest contributors to global warming.

Global Warming

There is still much uncertainty about the possible scale of global warming in the future and its likely direct and indirect effects. However, the scale of possible disruption to settlements and ecosystems and of increases in extreme weather events if there is a sustained trend towards atmospheric warming make curbs on greenhouse gas emissions particularly important. Although far more attention has been given to global warming over the more immediate environmental crises that have been described earlier – no doubt because the wealthy nations and households will also have to bear many of the costs – this should not mean the importance of curbing greenhouse gas emissions where possible should be neglected. The most important greenhouse gases are carbon dioxide (CO_2), halocarbons (that include CFCs), methane, water vapour and nitrous oxide; all but the halocarbons occur naturally in the atmosphere but human activities have been responsible for increasing their concentration. Carbon dioxide is the most important greenhouse gas. It is responsible for around 60 per cent of the greenhouse warming that has occurred since the beginning of the industrial revolution and is likely to continue being responsible for around this proportion of warming in the future.[27] Halocarbons were considered the second largest contributor to global warming but the warming to which they contribute may be off-set by the depletion they cause in stratospheric ozone.[28] A recent IPCC report suggested that their contribution was around 9 per cent with methane accounting for around 15 per cent.[29]

Atmospheric concentrations of the three most important greenhouse gases are increasing. For carbon dioxide, what is known is that there has been a significant increase in its concentration in the atmosphere – from 280 ppmv (parts per million (volume)) in pre-industrial times to 355 today. Human activities, especially the combustion of fossil fuels, have been a major contributor; deforestation also makes an important contribution. The increase in the concentration of halocarbons in the atmosphere is much more rapid, although this began from a lower base since virtually all halocarbons in the atmosphere come from their manufacture and use since the 1930s. The concentration of methane in the atmosphere has more than doubled since the 18th century, with annual measurements in recent years showing an upward trend in atmospheric concentration; natural wetlands and rice paddies, and enteric fermentation from animals are considered the main sources although methane emissions from gas drilling, venting and transmission, biomass burning, termites, landfills and coal mining are also important sources.[30]

There is evidence of an increase in the global average temperature over the last 120 years and many of the warmest years on record have been in the last 15 years. With few exceptions, glaciers, worldwide, are receding.[31] These are consistent with global warming induced by greenhouse gases released by human activities. However, there are uncertainties as to the extent to which the increase in global temperature is the result of human activities and the extent (and rate) at which it will continue. For instance, account must be taken of the contribution of non-human induced factors (for instance volcanic eruptions) and the extent to which the warming trend is part of a natural variation that may reverse itself. There is also the complication that other air pollutants associated with industrialization and high levels of fossil fuel consumption can counter the greenhouse effect. For instance, sulphate particles emitted into the air from burning coal (and heavy oil) in industries and power stations produces the haze that is often seen over urban and industrial concentrations; these also form clouds that help reflect sunlight and reduce warming.

ENVIRONMENTAL IMPACT OF CLIMATE CHANGE

Direct Effects

The most direct effects of global warming are higher global mean temperatures, sea level rises, changes in weather patterns (including those of rainfall and other forms of precipitation) and in the frequency and severity of extreme weather conditions (storms, sea surges). These can lead to major changes in the function and structure of ecosystems. They will also pose direct threats to human health and life, especially through increased incidence and severity of floods and storms and through decreased potential for crop production in particular areas.

Sea level rises will obviously be most disruptive to settlements on coastal and estuarine areas and this is where a considerable proportion of the world's population lives. Sea level rises will flood low-lying areas unless flood protection is built (and such protection may be prohibitively expensive for many settlements and societies). They will also bring rising ground-water levels in coastal areas that will threaten existing sewerage and drainage systems and may undermine buildings. Most coastal cities will need extensive and expensive modifications to their water supply and sanitation and drainage systems. Many of the world's most densely populated areas are river deltas and low-lying coastal areas. Many of the world's largest cities are ports that also developed as major industrial, commercial and financial centres and these will be particularly vulnerable to sea level rises. So too will the many industries and thermal power stations that are concentrated on coasts because of their need for cooling water or as the sea becomes a convenient dumping ground for their waste.[32]

Box 5.3 outlines the regions that are most vulnerable to the extreme weather events that are likely to be associated with climate change. Ports and other settlements on the coast or estuaries are also most at risk from any increase in the severity and frequency of floods and storms induced by global warming. For instance, in the unprotected river deltas of Bangladesh, Egypt and Vietnam, millions of people live within one metre of high tide.[33] The vulnerability of large sections of Bangladesh's population to floods can be seen in the fact that tens of thousands of people died from floods there in 1991.[34] The Maldives, the Marshall islands and coastal areas, archipelagos and island nations in the Pacific and Indian Oceans and the Caribbean are likely to lose their beaches and much of their arable land.[35] Global warming may also increase the incidence and severity of tropical cyclones and expand the areas at risk from them – bringing particular dangers to such places as the coastal areas of Bangladesh that are already subject to devastating cyclones.[36]

Global warming will also mean increased human exposure to exceptional heat waves. This is likely to cause discomfort for many and premature death for some. The elderly, the very young and those with incapacitating diseases are likely to suffer most.[38] Those living in cities that are already heat islands where temperatures remain significantly above those of the surrounding regions will also be particularly at risk. High relative humidity will considerably amplify heat stress.[39] Increased temperatures in cities can also increase the concentrations of ground-level ozone (whose health effects were discussed earlier), as it increases the reaction rates among the pollutants that form ozone.

Global warming will also bring changes in the distribution of infectious diseases. Warmer average temperatures permit an expansion in the area in which tropical diseases can occur. This is likely to be the case for many diseases spread by insect vectors – for instance global warming is likely to

Box 5.3 **Main Sectors Affected by Extreme Events and Vulnerable to the Effects of Climate Change**

Floods: Vulnerable regions are those hit by tropical cyclones such as typhoons and the lower reaches of large rivers such as the Mississippi (USA), Hwang Ho and Yangtze (China) and Nile (Egypt). Delta regions in South and Southeast Asia are particularly vulnerable.

Wind: Vulnerable regions include regions susceptible to tropical and outer tropical cyclones. Over the past 30 years or so, the average annual death toll from windstorms has been over 15,000.[37]

Heat waves and cold spells: Heat waves or cold spells may or may not become more common and severe if the climate warms. Climatologically, the most vulnerable areas in the northern hemisphere are the southern part of the temperate zone and the northern part of the subtropical zone. These are vulnerable to heat waves in summer and cold spells in winter.

Droughts: Droughts in the lower latitudes are intensified by prolonged dry seasons caused by anomalous monsoon circulation. In middle latitudes they are intensified by anomalies in cyclonic activities and the most vulnerable areas are those under the influence of subtropical anti-cyclones.

Wildfires: So-called 'Mediterranean climate' regions are most at risk because of their summer-dry climate. The risk of fire is very high in the summer months; the regions surrounding the Mediterranean Sea, California and Southeastern Australia have also suffered from severe fire damage recently. Fires are also frequent in the taiga regions of Siberia, Canada and Alaska. These tendencies are related to recent increases in resident population and tourism, shortages of labour in the timber industry, and lags in upgrading fire prevention systems. The risk of wildfires could be exacerbated by global warming.

High tides, storm surge, tsunami: Global warming results in sea level rise so the effects of 'normal' extreme events such as high tides, storm surges and tsunamis would become more severe. Multiple risks such as when storm surges and high tides coincide are of particular concern.

Acute air pollution episodes: Acute air pollution episodes are a result of high emissions and particular weather conditions that trap pollutants in the atmosphere and can cause exceptionally high concentrations of air pollutants. They are particularly serious where topographical features help trap pollutants - as in Los Angeles and Mexico City. Their health impact can be much increased if they occur during heat waves and high humidity. Warmer weather can also cause acute episodes of photochemical oxidant pollution.

Source: Drawn mainly from Scott, M J, 'Human Settlements; Impacts/Adaptation', Draft chapter for Working Group II of the Intergovernmental Panel on Climate Change, 1994. The information on the impact of acute air pollution episodes drawn from WHO, Our Planet, Our Health, *Report of the Commission on Health and Environment, Geneva, 1992.*

permit an expansion of the area in which mosquitoes that are the vectors for malaria, dengue fever and filariasis can survive and breed.[40] The areas in which the aquatic snail that is the vector for schistosomiasis can exist may expand considerably.

Indirect Effects

Increasing temperatures and changes in weather patterns will lead to changes in ecosystems that in turn impact on the livelihoods of those that exploit or rely on natural resources for their livelihoods. For instance, global climatic models suggest that global warming will also bring drier mid-continent areas.[41] Among the areas most likely to suffer decreases in rainfall and soil moisture are the Mediterranean, the Northeast of Brazil and parts of Southeast Asia. Forests and fisheries may also be subject to rapid change. Both traditional and modern agricultural practices may be vulnerable to the relatively rapid changes in temperature, rainfall, flooding and storms that global warming can bring. Traditional farming and pastoral systems have usually developed over long periods and become highly sophisticated systems for exploiting existing land and water resources within the variations of rainfall and temperature experienced. They often have a built-in capacity to cope with variation, although increasing population may have eroded this. But the speed of change arising from global warming may be too great for populations to adapt. Modern farming practices may be as vulnerable for different reasons. The problems are likely to be most serious in the countries or areas where the inhabitants are already at the limits of their capacity to cope with climatic events – for instance populations in low-lying coastal areas and islands, subsistence farmers and populations on semi-arid grasslands.[42]

In many instances, the additional stress placed on farmers and pastoralists by changing temperatures and weather patterns will be added to what are already serious stresses on ecosystems' carrying capacities. For instance, Latin American specialists have suggested that most of the areas in South and Central America experiencing rapid population growth in recent decades are within the more fragile eco-zones where sustainable exploitation of natural resources is problematic.[43]

One aspect of global warming is difficult to predict – the capacity and readiness of societies to respond to the changes that warming and its associated effects will bring. Societies have evolved a whole series of mechanisms to reduce risk from natural hazards – from those within traditional societies, where house design and settlement layout often includes measures to limit loss of life and property from earthquakes or storms, to those that have passed into law and statute books in industrial societies. These can be seen in the building and planning codes and in health and safety regulations, and the institutional measures developed to enforce them. Where these are appropriate to that particular society and its resources, and where they are enforced, they reduce risk and ensure that the built environment can cope with high winds, accidental fires or sudden heavy rainstorms. Their effectiveness can be seen in the great reductions achieved in accidental death and injury. For instance, even as late as the last

167

century, it was common for accidental fires to destroy large areas of cities in the North. This complex set of institutional measures and the built environment that they have influenced will have to change to reflect new hazards or a much increased scale of an existing hazard. There is the vast stock of buildings, roads, public transport systems and basic urban infrastructure that was built without making allowance for the changes that global warming will bring.

The very large economic, social and environmental costs that might occur and the relatively low cost of taking preventive action now suggest that all reasonable measures to limit greenhouse gases should be taken. A long-term programme initiated now can over time greatly reduce the emission of greenhouse gases that underlie global warming without high social and economic costs. Many of the actions needed to reduce the emissions of these gases have other social, economic or environmental benefits. The main difficulty in the more wealthy, urbanized societies where most greenhouse gas emissions currently take place is setting in motion a process that steadily reduces these emissions. The main difficulty in less wealthy societies is ensuring that a priority to economic prosperity and improved standards of living take place within resource-efficient, waste-minimizing settlements. Both require ways to ensure that individuals and enterprises revise the basis on which investment and consumption decisions are made so these take sufficient account of dangers that are most acute several decades into the future.

POVERTY AND THE LOSS OF ENVIRONMENTAL CAPITAL

Much of the writing about sustainable development has not only ignored the needs and priorities of low-income groups but also cast low-income groups as major causes of environmental degradation.[44] But low-income groups contribute very little to the depletion of at least three of the four kinds of environmental capital noted before. Their consumption per person of non-renewable resources is very low – which is not surprising, given the fact that they lack the income to own private automobiles and to own or use other resource-intensive capital goods. They generally use the least resource-intensive forms of transport – walking, bicycling and public transport. The levels of waste they generate per person are much lower than those of richer groups – and low-income households in rural and urban areas often re-use or recycle much of what wealthier households would throw away.* As the earlier section noted, their contribution per person to greenhouse gases and to stratospheric ozone depleting chemicals, both directly through their actions and indirectly through the goods they own or use, is very low in comparison to wealthier groups. The same is true for other non-biodegradable wastes.

---

* Some enterprises owned by low-income groups do create or contribute to serious problems of air pollution and liquid and solid wastes within their locality but this does not change the fact that low-income groups in general generate far less wastes than middle and upper income groups.

The only components of natural capital to whose depletion low-income groups may contribute is in certain renewable resources – for instance to soil degradation or the degradation of forests or the overuse of fresh water. But a large proportion of low-income households contribute little or nothing to this – for instance those living in urban areas or those who are landless in rural areas and who make a living through wage labour. The only basis for accusing 'the poor' of contributing to unsustainable resource use is that portion of 'the poor' who make their living as farmers (usually on smallholdings), pastoralists and forest users. But even these cannot be a major force for the degradation of soils or forests worldwide since their poverty is a result of them having so little land and such inadequate access to forests. Most deforestation and soil erosion takes place on land which the poor do not own and to which they do not have access. Wealthy farmers, landowners, commercial companies and governments own most of the worlds farmland and forests so it is difficult to see how the poor can be blamed for their overuse.

Thus, the discussion of the contribution of poverty to unsustainable resource use is only in regard to the very small proportion of the world's soils, forests, pastures and fisheries to which poor farmers, pastoralists, hunter gatherers and those who fish have access to. The fact that these people are poor will also mean that they generally have the most marginal or fragile renewable resources on which to draw their livelihoods. As such, of course they have most difficulties in sustaining production levels and are most likely to forsake long-term sustainability because of short-term survival. It is also common for many low-income households to be involved in deforestation on the agricultural frontier and to be expanding cultivation on land ill-suited to agriculture. But this does not mean that they are major contributors to unsustainable resource use on a global scale. And even if low-income households have to sustain themselves on inadequate land holdings and poor quality soil, as Chapter 4 described and as Chapter 6 will expand on, there is not necessarily evidence of environmental degradation and many examples of low-income groups involved in environmental protection and careful resource management. There are also many examples of 'low-income' communities whose indigenous knowledge and practices are far more oriented to long-term ecological sustainability than most modern farming and forestry practices.[45]

Earlier chapters have shown the enormous health problems that most low-income groups suffer because of very poor quality housing and living environments, but this is not the same as a depletion of environmental capital. The environment-related diseases and injuries that low-income households suffer are not depleting soils or forests or using non-renewable resources or seriously disrupting ecosystems.

LINKING GLOBAL AND LOCAL SUSTAINABILITY

There may be contradictions between ecological sustainability at global and at local level. At a global level, the world's economies cannot remain prosperous if the aggregate impact of their production and the consumption patterns which underlie them draws on environmental capital at unsustainable rates or levels. Most of the world's wealthiest nations have been relatively successful at meeting some sustainable development goals within their own nation or region (ie meeting basic needs within high quality living environments and protection of local ecosystems) but as noted earlier, this was by drawing heavily on the environmental capital of other regions or nations and on the global sink. In effect, they import environmental capital and deplete the world's stock of such capital; it is often their production and consumption patterns which underlie (or contribute significantly to) unsustainable forest, soil or water exploitation in poorer nations.

This implies the need for international agreements which set limits for each national society's consumption of resources and use of the global sink for their wastes. But it is also clear that most action to achieve sustainable development has to be formulated and implemented locally. The fact that each village, province or city, and its insertion within local and regional ecosystems, is unique implies the need for optimal use of local resources, knowledge and skills for the achievement of development goals within a detailed knowledge of the local and regional ecological carrying capacity. This demands a considerable degree of local self-determination, since centralized decision-making structures have great difficulty in implementing decisions which respond appropriately to such diversity. Nevertheless, some new international institutions are required to ensure that individual cities or countries do not take advantage of others' restraint.

National governments inevitably have the key role in linking local and global sustainability. Internationally, they have the responsibility for reaching agreements to limit the call that consumers and businesses within their country make on the world's environmental capital. Nationally, they are responsible for providing the framework to ensure local actions can meet development goals without compromising local and global sustainability. But there is little evidence of national governments setting up the regulatory and incentive structure to ensure that the aggregate impact of their economic activities and citizens' consumption is in accordance with global sustainability – although a few in Europe have taken some tentative steps towards some aspects.[46] Such an incentive and regulatory structure is relatively easy to conceive as an abstract exercise. Certainly, poverty can be greatly reduced without an expansion in resource use and waste generation which threatens ecological sustainability. It is also possible to envisage a considerable reduction in resource use and waste generation by middle and upper income households, without diminishing their quality of life (and in some aspects actually enhancing it).

The prosperity and economic stability that the poorer nations need to underpin secure livelihoods for their populations and the needed enhancement in the competence and accountability of their government can be achieved without a much increased call on environmental capital. However, the prospects for actually translating what is possible into reality both within nations and globally remains much less certain. Powerful vested interests oppose most, if not all, the needed policies and priorities. Richer groups are unlikely to willingly forsake the comfort and mobility that they currently enjoy. Technological change can help to a limited extent – for instance, moderating the impact of rising gasoline prices through the relatively rapid introduction of increasingly fuel-efficient automobiles and the introduction of alternative fuels derived from renewable energy sources. But if combating atmospheric warming does demand a rapid reduction in greenhouse gas emissions, this will imply changes in people's right to use private automobiles which cannot be met by new technologies and alternative (renewable) fuels – at least at costs which will prove politically acceptable. So many existing commercial, industrial and residential buildings and urban forms (for instance low density suburban developments and out-of-town shopping malls) have high levels of energy use built into them and these are not easily or rapidly changed.[47]

At the same time, in the South, the achievement of development goals which minimize the call on local and global environmental capital demands a competence and capacity by local governments which is currently very rarely present. The achievement of key development goals is also unlikely without strong democratic pressures and processes influencing decisions about the use of public resources.

Thus, perhaps the most critical environmental issue is how environmental problems can be addressed and development needs met within each locality in ways that respond to the particular needs and priorities of those living there, within each locality's unique local social, economic and ecological context – but in ways that ensure that the aggregate of all such actions in all such localities address the national and global issues in regard to sustainable development. In most nations in the South, this also has to be done with local governments that are usually weak and ineffective – and often unrepresentative. This is the issue considered in Chapter 6.

REFERENCES

1   This chapter expands and develops themes that two of the authors first wrote about with Jorge Hardoy in Chapter 6 of Hardoy, Jorge E, Diana Mitlin and David Satterthwaite (1992), *Environmental Problems in Third World Cities*, Earthscan, London.

2   See for instance *The Cocoyoc Declaration* adopted by the participants of the UNEP/UNCTAD symposium on 'Pattern of Resource Use, Environment and Development Strategies' in 1974 that was drafted by Barbara Ward and republished in *World Development*, Vol 3, Nos 2 and 3, Feb–Mar 1975. See also Ward, Barbara and René Dubos (1972), *Only One Earth: The Care and Maintenance of a Small Planet*, Andre Deutsch, London, Ward, Barbara (1976), 'The inner and the outer limits', The Clifford Clark Memorial Lectures 1976, *Canadian Public Administration*, Vol 19, No 3, Autumn, pp 385–416, and Ward, Barbara (1979), *Progress for a Small Planet*, Penguin – subsequently republished by Earthscan, London.

3   As noted in Barrow, C J (1995), 'Sustainable development: concept, value and practice', *Third World Planning Review* Vol.17, No.4, Nov, pp 369–386, the importance of the Brundtland Commission was not so much in its innovative ideas but in rekindling environmental interests within development. The economic crises of the early 1980s and the political realignments in the North had hindered action on what might be termed 'Brundtland-like' demands made during the 1970s.

4   WCED 1987, *Our Common Future*, Oxford University Press, Oxford, p 8.

5   Mitlin, Diana (1992), 'Sustainable development: a guide to the literature', *Environment and Urbanization* Vol 4, No 1, April, pp 111–124.

6   Ibid, p 111.

7   McGranahan, Gordon, Jacob Songsore, Marriane Kjellén, Pedro Jacobi and Charles Surjadi (1996), 'Sustainability, poverty and urban environmental transitions' in Cedric Pugh, *Sustainability, the Environment and Urbanization*, Earthscan, London.

8   Haughton, Graham and Colin Hunter (1994), *Sustainable Cities*, Regional Policy and Development series, Jessica Kingsley, London.

9   Haughton and Hunter 1994, op cit.

10 WHO (1992), *Our Planet, Our Health*, Report of the Commission on Health and Environment, WHO, Geneva.

11 Hardoy, Mitlin and Satterthwaite 1992, op cit.

12 Rees, William E (1992), 'Ecological footprints and appropriated carrying capacity: what urban economics leaves out', *Environment and Urbanization* Vol 4, No 2, Oct, pp 121–130.

13 Haughton and Hunter 1994, op cit.

14 von Amsberg, Joachim (1993), *Project Evaluation and the Depletion of Natural Capital: an Application of the Sustainability Principle*, Environment Working Paper No 56, Environment Department, World Bank, Washington DC.

15 Haughton and Hunter 1994, op cit.

16 Serageldin, Ismail (1993), 'Making development sustainable', *Finance and Development*, Vol 30, No 4, Dec, pp 6–10.

17 Serageldin 1993, op cit; Winpenny, J T (1991), *Values for the Environment: A Guide to Economic Appraisal*, HMSO, London.

18 See for instance Serageldin, Ismail (1995), *Sustainability and the Wealth of Nations: First Steps in an Ongoing Journey*, Paper presented at the Third Annual World Bank Conference on Environmentally Sustainable Development.

19 Serageldin 1995, op cit.

20 UNCHS (1996), *An Urbanizing World: The Global Report on Human Settlements 1996*, Oxford University Press, Oxford.

21 Newman, Peter W G and Jeffrey R Kenworthy (1989), *Cities and Automobile Dependence: an International Sourcebook*, Gower Technical, Aldershot.

22 Nishioka, Shuzo, Yuichi Noriguchi and Sombo Yamamura (1990), 'Megalopolis and climate change: the case of Tokyo' in James McCulloch (Ed), *Cities and Global Climate Change*, Climate Institute, Washington DC, pp 108–133.

23 WHO 1992, op cit.

24 UNEP (1991), *Environmental Data Report, 1991–2*, GEMS Monitoring and Assessment Research Centre, Blackwell, Oxford and Massachusetts.

25 WHO 1992, op cit.

26 UNEP (1991), *Environmental Effects of Ozone Depletion: 1991 Update*, UNEP, Nairobi.

27 IPCC (1990), *Climate Change: the IPCC Scientific Assessment*, J H Houghton, G J Jenkins and J J Ephraums (Eds), Cambridge University Press, Cambridge, 1990.

28 Ramaswamy, V and others (1992), 'Radiative forcing of climate from halocarbon-induced global stratospheric ozone loss', *Nature*, Vol 355, No 6363,

pp 810–812, quoted in WRI (1994), *World Resources 1994–95: A Guide to the Global Environment: People and the Environment*, Oxford University Press, Oxford.

29 WMO/UNEP (1990), *Scientific Assessment of Climate Change*, Report prepared for the Intergovernmental Panel on Climate Change by Working Group I, World Meteorological Organization, Geneva, and UNEP, Nairobi.

30 WMO/UNEP 1990, op cit.

31 UNEP (1993), *Environmental Data Report, 1993–94*, GEMS Monitoring and Assessment Research Centre, Blackwell, Oxford and Massachusetts.

32 Parry, Martin (1992), 'The urban economy', presentation at *Cities and Climate Change*, a conference at the Royal Geographical Society, 31 Mar.

33 Scott, M J (1994), Draft paper on Human Settlements – impacts/adaptation, IPCC Working Group II, WMO and UNEP.

34 UNEP 1993, op cit.

35 Scott 1994, op cit.

36 WHO 1992, op cit.

37 Smith, D K (1989), *Natural Disaster Reduction: How Meteorological and Hydrological Services can Help*, Report No 722, World Meteorological Organization, Geneva, quoted in UNEP 1993, op cit.

38 WHO 1992, op cit.

39 Ibid.

40 Ibid.

41 Scott 1994, op cit.

42 Scott 1994, op cit.

43 Di Pace, Maria, Sergio Federovisky, Jorge F Hardoy, Jorge E Morello and Alfredo Stein (1992), 'Latin America', Chapter 8 in Richard Stren, Rodney White and Joseph Whitney (Eds), *Sustainable Cities: Urbanization and the Environment in International Perspective*, Westview Press, Boulder, pp 205–227.

44 See for instance UNDP (1991), *Human Development Report 1991*, UNDP, Oxford University Press, Oxford and New York which claims that 'significant environmental degradation is usually caused by poverty in the South' (p 28). Poverty is also considered as a major factor in environmental degradation in: Holmberg, Johan (1992), *Poverty, Environment and Development: Proposals for Action*, Swedish International Development Authority, Stockholm; Leonard, H Jeffrey (1989), 'Environment and the poor: development strategies for a common agenda', in H Jeffrey Leonard and contributors, *Environment and the Poor: Development Strategies for a Common Agenda*, Overseas Development Council, Transaction Books, New Brunswick (USA) and Oxford (UK), pp 3–45 and many publications by the Worldwatch Institute.

45 Ecologist, The (1992) *Whose Common Future: Reclaiming the Commons*, Earthscan, London.

46 See for instance UNCHS (1996), *An Urbanizing World: The Global Report on Human Settlements 1996*, Oxford University Press, Oxford and New York.

47 Gore, Charles (1991), *Policies and Mechanisms for Sustainable Development: the Transport Sector*, mimeo.

6

Primary Environmental Care[*]

INTRODUCTION

A large and growing number of case studies show how particular communities or groups of people recognize their dependence on natural resources and systems and act collectively to maintain their integrity and defend them (and their right to manage them) against outside encroachment.[1] Many such case studies highlight the sophistication in such environmental management. There are also many case studies describing how the inhabitants of a particular settlement act collectively to improve their living environment or to limit or control particular environmental hazards in the home and neighbourhood.[2] An increasing number of agencies involved in environmental or development issues have recognized this capacity of local groups to act collectively. They include local and national governments, international agencies and many national or local NGOs. Some recognize that this can form the basis for more effective development and environmental management than conventional, external-agency directed initiatives.

Primary environmental care (PEC) was the term given to this community or collective environmental management during preparations for the Earth Summit (the UN Conference on Environment and Development in Rio de Janeiro in 1992). It was used to emphasize the knowledge and capacity of local groups to act and to promote their right to do so and to highlight how external forces were often ignoring or undermining their efforts. It was also used to ensure that the environmental problems described in

* This chapter draws heavily on earlier works on primary environmental care - especially on Pretty, J N and Irene Guijt (1992), 'Primary environmental care: an alternative paradigm for development assistance', *Environment and Urbanization* Vol 4 No 1, April, pp 22–36. Some of the text and the headings are drawn direct from this paper. This chapter also draws on DGCS (1990), *Supporting Primary Environmental Care*, report of the PEC workshop, Siena, to OECD/DAC Working Party on Development Assistance and the Environment, Ministero degli Affari Esteri, Direzione Generale per la Cooperazione allo Sviluppo, Italy; Borrini, G (ed) (1991), *Lessons Learned in Community-Based Environmental Management*, ICHM, Rome; Pretty, J N and R Sandbrook (1991), *Operationalising Sustainable Development at the Community Level: Primary Environmental Care*, Report to the DAC Working Party on Development Assistance and the Environment; and Bajracharya, Deepak (1993), 'UNICEF and the challenge of sustainable livelihood; an overview', presented at the UNICEF Preparatory Meeting for the Inter-Regional Consultation on PEC and the UNICEF Programming Process, Villa de Layva.

earlier chapters of this book received greater attention, and to prevent the Earth Summit's agenda being dominated by global issues such as global warming. The attention given to PEC can be seen as part of the wider movement to promote a greater decentralization of decision-making and to permit greater citizen participation.

This chapter describes the characteristics of PEC and how it can form the basis for a more successful tackling of environment and development issues at local level than the conventional environmental and development initiatives of governments and aid agencies. The focus is *not* on *children* but on the means by which the *households* in which most of the world's sick and malnourished children live can acquire a more stable and sustainable basis for their livelihoods and a safer living environment. Chapter 7 concentrates on children's involvement in environmental education and action.

THE CONCEPT

Primary environmental care is a term given to the process through which local groups apply their knowledge and management capacity to address their own development needs, within systems of environmental management that are ecologically sustainable.[3] Although the term is relatively new, it certainly encompasses many traditional or long-established systems of community-based resource management. It also includes many instances of where local populations acquire (or recapture) the power to do so, often supported by new crops or new technologies and sometimes with external support.

The basic ideas behind PEC draw from more than 40 years of dissatisfaction with the conventional, top-down development policies of governments and international agencies. It integrates three central elements:

- meeting the livelihood and health needs of all household members;
- the sustainable management and optimal use of the environment and natural resources; and
- the empowering of groups and communities for self-directed development.

Box 6.1 provides a simple, schematic diagram to highlight these three elements.

PEC's focus is thus on combining ecological sustainability with meeting development needs – especially those relating to livelihoods and to health. In most areas of the South where agriculture, forestry and fishing are not heavily commercialized, most local actions have always integrated environmental management with livelihood and never considered environment and development as separate.[4] For those whose living depends on agriculture, forestry or fishing, environmental management is usually a necessary condition for sustaining or strengthening their livelihoods while stable and adequate livelihoods make possible greater attention to environmental management.[5] This stress on combining ecological sustainability

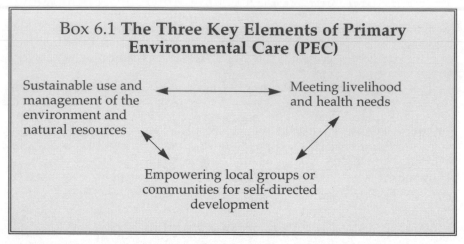

Box 6.1 **The Three Key Elements of Primary Environmental Care (PEC)**

Sustainable use and management of the environment and natural resources

Meeting livelihood and health needs

Empowering local groups or communities for self-directed development

with meeting development needs is similar to most policies and initiatives promoting 'sustainable development' but the critical difference is the extent to which this remains under local control. In urban areas, local action also combines environmental issues and livelihood issues, although the environmental focus is often more on environmental health than on natural resource management. One important and common exception to this is urban agriculture and/or forestry where local action usually combines access to land and water, including protecting it from encroachment, and soil and water management.

The concept of PEC has received greater attention from many governments, NGOs and international donors as more case studies have shown that a local population that relies on particular resources for their livelihoods are often better managers of these resources (and of the ecosystems on which they depend) than governments or external 'experts', especially if supported by appropriate legal frameworks, technical advice and economic incentives. While most of the early case studies on PEC were in rural areas, and associated with natural resource management, a growing number are now from urban areas and centre on improved provision for water supply, sanitation, drainage or other measures associated with improved environmental management and the reduction of environmental hazards.

Although PEC is receiving increased attention from external agencies,[*] it aims to reduce the power and influence of such agencies at local level and to change their role. But it often implies more changes 'upstream' of any local intervention – to change laws, regulations or institutions that inhibit or remove the possibility of people working together for collective goals and to greatly increase the possibilities for the inhabitants in each locality to obtain support for their own PEC initiatives. It also implies major changes in many national and international agencies whose structure and

---

[*] In this chapter, 'external agencies include all agencies working in some area of development or environmental management that are *external* to community level actions or initiatives. They include agencies of local, regional and national governments, regional and national NGOs and international agencies (including multilateral development banks, official bilateral agencies and all manner of international NGOs or private voluntary organizations).

'project-cycle' are too centralized and too oriented to supporting conventional projects to be able to support a large number of small, diverse, citizen-initiated or directed initiatives. These are issues to which this chapter will return, after describing the characteristics of PEC in more detail.

THE RATIONALE

The need for new approaches that combine environmental management with more stable, secure and adequate livelihoods and much reduced environmental hazards is hardly in doubt. First, there is the failure of 'development' to improve conditions for a high proportion of the population in the South. Second, there is the widespread evidence of serious environmental degradation described in earlier chapters. Third, there is the evidence from many case studies that a new approach can address both these problems.

On the first of these, despite the rapid expansion in the world's economy (and in the per capita income of most countries in the South) the number of children and adults living in extreme poverty is probably increasing. Chapter 4 noted the most detailed recent estimate for the scale of rural poverty – the 940 million people who were either landless or who had too little land to provide them with an adequate livelihood in 1988.[6] This represents a third of the entire rural population in the South. Estimates for the scale of absolute poverty in urban areas of the South around 1990 vary from between 300 and 600 million, depending on the criteria used to make the estimate; this means that between one fifth and two fifths of the urban population live in absolute poverty.[7]

But the lower estimates are derived from setting a single, international income-based poverty line for both rural and urban areas that does not take into account the higher cost of living in major cities and also ignores all aspects of deprivation other than low income. An estimate in 1990, based on dozens of national and city studies, suggested that at least 600 million urban dwellers in Africa, Asia and Latin America live in 'life and health-threatening' homes and neighbourhoods because of the very poor housing and living conditions and the inadequate provision for safe and sufficient water supplies and for sanitation, drainage, the removal of garbage, and health care.[8] If these 600 million urban dwellers are considered 'poor' – for it is largely their lack of income and assets that makes them unable to afford better quality housing and basic services – it greatly increases the scale of urban poverty when compared to conventional income-based poverty lines.

In most cities, low-income individuals and households are simply priced out of all possibility of safe and healthy living environments as good quality housing or land sites on which housing could be built is too expensive and there is little or no public provision for infrastructure and services for homes and settlements in which they live.[9] The hundreds of millions of urban and rural dwellers who still suffer huge health burdens from diseases and injuries that are easily and cheaply prevented or cured (as described in earlier chapters) is in itself one of the most damning indictments of the last 40 years of development assistance and of governments' own priorities in development expenditures.

Table 6.1 *Priority given by Aid Agencies and Multilateral Banks to Improving Housing and Living Conditions and Basic Services in the funding commitments, 1980–1993*

Agency	Total funding (US$ billion)	Proportion of total project commitments					Percentage of total commitments	
		Housing and housing finance	Water and sanitation	Primary health care	Basic education	Poverty reduction and jobs	1980–93	1992–93
Aid (Concessional Loans or Grants)								
International Development Association								
Africa	27.9	1.2	3.6	2.7	4.3	1.9	13.9	16.4
Asia	38.6	1.3	5.5	5.3	2.7	1.4	16.3	36.2
Latin America & Caribbean	1.9	1.4	3.8	3.5	1.8	7.6	18.2	11.8
African Development Bank	10.2	0.4	7.3	2.7	4.3	1.3	16.3	15.3
Asian Development Fund	14.3	1.0	4.4	1.6	1.7	0.3	8.9	22.6
Inter-American Development Bank	6.5	3.4	18.0	1.4	3.1	1.3	33.0	42.2
Caribbean Development Bank	0.7	1.2	4.1	–	–	0.5	6.1	2.8
UNICEF	6.6	0.0	13.7	33.5	7.9	–	55.1	47.9
Overseas Economic Cooperation Fund, Japan (1987–91)	36.5	0.9	3.8	–	0.4	–	5.4*	
Non Concessional Loans								
International Bank for Reconstruction and Development (IBRD)								
Africa	29.6	3.3	8.0	1.2	0.9	0.1	13.7	24.3
Asia	90.6	2.3	3.3	0.9	0.9	0.04	7.4	6.6
Latin America &								

Caribbean	68.7	3.8	5.1	1.6	2.1	0.0	12.7	15.6
African Development Bank	17.6	0.1	9.0	0.4	1.6	0.4	11.6	14.5
Asian Development Bank	30.9	1.2	4.5	1.0	–	–	6.8	0.7
Inter-American Development Bank	41.7	2.1	6.3	0.3	0.3	0.6	9.6	18.2
Caribbean Development Bank	0.5	1.0	6.7	0.0	0.0	0.0	7.7	0.5

* 1987–91

Notes: These funding flows only apply to commitments to countries in the South – for instance, they do not include World Bank commitments to East and Southern European nations. Housing projects include slum and squatter upgrading, serviced site schemes, core housing schemes and community development projects which include housing improvement. Water and sanitation are part of Primary Health Care so the column headed Primary Health Care includes all its components other than water and sanitation. Basic education is taken to include primary education, literacy programmes and basic education programmes. UNICEF figures are for disbursements, not commitments so they are not directly comparable; they are included here to give an idea of the scale and relative importance of UNICEF funding in this project category. The disbursements for basic health care include support for child health and nutrition and for child and family basic health services. The funding totals noted above include funding for both rural and urban projects. For the totals reported here for water supply, sanitation and drainage, these only included projects whose main focus was delivering or improving these for residential areas. City–wide investments in improved drainage and investments in water supplies whose main focus was not improving supplies to residential areas are not included. The figures are drawn from two computer data-bases. The first contains each agency's total annual commitments to each nation, with total commitments converted into US$ at their 1990 value. The second database is an aid project database with details of all human settlement projects or projects with human settle-ments components. Both have been developed by IIED's human settlements programme with the information drawn almost exclusively from each agency's own official publications

Source: *Satterthwaite, David (1995), 'The scale and nature of international donor assistance to housing, basic services and other human–settlements related projects', Paper presented at the UNU/WIDER Conference on 'Human Settlements in the changing global political and economic processes', Helsinki.*

Conventional development programmes are rarely addressing the needs and priorities of small-scale farmers, agricultural labourers, pastoralists and low-income households in urban areas. In addition, improved health or environmental health receive a low priority from most agencies. For instance, an analysis of funding priorities covering the period 1980–1993 found that very few development banks or official bilateral agencies allocate as much as 10 per cent of their funding to the kinds of projects that bring the most direct health benefits to low-income groups: primary health care, water, sanitation and drainage, and support for improving housing quality.[10] This analysis also found that it was also rare for primary health care to receive more than a few per cent of an agency's funding while projects aimed specifically at poverty reduction or employment provision for those with inadequate or no incomes usually received less than 1 per cent of funding – see Table 6.1.[11] Primary education and literacy programmes also rarely received more than 1 or 2 per cent of funding – and in many agencies, they receive less than 1 per cent.[12] Although many agencies increased the proportion of their funding going to health care, environmental health, basic education and poverty reduction projects during the period 1990–1993, these still remained relatively low priorities for most agencies.

Conventional development projects are also largely designed by people with little knowledge of the specifics of each locality. The knowledge of outsiders – government agencies, international agencies, NGOs and researchers – about the specific environmental pressures within each locality and the ways in which poorer households' livelihood strategies are integrated with attempts to come to terms with such pressures is usually extremely limited. External agencies rarely fully grasp their complexity. Environment and development are often considered as separate[13] so they fall under the responsibility of different agencies. Development-oriented agencies may not feel that environmental management is their responsibility while agencies concerned with natural resource management may feel no responsibility for creating or supporting livelihoods for those with low incomes and/or few assets.

Mike Douglass notes how the division of planning into bureaus, each with their own access rules and each competing with and often contradicting the policies of others, further diminishes chances of a coordinated public effort toward the resolution of environment and poverty issues.[14] As each agency imposes its priorities, these often do not match the priorities of the inhabitants, or they are too sectoral to address multiple needs – for instance supporting only environmental management when more adequate and secure livelihoods are needed to permit improved environmental management.

One of the best documented examples of this is the many 'improved stoves' projects that international agencies supported, with the claim that these would reduce deforestation by improving the efficiency of wood and charcoal burning stoves. Not only did many of the stoves that these projects promoted fail to meet the needs of their intended users but they also failed to make any significant impact on deforestation. Madhu Sarin describes how major stove projects of the 1970s and early 1980s were based on assumptions that were wrong or inaccurate:

> *'An emphasis only on energy saving stoves as a solution to deforestation and the rural energy crisis may misinterpret the causes of deforestation and the needs and priorities of those most affected by the crisis ... an account of the experience of an NGO working with village communities in southern Rajasthan (India) ...shows how there are important underlying causes of the energy crisis which improved stoves did little to counteract – for instance forests cut down when their management, previously controlled by villagers and princely rulers, became the responsibility of government who permitted their exploitation by the urban industrial sector. Improved stoves are only meaningful where a more equitable access to natural resources is established with local management and control of such resources.'[15]*

Box 6.2 draws from Sarin's work in illustrating the limitations of the improved stoves in one particular instance.

If external interventions are to address people's needs and improve environmental management, they will have to draw on the knowledge and skills of the people who know most about their own livelihood systems in decisions about how natural resources are to be managed, including who has rights of use and the terms under which use is permitted. They will have to value and develop their knowledge and skills, and put into their hands the means to achieve self-development and environmental management. This will require a reshaping of thinking and practices associated with development assistance for both external donors and for local and national government agencies.

PRECONDITIONS FOR PRIMARY ENVIRONMENTAL CARE

The growing number of well-documented case studies of PEC when considered together, suggest some necessary conditions for successful local action for sustainable development.[16] There are also certain external conditions that encourage or support PEC approaches – or that may be necessary conditions for PEC approaches to be possible – and these are discussed in the section on 'scaling up'.

PEC approaches generally have the following characteristics:

- process oriented and, as such, adaptive to changing circumstances;
- promoting a rapid return for poorer groups;
- building on local systems of knowledge and management of women and men of all ages, classes and ethnic backgrounds;
- strengthening community-level institutions and social organization;
- emphasizing the use of locally available resources and technologies;
- ensuring the participation of local women and men in all stages of planning, implementation, management and monitoring; and
- recognizing the diversity of need and priority within each locality and

Box 6.2 **The Mismatch Between Household Needs and External Agency Solutions: improved stoves in South Rajasthan**

In a project to introduce the 'Nada Chula' stove in south Rajasthan, women were selected for dissemination as the local stove users are almost exclusively women. In this area, collection of firewood is also exclusively women's work in the traditional division of labour between women and men. Earlier experiences in Haryana and Himachal Pradesh had made it clear that biomass energy saving was only one of rural women's priorities. They were equally or more interested in removing smoke from the kitchen, reducing cooking time, having cleaner cooking pots to minimize the daily chore of scrubbing them, being protected from fire heat during the hot summer months, having cleaner kitchens and, above all, increased personal comfort while cooking. In other words, the women were more concerned about saving their own energy on cooking related-tasks than on simply reducing cooking fuel consumption. In places where fetching firewood was an arduous task, reducing firewood consumption was a major priority, but this was not so in areas where forest cover was still good.

However, the failure of three successive monsoons after 1985, brought the project face to face with the really critical issues in the area and showed how peripheral the fuel savings achieved through the stoves were to these issues. Failure of the rains resulted in the total failure of crops crucial for sustaining the subsistence economy. Due to the destruction of the forests, the lack of rain also resulted in the drying up of wells, streams and ponds, which caused acute scarcity of even drinking water for people and livestock. Whereas in earlier times, people could rely on the forests for food, fuel and fodder during such periods, now such goods were not available. Few alternative employment opportunities have been created in the area and the only option for people was to work in the drought relief works started by the government for daily waged employment. These were inadequate for the people, and large numbers of men, women and, in some cases, entire families were forced to migrate to other areas in search of work. The public distribution network of the government ensured the availability of foodgrains to the people but could not provide adequate fodder for the cattle. Cattle died in enormous numbers, and people suffered from extensive malnutrition and disease.

Some of the well-functioning stoves collapsed during this period. The old, the sick and the infants left behind could neither maintain them nor use them properly. Even where the woman of the house had not migrated, she was unable to attend to the stove as she was barely at home. The search for wages, water, fodder and firewood took most of her energy together with caring for the children and other household tasks. If the husband had migrated in search of work, she also had to complete the work usually done by him. Increased illnesses meant that the little income coming in had to be spent on medicines instead of food, and care of the sick became an added burden. The extent of the scarcity of basic essentials can be shown by the fact that the small amounts of water and chopped straw required for preparing the mud mixture for the stove were not always available. Due to the absence of an alternative income source, many families were forced to cut down trees from the few remaining patches of forests to sell firewood in the towns. The destructive circle was complete. Talking only about stoves under such circumstances started to feel more and more irrelevant.

Source: Sarin. Madhu (1991), 'Improved stoves, women and domestic energy',
Environment and Urbanization, *Vol 3, No 2, Oct, pp 51–56.*

the obvious fact that there are usually conflicting interests within 'communities' and virtually always powerful interests outside the community opposed to PEC initiatives there.

More details are given about each of these points below, with case studies used to illustrate them.

Process Oriented Projects

There is still a tendency within development planning or project planning for governments or aid agencies to use 'blueprints' for the design of a project. The agency concerned selects the most cost-effective designs for achieving particular outcomes based upon data derived from pilot projects and other studies or on what was judged to have been successful elsewhere. Much as a building contractor would follow construction blueprints and schedules, implementing organizations faithfully execute the plan or project cycle, not least because those involved in implementation know that a large part of any evaluation of their work will be based on whether what was originally planned was implemented. Once implementation is complete, evaluators may measure actual changes in the target populations (or simply whether initial goals were achieved) and report on actual versus planned changes at the end of the project cycle. The blueprints can then be revised before being reapplied elsewhere. The external agency then usually withdraws from that particular locality to implement other projects in other locations.

Such an approach is *inappropriate* when planning for the management of natural resources in which many complex interests are involved, where there is a considerable diversity of objectives among the different interest groups, and where there are rapid changes in stocks. The external agency's knowledge of these complexities is usually severely limited, yet the conventional approach assumes that this knowledge is nearly perfect. It also assumes that development actions produce benefits which will be sustained after project completion, with the withdrawal of the implementing agency, even though many projects give little attention to developing local organizations' capacity to ensure that this happens.

Such an approach is also *inappropriate* to settlements where there are multiple needs for improved environmental management within a village or urban neighbourhood and where what is needed is a continuous process through which different problems are addressed and the capacity and confidence of local inhabitants strengthened by each particular initiative. Thus, as one problem is addressed – for instance improved water supply and drainage – so the organizational and management framework within the settlement developed to achieve this can move on to address other problems or new problems. Yet, external agencies often refuse to support more than one 'project' in a particular village or urban neighbourhood. Or they will only support water supply and cannot respond to the request of community organizations for help in developing a health care system, after working with this organization to improve water supply. What the inhabitants of most villages and low-income urban neighbourhoods need is the possibility of calling on financial support or technical advice, as their capacity and competence to address their own needs and priorities grows with each initiative they undertake. They often require far less funding than the external agencies find convenient. But they may need small amounts of funding for different initiatives over a long period – which, again, rarely fits well with external agencies' structure for project identification, funding and management.

For PEC to succeed, projects must also centre upon a learning process rather than blueprints.[17] Projects usually start small and with little cost. Their design is uncomplicated and they do not try to over-innovate. A common feature of successful projects has been an early period of experimentation and of building local capacity. This period of continual dialogue allows outsiders to learn, plan and replan with the local people. Box 6.3 provides an example of a Pakistan NGO in Karachi whose support for community-based sewer/drainage installation responded to community demands and ensured that the inhabitants themselves retained control over the processes by which the sewers/drains were planned, implemented and maintained. It also shows how once the new sewers had been successfully installed, new initiatives were developed in health and other areas.

Promoting a Rapid Return for Poorer Groups

At the outset, PEC focuses on what people within the locality articulate as their most important priorities. This may mean starting with activities that are not central to the project remits of external agencies, and this implies the need for such agencies to be flexible in what they can fund. The technologies that generally work best when introduced into areas for the first time are low risk, easy to learn, and tested under local conditions. They also offer those involved in the project the prospect of clear, on-site benefits in the coming season or year.

Projects developed by external agencies that aim at improving natural resource management have often given too little attention to meeting the immediate needs of the groups with the lowest incomes and/or the least access to natural resources. This may be one reason for their high rate of failure.

Box 6.3 **The Orangi Pilot Project in Karachi, Pakistan**

Orangi is an unauthorized settlement with over 800,000 inhabitants extending over 8000 hectares. Most inhabitants built their own houses and none received official help in doing so. There was no public provision for sanitation; most people used bucket latrines which were emptied every few days, usually onto the unpaved lanes running between houses. More affluent households constructed soakpits but these filled up after a few years. Some households living near creeks constructed sewage pipes which emptied into the creeks. The cost of getting local government agencies to lay sewage pipes in Orangi was too much for local residents – who also felt that these should be provided free.

A local organization called the Orangi Pilot Project (OPP) was sure that if local residents were fully involved, a cheaper, more appropriate sanitation system could be installed. Research undertaken by OPP staff showed that the inhabitants were aware of the consequences of poor sanitation on their health and their property but they could neither afford conventional systems nor had they the technical nor organizational skills to use alternative options.

OPP organized meetings for those living in 10–15 adjacent houses each side of a lane and explained the benefits of improved sanitation and offered technical assistance. Where agreement was reached among the households of a lane, they elected their own leader who formally applied for technical help. Women were very active in local groups and many were elected group leaders. Their site was surveyed with plans drawn up and cost estimates prepared. Local leaders kept their group informed and collected money to pay for the work, and it was often women who found the funds to pay out of household budgets. Sewers were then installed with maintenance organized by local groups. The scope of the sewer construction programme grew as more local groups approached OPP for help and the local authorities began to provide some financial support.

Over the last eight years, households in Orangi have constructed close to 69,000 sanitary pour-flush latrines in their homes plus 4459 sewerage lines and 345 secondary drains – using their own funds and under their own management. One indication of the success of this work is shown by the fact that some lanes have organized and undertaken lane sewerage investments independently of OPP; another is the households' willingness to make the investments needed in maintenance.

OPP's research concentrated on the extent to which the cost of sanitary latrines and sewerage lines could be lowered to the point where poor households could afford to pay for them. Simplified designs and the use of standardized steel moulds reduced the cost of sanitary latrines and manholes to less than one quarter of the contractors' rates. The cost of the sewerage line was also greatly reduced by eliminating the profits of the contractor. The average cost of the small bore sewer system is no more than US$66 per house.

Despite women's active involvement in the local decision making and financing, they had difficulty visiting health centres since custom dictates that they should stay at home. OPP developed a health programme, working through women's groups, also at the level of the lane, with advice provided on hygiene, nutrition, disease prevention, family planning and kitchen gardens. There is also an income genera-tion programme which provides credit and advice to small businesses and a project to help upgrade physical conditions and academic stan-dards in schools in Orangi. Local building technology has also been improved through the use of machine made bricks to replace those made by hand.

Sources: Arif Hasan, 'A low cost sewer system by low-income Pakistanis' in Bertha Turner (Ed), Building Community: a Third World Case Book, *Habitat International Coalition, 1989; Hasan, Arif 'Community organizations and NGOs in the urban field in Pakistan'* Environment and Urbanization *Vol 2, No 1, April 1990, pp 74–86; and Khan, Akhter Hameed,* Orangi Pilot Project Programmes, *Orangi Pilot Project, Karachi, 1991*

There are many examples of regions or districts where serious degradation and increasing levels of poverty were reversed and where a decentraliza-tion of responsibility to the local level and a participatory approach were key innovations. Box 6.4 gives an example of the reclamation of saline land in Hebei province in China. The example has considerable relevance, given the large areas of land worldwide that were once among the most produc-tive farmlands and which are now too saline because of poor irrigation and agricultural practice.

Building on Local Systems of Knowledge and Management

As noted earlier, in both rural and urban areas, the livelihoods of most poorer households draw from diverse sources. Many rural and some urban households rely on a mix of crops and livestock for their own consumption (with perhaps some for sale), the gathering of wild plants, remittances from one or more household member working elsewhere, wage labour and trad-ing. Households often diversify the sources of livelihood in response to changing environmental or economic conditions. And livelihood strategies often have to adapt rapidly in response to unpredictable environmental and economic change.

Households have to continually adjust to satisfy new needs, address new contingencies and grasp new opportunities. Where there is such spatial and social diversity in households' livelihood strategies, it is impossible for external agencies to predict the needs and preferences of households. There is also the fact that different household members have different priorities – and those of women and of children who have important roles in livelihood

---

Box 6.4 **Reclamation of Saline Land in Hebei Province, China**

The Hebei Agricultural Development Project in China has combined a rehabilitation of poor and saline soils with other improvements which ensure higher agricultural production that is ecologically sustainable, and higher incomes and improved services. Drainage and irrigation canals were constructed as well as deep and shallow tubewells to bring up fresh water to leach out the salt residues. This greatly reduced the area of highly saline soils and lowered the water table to acceptable levels. The area under irrigation increased and 25,000 hectares of land subject to waterlogging were reclaimed. Some 5000 hectares of wasteland were turned into forests and orchards and 3000 kilometres of shelter belts planted. This helped contribute to a more favourable microclimate in the region. Drinking water supplies were also improved. The removal of salt from the top layers of the soil combined with the levelling of the land has helped increase agricultural production. Grain production has more than doubled and cash crop production has quadrupled. Average incomes have nearly doubled and the combination of improved drinking water and greater diversity of diet (with increased consumption of meat and eggs) has also improved health.

Although factors such as a decentralized management system were important, participatory development with a strong response from the villagers was the key to the project's success. To improve their livelihoods, the entire workforce of the village – men, women, children, farmers and non-farmers – excavated the drains using manual labour. They are now operating and maintaining the irrigation systems, either individually or through village communities. They paid for the costs of deep and shallow wells and of levelling the land and planting the trees. In all cases, they undertook the construction of farm irrigation facilities and the leaching of the salt from the land. They also took full advantage of the resources made available by the project in the form of credit, fertilizer, agricultural machinery and improved seeds.

Source: Jazairy, Idriss, Mohiuddin Alamgir and Theresa Panuccio (1992), The State of World Rural Poverty: an Inquiry into its Causes and Consequences, *IT Publications, London*

---

strategies are often forgotten or not understood by external agencies. In all households' livelihood strategies, there is a division of labour by gender and by age in which female and male household members of different ages have different access to and control over resources in their different tasks.

There are no prescriptions for designing PEC to ensure it meshes with the diversity of physical and socio-economic circumstances, except that these prescriptions are developed in constant dialogue with both the women and the men and their organizations. It is also important to involve older children in this dialogue, both as important contributors to livelihood strategies and as children who must experience and learn from participatory decision-

making processes.[18] It is difficult to imagine children developing a support
for and an understanding of democracy at work, if there is little or no
evidence of democratic processes within their own communities.[19]

PEC initiatives have to begin with those who know most about local
conditions. The imposition of outside solutions often not only fails to build
upon indigenous knowledge and techniques, but may even obliterate them.
Box 6.5 gives an example of soil conservation that was based on local self-
help groups and drew on traditional techniques and work organization.

Box 6.5 Soil Conservation using Local Self-help Groups

In the Machakos district of southeast Kenya, more than 70 per cent of
farmed land is now terraced which has brought better and more reliable yields of maize. The National Soil and Water Conservation Project
initiated fieldwork in 1979 and on the basis of its success there, it has
been expanded since 1986 to cover the entire country. Funded by the
Swedish International Development Cooperation Agency (formerly
the Swedish International Development Authority) which has
provided long-term support, this project provides an example of the
potential of working with local groups in building upon locally known
techniques for stemming soil erosion in a densely populated area. The
main technique for soil conservation is an improved version of the
traditional *fanya juu* terrace, constructed by communal work groups,
largely made up of women.

*Source: Critchley, W Looking After Our Land; New Approaches to Soil and
Water Conservation in Dryland Africa, OXFAM and IIED, London, 1991,
quoted in Toulmin, Camilla, Ian Scoones and Josh Bishop, 'Drylands' in Johan
Holmberg (Ed), Policies for a Small Planet, Earthscan, London, 1992*

Initiatives should also start with what people know and what they already
do well. Where projects have done this, the economic benefits can be
remarkable. One study of 68 multilateral projects found that those sensitive
to local skills and knowledge had an economic rate of return that was
double that of insensitive ones.[20] Box 6.6 gives an example of how a local
NGO worked with villagers in designing an action plan which achieved
agreements on issues which were a potential source of conflict between
different social groups. It also describes a watershed development
programme that was based on local knowledge.

In urban areas, there are many examples of initiatives that incorporated
the knowledge, resources and capacity of low-income groups to produce a
wide range of benefits. These include: the installation of community water
and sanitation systems in low-income settlements at costs per household
served that were much less than would have been achieved by government
agencies or private contractors; the design and implementation of cheap
and effective drainage and garbage collection systems; the design and

Box 6.6 **Building on Local Knowledge and Skills for Watershed Development: the Approach of SPEECH in Tamil Nadu, India**

The NGO SPEECH was established in 1987 and operates in 25 villages in the Kamarajar District of Tamil Nadu. This district is one of the most disadvantaged in terms of health, literacy, rainfall, agricultural production, environment and basic livelihoods. The living conditions (especially of the women and children) are very poor.

In late 1990, SPEECH conducted a Participatory Rural Appraisal in Paraikulum village. The action plan designed by the villagers included gully plugs, *nullah* treatment, fruit trees just inside the *bunds*, field *bunds* and spillways on the boundaries and contour ploughing. The landowners agreed only to plant trees on two sides of each of their fields, so as not to compete with neighbours. A water diviner identified a site for a communal well (a fifth of a hectare was needed) and other farmers compensated the landowner for the loss of this land. The landless have been involved in working on the gully treatment and the well-digging. There is also an agreement to give them the marketing rights for the fruit when it is harvestable. In one year, the watershed has undergone a remarkable transformation with net family income rising four fold between 1990–91 and 1991–92 and more employment opportunities for the landless.

The watershed was formerly degraded with a hard crust and only sparsely covered with a few grasses. But where the protection measures are in place, the yield for the first crop of beans was around one tonne per hectare. The survival rate for the mango, guava, custard apple, cashew and pomegranate tree seedlings is about 80 per cent. The *nullah* will have tamarind on the outside, and napier grass along the inside. The farmers have planned pulses for the first two years, since they are drought resistant, and require no fertilizers. During the second year, they will start applying silt from the tank to the land and further develop compost pits. In the third year, they plan to upgrade the road and build a percolation pond. The ground has been laid for economic benefits to flow to the whole community.

Source: John Devavaram, personal communication quoted in 'PEC: an alternative paradigm for development assistance', Jules N Pretty and Irene Guijt, Environment and Urbanization Vol 4, No 1, April 1992

construction of housing more appropriate for comfort, safety and control of disease vectors; and the acquisition and development of land for housing at costs affordable to relatively low-income households.[21]

Strengthening Local Institutions and Social Organizations

Most development efforts by external agencies have long ignored the formal and informal institutions which operate within particular settlements, neighbourhoods or localities. Many governments or political parties have an interest in limiting their development or their influence. Yet the cooperation and full involvement of these local organizations is often a key to sustainable resource use and development because they can act to ensure that resource management and control responds to the specifics of the local context and that management continues after the withdrawal of external agency support. In many contexts, they should be strengthened and developed, not ignored. Such groups include: traditional leadership structures, water management committees, water users groups, neighbourhood groups, youth groups, women's groups, housing societies, informal beer-brewing groups, farmer experimentation groups, burial societies, church groups, mothers' groups and grazing management groups.[22] There are often women's groups that have particularly important roles, some organized around specific issues such as mothers' groups or groups based on homeworking. Formal or informal youth groups are often present and may have considerable potential to act and to organize, with appropriate support.

Effective local groups and organizations rarely involve whole communities. PEC approaches are most successful when dealing with groups in which members have similar interests, values and needs. These different groups have different needs and perceptions which they may not articulate in large assemblies. This diversity of social groups in each locality is a feature of rural and urban communities commonly missed by outsiders. In rural areas, large cooperatives, in which the needs of different members vary enormously and which are too large for widespread participation, are often managed by small groups, usually the most wealthy men, to whom decision making has been delegated. Inevitably, they are less effective in meeting the special needs of the poor women and men. The same may be true in large low-income settlements in urban areas where local organizations may have an over-representation of certain interest groups or have become too coopted by a particular political party or influential individual to represent the needs of all inhabitants. Box 6.7 gives an example of a squatter settlement where a representative organization slowly developed, with the support of an external agency. But what has become a long-term programme to improve water, sanitation, drainage and housing, to provide day care, to acquire tenure of the land and to support a range of other activities, began when the external agency responded to the specific requests of a small group of women.

Emphasizing the Use of Locally Available Resources and Technologies

Most rural and urban development assistance has been based on the assumption that external resources will be needed. For many poor people and communities, this is not a viable option. They can neither command

Box 6.7 **Barrio San Jorge, Argentina**

The Barrio San Jorge project is a long-term programme of support for a low-income district in the suburbs of Buenos Aires provided by IIED-America Latina. It is unusual in that it began within a squatter settlement in which there was no representative community organization. Most external support for community action to improve housing and living conditions is for settlements in which a community organization had already been formed, since this makes it easier for external agencies to negotiate with the inhabitants and obtain rapid implementation.

Barrio San Jorge is located in San Fernando, one of the municipalities on the periphery of Buenos Aires metropolitan area and some 35 kilometres north of the city centre. It covers a site of less than ten hectares located in the middle of a neglected environment of flat lowlands with few trees and is subject to flooding from polluted water. Two narrow streams, which form the east and west boundaries, are full of garbage – much of it put there by local residents because of the inadequate garbage collection service. There are 630 households; a high proportion of the inhabitants are infants, children and adolescents and there are few elderly people.

Since 1987, various community projects have been implemented to improve conditions, with funding raised from a variety of local, national and international sources. They include the construction and development of a mother and child crèche/day care/health centre and a conversion of an existing house into a community centre (the house of the *barrio*), the provision of a piped water and sanitation system, a health education programme, a sewing and clothing workshop; and the surfacing of some internal roads. A community-managed building materials store has also been opened to lower prices and to make it easier for the inhabitants to obtain materials.

When the construction of the mother and child centre began in September 1987, only 16 people in San Jorge (mostly women) were interested in community activities. The great majority of the population looked upon the construction of the centre with scepticism. In late 1989, residents became more interested in the activities being introduced in the Barrio. Attendance at meetings increased; so too did participation in decisions about work priorities. But few people were prepared to contribute to building tasks unless they received payment. During the first half of 1990, the consolidation of a community organization continued. In August 1990, elections were held in the Barrio to choose representatives from the community to join a commission which was to develop a long-range plan and a programme for the improvement and integrated development of the Barrio. This long-term programme has included negotiating secure tenure for the inhabitants and obtaining an extra seven hectares of land that is adjacent to the barrio on which to resettle some of the inhabitants and reduce the overall density.

Source: Barrio San Jorge, Annual Reports 1989/90 and 1990/91; Hardoy, Ana, Jorge Hardoy and Richard Schusterman (1991) 'Building community organization: the history of a squatter settlement and its own organization' Environment and Urbanization, Vol 3, No 2; UNCHS (1996), An Urbanizing World: The Global Report on Human Settlements 1996, Oxford University Press, Oxford and New York

capital nor have access to necessary generators of value, such as machinery, agricultural chemicals, water pumps or building materials. Although there is an obvious role for outside support in securing initial funds, PEC gives preference to local, appropriate technologies by emphasizing the opportunities for intensification (or better use) of available resources. Provided that groups or communities are involved in the identification of technology needs and of the technologies themselves (the design of testing and experimentation, the adaptation to their own conditions, and the extension to others), then sustainable and cheap solutions can often be found.[23]

Resource-poor rural areas that lack infrastructure, which are far from roads and markets, and which have risky climates and poor soils, typically produce in the order of five times less food per unit area than irrigated and lowland areas near to cities.[24] Yet there is enormous potential for increasing incomes and making livelihoods more stable, without recourse to high levels of fertilizer and pesticide use and increasing reliance on external suppliers. The development of appropriate agro-ecological pest, nutrient and water management practices commonly leads to 50–100 per cent increases in the yields of crops, livestock and trees. These increases bring greater self-reliance coupled with reduced dependency on outside suppliers of pesticides, fertilizers and seeds.

In urban areas, the options affordable by low-income groups who wish to build or develop their own homes and work together to address problems of water supply, drainage, street paving and health care is usually limited, as most materials and components are beyond their price range. They usually make do with what is available. Yet if they are fully involved in the design, implementation and maintenance phases of projects designed to meet housing, sanitation, water and garbage collection needs, then the results are more sustainable and effective than those imposed by outside professionals and there are often major costs savings.[25] Locally-developed initiatives for building material production or the design and implementation of infrastructure have often produced much more cost-effective solutions, although their implementation is often hindered both by the attitudes of local authorities and unrealistic building and planning norms, codes and regulations.

One major theme for PEC in urban areas is community-based schemes to manage solid wastes that achieve the objective of efficiently removing household wastes while also promoting resource conservation, reclamation, re-use and recycling. There are many recently documented examples of initiatives undertaken by local NGOs or community-based organizations which combine environmental and social objectives such as better returns and lower health risks for garbage pickers and recyclers.[26] Box 6.8 gives an example of an initiative in Manila which promoted resource recovery from the wastes of homes and schools and created work for some 200 eco-aides.

Local Participation in Planning, Management and Monitoring

In conventional rural and urban development projects, there is little participation in the sense of those who are within the project area or affected by

Box 6.8 **The Garbage Recycling Project in Metro Manila**

The garbage recycling project in metro Manila has evolved over a decade from the inspiration of one woman, backed by a large and well-funded national NGO, the Metro Manila chapter of Women Balikatan Movement. Leonarda Comacho, now the chair of the Metro Manila chapter, spent a year in Switzerland in the early 1980s and was impressed by the cleanness of Swiss towns and by people's habit of keeping recyclables separate from their refuse and depositing them for the municipal authorities to collect and distribute to recycling firms. On her return to Manila, she engaged the Quezon City chapter of Balikatan in the mounting garbage problem. From clean-up drives in San Juan city in metro Manila, they moved to discussions of the root causes of solid waste problems. Leonarda suggested that local traditions of householders separating newspapers, bottles, cardboard and the like could be supported and extended.

The possibility that a materials separation and trading project could benefit the 'barrow boys' who mainly obtain recyclables by picking from mixed wastes was seen as a social benefit from the beginning. There had been an attempt funded by the government for a 'Cash for Trash' project that established waste materials purchasing centres and tried to bypass the traditional junk dealers in the mid-1980s. Its failure persuaded Leonarda Comacho that a viable approach to household resource recovery had to have the cooperation of junk shop dealers. The project, originally called *Linis-Ganda* (Clean-green) was originally based in San Juan and Quezon City only and focused on: gaining the cooperation of neighbourhood waste dealers to employ door-to-door buyers (eco-aides) issued with photo identity cards by Balikatan; mobilizing the support of households for separation and sale; and aiding dealers in technical and business development.

By 1994, there were 21 dealers in the project with 200 eco-aides who were purchasing some 50 kg of materials each day (mainly cardboard, bottles, plastics and metals). Since Sept 1992, 25,000 households in Quezon City and San Juan are taking part and the concept is now being implemented in other places of the three cities and 12 towns of Metro Manila, mostly by Balikatan chapters although other citizen groups support the effort.

The project had 300 volunteers working for various components: motivation for source separation, assistance to junk shop dealers, training of eco-aides, work in schools and monitoring. Officers from the Metro Manila chapter of the Women Balikatan Movement contribute to the planning and monitoring of the project and it is this organization's support that has been crucial to the initiation and continuation of the work; no funds have been received from international agencies.

A recent development has been the organization of cooperatives for the dealers who were experiencing difficulties in obtaining loans to expand their businesses. They needed to expand as a result of greater volumes of materials brought in by eco-aides but loans were difficult to obtain as they do not own their premises. By forming a cooperative, they can obtain a loan at 7 per cent interest from the government's Department of Trade and Industry. There is also a considerable involvement of schools; in all, some 3000 students at 116 public and 50 private schools sort their dry wastes and sell them to eco-aides, while the composting of food wastes from the canteens is being tried in some places.

This is an example of a predominantly environmental project emphasising community participation in source separation, with social assistance focused on waste dealers rather than waste pickers. There is no requirement that dealers employ street pickers as itinerant buyers and no records of how many eco-aides are former pickers. Dealers are doing well out of public cooperation and cooperative membership. Balikatan is an affluent organization with many volunteers and support from private corporations. For these reasons, the project does not face the problem of welfare subsidies usually needed by groups dealing with poor waste pickers.

Source: Furedy, Christine, 'Socio-environmental initiatives in solid waste management in Southern cities: developing international comparisons', Paper presented at a workshop on 'Linkages in Urban Solid Waste Management', Karnataka State Council for Science and Technology, University of Amsterdam and Bangalore Mahanagara Palike, 18–20 April, Bangalore, 1994

it having the right to influence priorities, project design and implementation. In fact, 'participation' may be no more than external agencies informing the recipients about what is going to happen. Or it may simply be encouraging local people to sell their labour in return for food, cash or materials, during project implementation. Yet these incentives distort perceptions, create dependencies, and give the misleading impression that local people support the project.[27] Such paternalism undermines the possibility of sustaining the beneficial impacts of the project after it has been completed. As little effort is made to build local skills, interests and capacity, local people have no stake in maintaining structures or practices when the flow of incentives stops.

Box 6.9 gives an example from Indonesia where the government's water agency incorporated local populations (their customers) in the planning, implementation and maintenance of water supply. However, as the authors who documented this case study note, this is an example of community participation as a means to reach an externally-defined, though important goal. It was not community participation as a fully empowering process because it lacked the involvement of the population in the problem-identification phase.[28]

What can be termed the PEC approach is for external institutions to enter into partnerships with communities for all phases of planning, management and monitoring. New research techniques and methods have been developed which respond to the need for 'ways of researching ...

Box 6.9 **Community Involvement in Planning and Maintaining Water Supply in Small Towns in West Java**

A piped water supply programme currently underway in small towns in West Java province in Indonesia has sought to fully involve households in determining the level of provision and the location of supplies and in setting up the means to ensure that public taps are managed and maintained. Initial results suggest that active community involvement produces more appropriate and effective water provision but also makes for more efficient implementation and maintenance, and greater likelihood of cost recovery. The piped water programme is for 44 towns in West Java province and seeks to reach some 300,000 people with improved supplies. In a first phase, work concentrated on supplying water to a water storage basin within the house or to public taps. A review of this work found that the public taps did not provide the service to the lower-income groups to the degree anticipated and some public taps were hardly used at all, usually because they were poorly sited, with sites chosen by contractors in consultation with local government but with no community involvement. The standard set for water quantity often proved to be well below actual demand.

The agencies concerned changed their procedures to include greater flexibility in what was provided (for instance a staggered construction schedule that allowed for adjustments), a community involvement programme (that included a community self-survey) and greater emphasis on training and institutional support. The community self-survey is conducted by local community members, usually with considerable involvement of existing local organizations, with guidance from the implementing agency's project staff. This survey determines customer preferences (for instance which households want house connections and which want shared taps) and the data it gathers forms the basis for the installation of the water system and associated facilities. It determines the location of public taps and permits the formation of a public tap user group to ensure maintenance and payment. Each public tap user group can organize its own system for payment and maintenance and the plan is also to provide them with practical guidance on day-to-day organization and problem solving. This represents an important change in the attitude and mode of operation of public water authorities towards a more customer-oriented approach. It is also likely to produce tangible benefits for the water authorities in a higher level of customer satisfaction, better utilization and maintenance, and higher revenues. Certain problems still remain – including the failure to integrate environmental sanitation into the scheme and the relatively high proportion of households who express no interest in a house connection or a public tap. In addition, this is an example of community participation as a means to reach a stated goal and not community participation as a potentially empowering process for human development.

Source: Britha Mikkelsen with Yanti Yulianti and Anton Barré, 'Community involvement in water supply in West Java', Environment and Urbanization *Vol 5, No 1, April 1993*

which combine finding out about complex and dynamic situations with taking action to improve them, in such a way that the actors and beneficiaries of the action research are intimately involved as participants in the whole process.'[29] Institutions committed to supporting PEC initiatives have, through repeated practice, developed a large number of approaches for collaborative research, planning, implementation and monitoring which fall under the general heading of 'participatory inquiry' (see Box 6.10).

Much work needs to be done on developing the means by which there is a devolution of planning and monitoring phases to project participants. In PEC activities, men, women, girls and boys in rural and urban communities should not be seen simply as informants for project design, but as teachers, extension agents, activists, and monitors of change. In rural contexts, these specialists, or para-professionals, might include village energy workers, villager extension agents, pest control experts, village game wardens and veterinarians.[30] In urban areas, they may include local community leaders (including religious leaders), women's groups (for instance formed for childcare, community kitchens or some other common purpose), inhabitants working in local government and para-medical staff from health care clinics and local school personnel. As described in more detail in Chapter 7, there are important roles for children in designing and implementing PEC initiatives and in investigating environmental issues within their own locality.

In this, as in many other aspects, there are themes in common with primary health care. Many primary health care systems have also sought to ensure the participation of local women and men in planning, implementation and management. Primary health care and primary environmental care also have a common agenda in improving environmental health and this needs the incorporation of local residents' knowledge. There has to be a dialogue between health professionals and local inhabitants and their community organizations about disease which develops into the full involvement of local residents as 'community-based epidemiologists'.[31]

There are many examples of how such a dialogue revealed the misunderstanding or inaccurate diagnosis of external health professionals. One given by May Yacoob and Linda Whiteford was of women working in various positions in the peri-urban areas around Quito who complained of frequent chronic bladder infections. North American male physicians and biomedical health workers attributed this problem to the possibility of multiple sexual partners because of the women's socio-economic group. Interviews with the women found that following pregnancies, they were forced out of their jobs. They had to work in the informal sector so they could also bring their children. But because the markets and roadsides where they worked had no toilet facilities for women, they were forced to go all day without urinating which makes them more vulnerable to bladder infections. What was needed was the personal accounts of the women themselves to permit an accurate diagnosis that then allowed this particular problem to be addressed.[32]

There are also examples of environmental health improvements and improvements in primary health care provision whose effectiveness and

Box 6.10 **Participatory Inquiry**

Participatory Inquiry is an action/research methodology based on principles of multiple perspectives, group enquiry, context specificity and flexibility. At its core are several themes:

- defined methodology and systematic learning process utilizing a range of techniques and methods – the focus is on a cumulative learning process by all those involved;
- acceptance of diversity and need for multiple perspectives to arrive at understanding of this diversity; participatory inquiry implies a group inquiry process involving local people and outsiders from different sectors and disciplines;
- context specific; a range of techniques and methods used in participatory inquiry where the methods and the mix of methods used must be flexible enough to be adaptable to the particular conditions and processes within each context. Knowledge and associated technology seen as contextual in time and space, and so limited in their transferability, while ways of learning have wider validity;
- leading to action; the inquiry process is to produce agreement about needed actions and motivate their implementation;
- the future recognized as uncertain and indeterminate so the inquiry process has a built-in and continuous monitoring and evaluation process involving all actors to permit basis for changes in approaches;
- role of external 'experts' much more as facilitators than advisors.

Participatory inquiry uses a range of methods which fall into four general categories: group and team dynamics (which include a range of workshop and field methods to help in formation of groups and support of community-level shared discussions); sampling methods to ensure multiple perspectives are investigated and represented (including social maps, interview maps and transect walks); interviewing and dialogue (which include semi-structured interviews, focus groups, key informants and local stories and oral histories); and visualization and diagramming (including group-developed maps, calenders and models).

Participatory Inquiry techniques come under many names including Participatory Rural Appraisal, Rapid Rural Appraisal, Action Research, *Méthode Accélérée de Recherche Participative*, GRAAP, Farmer Participatory Research and many more.

Source: Pretty, Jules (1993), 'Participatory inquiry for sustainable agriculture', IIED, London, mimeo (draft) and RRA Notes 1988–1992, Issues 1–14, Sustainable Agriculture Programme, IIED, London.

low costs were largely due to the involvement of community representatives in problem identification and monitoring, health promotion and health care. One example of this is the work of the *Reproinsas* (community health promoters) in Guatemala City. These are elected by low-income communities from among their own inhabitants and, with the advice of technical teams, help identify the most pressing health and environmental problems, help address them (for instance administering vaccines and advising on how to treat diarrhoeal diseases and avoid parasitic infections) and monitor progress.[33] More details of their work and of other community-based initiatives in Guatemala City are given later in this chapter (in Box 6.20) as an example of the kind of support that an international agency can give to community-based initiatives.

Methods used in PEC reduce lags in information flows, as feedback occurs during the 'project cycle' for any particular initiative. But it is still more common for local populations to be involved in the planning than in the other phases, and there remains a tendency for monitoring and evaluation to be conducted by outside professionals at intermittent intervals. A study of the views on participation of some 230 African organizations found that though participation in planning was relatively common, monitoring and evaluation is still largely conducted by outside organizations.[34]

Recognizing the Diversity of Need and Priority within each Locality

Recognizing that local specialists come from among women and men in all sectors, classes and ethnic groups in the community facilitates the integration of groups that are excluded from most public programmes. It also allows their skills and knowledge to influence development priorities. External agencies tend to assume that there is a 'community' within a village or low-income urban settlement, without understanding what are often complex power structures and divergent interests.

There are also the obvious differences in people's priorities arising from different asset bases. For instance, landowners, tenants and agricultural labourers will often have very different needs and priorities in rural areas. Owners* and tenants living in the same neighbourhood in urban areas also generally have different priorities. Or they may be conflict over the use of common property or public resources, as different villages or settlements compete with each other. Box 6.11 gives some examples from Orissa in India where some 2000 villages are actively engaged in protecting some 15,000 hectares of forest.[35] Here, as in most other examples in this section, management of the resource becomes possible as local people reach consensus on use and management, with systems set up to ensure implementation and the control or prevention of use by outsiders. But the example also illustrates how problems with equity often have to be addressed, either within the community or between communities as one village takes control of a forested area which those from other villages had previously used.

---

* Squatters may also be considered de facto owners if they are unlikely to be forced off the land.

Box 6.11 **Community Management of Forests in Orissa, India**

Community initiatives for forest protection arise largely from a desire to save forests which have become degraded and from a desire on the part of a village to assert control over the use of local forests from other users. Forest protection usually begins with patches that are seriously degraded but which have their rootstock intact – and such areas, when protected, regenerate rapidly. Hardship arising from a scarcity of forest products is the main reason given by villagers for beginning such initiatives, although the environmental effects of degradation such as loss of soil fertility or drying-up of streams are also significant. In some cases, large-scale farmers initiated protection measures after plots at the foot of denuded hillsides were found to be losing soil fertility.

Traditional village-level organizations that exist in many parts of Orissa provide a forum for discussing and then acting on forest protection. Traditionally, village organizations are responsible for other common areas such as ponds and temple lands – and they also act to resolve conflicts. It is relatively easy to extend the principle of community management to forests.

Village initiatives protect forests both in 'reserve forests' which are in theory managed by the government forest department and in non-reserve forest areas. Protected forest land belongs to the government's revenue department but its management is the responsibility of the forest department which usually fails to provide the needed management. Local initiatives to protect or regenerate forests have proved most effective in areas of only moderate forest scarcity, with villagers able to meet their needs while also letting the protected patch regenerate. Community protection of a patch of forest involves bringing an unmanaged area under a protection system with well-defined rules and penalties. Once a village has asserted its control over part of a forest, people from surrounding villages are excluded from sharing the benefit and they often take up protection of other degraded forest land to ensure their own needs can be met.

Once villagers decide to protect a forest area, they demarcate it and inform nearby villages of their intent to protect that area. At first, there is opposition from nearby villagers who formerly had free access to that area – but where the area is severely degraded and other forested areas are available, there is often very little opposition.

Forest protection involves partial or total controls on its use by village members and denial of access to outsiders. Villages engage people to keep watch or set up a voluntary patrolling system. They also draw up their rules and penalties and in some instances, these are written down and records maintained. Often, grazing is banned in the initial years to allow young plants to grow and the removal of small timber is restricted and the felling of green trees prohibited. In some cases, even entering the area without permission is prohibited.

Institutional arrangements are made by such community-level organizations as a youth club or an informal village forest protection committee or even a committee formally set up by the state forest department. These groups are not always equitable and may be controlled by dominant social or caste interests.

Some support is now coming from the state government for community protection of forests:

> 'Community-based management systems ... have shown they can effectively manage local resources, but they need support because well-established systems can resolve community conflicts and contradictions.' (p 28)

> 'As in any group endeavour, forest protection by rural communities has its own problems ... In many cases, the protection system breaks down after a few years due to conflicts within and between communities. Once the forest grows and trees are larger, the temptation to cut them down increases. In a few instances, a cyclical process of protection has occurred; clear-felling after six or seven years followed by a renewal of protection. Often conflicts arise because villages with foresight take up large areas of the forest for protection. While the forest is still completely degraded, it might not attract attention, but once regeneration occurs, neighbouring villages demand a share, which the protecting village justifiably refuses. Such situations lead to conflict and raise the issue of equity. Community management of forests has to be an integral part of overall forest management. Yet the simplistic assumption that merely handing over forests to communities will solve all problems does not hold good. Any number of issues can threaten community systems, particularly equity within and between villages and demand and supply for forest products. Such issues have to be resolved if community management is to become a sustainable forest management alternative.' (p 28)

Source: Singh, Neera M and Kundan K Singh (1993), 'Saving forests for posterity', Down To Earth 15 April, pp 25–28

One of the most important divergences in priorities between the inhabitants of any locality is related to gender, as women and men have different needs and priorities, based on their particular roles in income earning, child-rearing and household management. In most societies, women's needs and priorities are not given equal status to those of men, and women face particular constraints in gaining access to political structures to voice these differences and imbalances.[36] Yet women often take a central role in community organizations both to work collectively to address common problems and to organize collectively to obtain external resources or oppose external plans that threaten their livelihoods or homes.

Meeting the Gender-defined Needs of Adults and Children

New approaches must systematically integrate a *gender* perspective into their concerns and methodologies. In many societies, this may be one of the main potential sources of conflict between the goals of PEC and traditional systems of resource ownership, use and management. In virtually all societies, females and males of different ages perform different roles and have different access to and control over resources. For this reason, they have different needs that are defined by the gender division of labour and gender relations in different societies.[37] Moreover, they hold different knowledge and experience of the environment. The particular roles they take will also expose them to particular environmental hazards or to a greater level of risk from more general hazards. As Chapter 3 described, there is usually considerable differentiation in the level and nature of risk from environmental hazards by gender and by age.[38]

Thus, support for PEC must address the practical needs of women and men of different ages in resource use and management. Many agricultural and rural development programmes have ignored or misunderstood the roles played by women and men, and girl and boy children because they have been based on faulty assumptions about gender relations and gender-defined roles. One result is that they have given little or no attention to the ways and means by which improved resource management and labour-saving technologies can lessen the workloads of women. Even though it is common for women and children to have a major role in crop production and/or livestock management and resource conservation in both rural and urban areas, there is often no consideration within official support programmes (including agricultural extension programmes) of the support they need and the technologies they would find useful.[39] Indeed, many of the subsistence activities in which women engage may be considered illegal.[40] Women rarely have equal access to inputs and credit as men, even where women have total responsibility for farming as sole income earners or because their partners have migrated out of the village to obtain wage labour. Fuelwood collection is often an onerous burden for women and/or children yet too little attention has been given to ensuring that they can obtain the fuel they need without deforestation and to decreasing the labour, time and physical effort needed for its collection.

In a recent paper on 'the struggle to legitimize subsistence; women and sustainable development', Lee-Smith and Trujillo note that:

> *'the right to survive, to subsist, is being claimed by women on behalf of their families in rural and urban poor communities world-wide, in the face of development pressures which make it increasingly impossible for them to eat, clothe and shelter themselves.'[41]*

In recognition of this, a range of possible mechanisms is needed for ensuring the participation of women as well as men in organizations to deal with environmental management. In describing the new village institutions that are needed in India to promote resource conservation and management, Agarwal and Narain point to the need for separate women's groups (*Mahila mandals*) within each village unit, with their own clearly defined roles, rights, and access to funds. 'Experience in India shows that women take an active interest in programmes designed to improve ecological conditions because of their culturally determined role as fuel, fodder and water carriers'.[42] In other societies, it may be more appropriate to bring women and men together in the same organizations.

One other area that deserves special attention is the role of both formal and non-formal education. The importance of utilizing traditional knowledge about resource use, management and conservation has already been noted. So too has the fact that this is recognized by increasing numbers of agricultural specialists and is being incorporated into agricultural extension services. But comparable changes are needed in education, where both the formal curriculum and teachers may not only ignore traditional knowledge but actually discredit it. Schools and higher education institutes which actively encouraged the rescue and recording of traditional and gender disaggregated knowledge on resource use, management and conservation from their area would be a more appropriate basis for supporting PEC.

THE NATURE OF PARTICIPATION; FROM PASSIVE PARTICIPATION AND MANIPULATION TO SELF-MOBILIZATION

Whenever the issue of people's right to participate in environment and development projects is raised, inevitably, there is discussion as to what such participation implies. In addition to the dimension of who participates, the spectrum of 'participation' for such people stretches from, at one extreme, simply being told what will happen (with no capacity to influence this) or even symbolic 'participation' with no substance, to, at the other extreme, having the capacity to initiate projects themselves and acquire resources and technical advice from external agencies on terms in which they have the central role. In most 'participatory' projects or initiatives, the form of participation falls somewhere between these two extremes – although there are good grounds for suggesting that there is no legitimate 'participation' where people are simply told what will be done by external agencies in advance or are required to contribute time and labour to some externally designed and directed project. Box 6.12 highlights the different levels of participation that can be part of any environment or development project.

Primary environmental care and the participatory methods and techniques used by external agencies in developing action programmes with local populations imply greater decision-making power and more fundamental roles for a multiplicity of local groups. Emphasizing the role of local people in determining key indicators of local sustainable development and providing early warning of resource-degrading change is also an area being developed by some PEC initiatives.

Box 6.12 Different Levels of Participation within any Environment or Development Project

Self-mobilization
Project initiated by the population themselves who develop contacts with external institutions for resources and technical advice they need, but retain control over how resources are used. Can 'go to scale' if governments and NGOs can provide the 'enabling' framework to support a wide range of such initiatives. Also, within any low-income settlement, this is less of a project and more part of a process by which people organize to get things done and negotiate with external agencies for support in doing so.

Interactive participation
Project initiated by external agency working with local population (and often in response to local people's demand). Participation seen as a citizen's right, not just as a means to achieve project goals. People participate in joint analysis, development of action plans and formation or strengthening of institutions for implementation and management. As such, they have considerable influence in determining how available resources are to be used.

Functional participation
Participation seen by external agency as a means to achieve project goals, especially reduced costs (through people providing free labour and management). For instance, people participate by forming groups to meet predetermined objectives but after major decisions have been made by the external agency. At its worst, the population is simply coopted to serve external agency's goals which accord little with their goals. However, this limited form of participation has brought real benefits to 'beneficiaries' in many instances.

Participation for material incentives
People participate but only in implementation in response to material incentives (eg contributing labour to a project in return for cash, food or other material incentives; building a house within a 'self-help' project as a condition for obtaining the land and services).

Consultation and information giving
People's views sought through a consultation process whose aim is to elicit their needs and priorities but this process is undertaken by external agents who define the information gathering process and control the analysis through which the problem is defined and the solutions designed. No decision-making powers given to the population and no obligation on the part of the project designers to respond to their priorities. Great variety in extent to which people's

> views are accurately elicited and incorporated into
> project design and implementation.
>
> **Passive**   People are told what is going to happen but without
> **participation** their views sought and with no power to change what
> will happen.
>
> **Manipulation** Pretence of participation – eg with 'peoples' represen-
> **and**   tatives on official boards but who are not elected and
> **decoration**   have no power.
>
> *Sources: Drawn from Pretty, Jules (1993), 'Participatory inquiry for sustainable agri-*
> *culture', IIED, London, mimeo (draft), and Hart, Roger A. (1992),* Children's
> Participation; from Tokenism to Citizenship, *Innocenti Essays No. 4, March,*
> *UNICEF International Child Development Centre, Florence*

FUTURE NEEDS – SCALING UP[43]

As PEC projects usually start small and many remain small, considerable attention must be paid to supporting a multiplication of initiatives so a large impact is achieved through the aggregation of many initiatives.[44] Two strategies are needed to encourage this. The first is to ensure that all agencies external to a locality with a role in development and/or environmental management (including government agencies, international agencies of all kinds and NGOs) have the knowledge and capacity to help advise and support new initiatives. This is the focus of this section. The second, considered in the next section, is to provide the conditions at regional, national and international level that allow a great variety of local PEC initiatives to develop – ie to encourage self-mobilization as described in Box 6.12. This includes the need to address the political, legal and financial constraints on such initiatives at local, regional (state), national and international level.

The Role of External Agencies

For external agencies to 'go to scale' by stimulating and supporting large numbers of communities to develop their own PEC initiatives – which is not replication since this implies the use of a standard model – considerable attention will have to be given to operational policies and frameworks. Some of the key aspects of this are discussed below: training, financial support, and working with NGOs and other intermediary institutions.

In regard to *training*, support for PEC implies new roles and attitudes for project staff. The idea that educated professionals may have something to learn from low-income groups remains for many an awkward notion, not least because their education stressed the validity of their 'specialist knowledge'. Where the professionals cannot understand and speak the same language as project participants, the possibility of two-way learning processes is further diminished. The success of many PEC projects has been shown to depend on changed attitudes by outside 'experts'.[45] Many development projects fail not because they were the wrong projects but because of the inadequacies in the knowledge of the implementors as to the local context and the needs and priorities of local women and men of all ages, classes and ethnic backgrounds. As many outsiders continue to impose their own ideas and have not been trained to acknowledge and elicit the views of poor women and men of all ages, individually or collectively, training is essential.

Project professionals must learn to work closely with rural and urban dwellers as well as with colleagues from different disciplines or sectors. This will mean emphasizing judgement and communication skills through the use of participatory methods. Where the skills are lacking, the success of PEC may be threatened. Or the scaling up of support for PEC may prove particularly problematic because too few staff know how to work with low-income communities.

In such cases there is a role for training and the better dissemination of new ideas. Training and education in interpersonal skills must also be accompanied by the use of new economic, environmental and social assessment tools. It is very common for benefit-cost ratios and economic rates of return to be overestimated at a project's inception, largely because appropriate tools for valuation are not available and because unrealistic growth rates are set.[46] Environmental and social impact analyses often fail to anticipate major problems. Professionals also need regular training and involvement in the application of flexible methods for assessment, to allow them to be responsive to the dynamic nature of the participatory process and hence the changing nature of the intervention.

The impact of attitude change on NGOs and government bureaucracies has been significant. The adoption of PEC methods by institutions has challenged corrupt and unaccountable bureaucrats, narrowly focused specialists, unfocused activists, and top-down planners there.[47] It has also been shown that such an approach can effectively substitute for shortages in external capital and technology by catalysing the release of many local unused or underutilized local resources and enhancing the synergy between different sectoral actions – see below.

External agencies should also support *community-to-community exchanges*. The best educators are often the rural or urban women and men who developed PEC initiatives in other locations, so innovative extension methods promote group demonstrations, visits, workshops and farmer-to-farmer, organizer-to-organizer and builder-to-builder extension to achieve effective multiplication. For instance, in Barrio San Jorge, described in Box 6.7, elected community leaders are working with IIED-América Latina's technical support team in advising those living in other low-income settlements nearby about initiating comparable development programmes. Another example of a community-to-community exchange is one between representatives from community organizations in South Africa and Bombay, India. They have spent time in each other's city to learn from each other about how to address housing problems in urban areas. This exchange has been between members of the People's Dialogue in South Africa, a national network linking representatives from illegal and informal settlements and the National Slum Dwellers Federation and *Mahila Milan* (a federation of women's collectives) in India.[48]

Project staff can take on the role of bringing interested groups together and facilitating the process of information exchange.[49] Within urban centres, informal or formal coalitions or federations of community organizations have also contributed to this. This provides crucial leadership experience for villagers and urban dwellers and sets examples for future cooperation and extension practice.

Financial Assistance

For governments and aid agencies, providing financial assistance to PEC initiatives does not necessarily imply increased funding commitments but it does imply changes in the ways in which choices are made (and who is involved in making choices), resources are marshalled and deployed, and how external funding is used. Interventions that are so often considered 'too expensive' by external funding agencies turn out to require much less funding than they thought, as local knowledge and local contributions reduce the costs of construction, operation and maintenance and local organizations negotiate support from local sources. In addition, as costs per person come down, so too do the possibilities of partial or total cost recovery, even from low-income beneficiaries. This is especially the case in initiatives that bring obvious and immediate benefits in terms of improved health and reduced work-loads, as well as initiatives that increase incomes, and where repayments for capital costs can be spread over extended periods. The examples in this subsection are drawn primarily from initiatives to improve housing and living conditions and basic services, such as water and sanitation, as these are often considered by external agencies to be too expensive for them to fund.

In general, PEC initiatives keep down the need for external funding by:

- making maximum use of local resources;
- keeping down capital costs;
- drawing on local willingness to pay;
- ensuring that repayment schedules and procedures are affordable and flexible;
- supporting increased incomes; and
- reducing the costs of operation, maintenance and repair.

Making maximum use of local resources
Perhaps the most critical resource for PEC is the commitment, energy, innovation and managerial capacity of local groups. The scale of funding that low-income households and their local organizations can bring to any new initiative will inevitably be limited, but the monetary value that they are able to contribute can be very large, if one considers the costs saved by not having to pay consultants, contractors and government or aid agency staff to do the tasks they can undertake, provide the knowledge they can bring, provide the mass labour inputs they can organize for specific tasks needing such inputs, and provide the management for many aspects of the construction, operation and maintenance.

Many of the successful initiatives described in boxes in this chapter did not draw on aid budgets at all but relied on resources that the local inhabitants could contribute and achieved significant improvements in liveli-hoods and health and in environmental management without external funding. In other instances, the capital required from external sources was much lower than in conventional, externally funded projects. For instance, the cost of the lane sewers per dwelling served described in Box 6.3 that were constructed by the inhabitants of Orangi with technical support from the local NGO, the OPP was one-fifth to one-sixth of the cost, if these sewers had been installed by the Karachi Municipal Corporation.[50] These savings were achieved through a number of factors. Lane committees of local resi-dents organized the collection and finance and managed the work, absorbing any associated management costs. The technology (designed by the OPP) was low-cost and could be implemented by local construction workers. The lane committees employed workers from the settlement (or completed part of the work with voluntary labour) and negotiated in order to keep costs down. Ten years after some of the first lane sanitation was installed, OPP monitoring has shown that the residents regularly clean and maintain their investment.[51]

When funding is needed from external resources, the amount of such funding can be reduced either through contributions made by the inhabi-tants or contributions negotiated from local sources. For instance, the funding needed from aid agencies to support the many initiatives in Barrio San Jorge (Box 6.7) has been much reduced by the contributions made by local inhabitants in construction, organization and management and by the growing capacity of the settlement's organization to negotiate resources from local authorities and other sources in Argentina. In the pre-school education component of the Slum Improvement Programme in Indore (India), the parents of all children contribute to the costs. In a small number of settlements, the neighbourhood committee has taken over responsibility for financing and managing the direct costs of the pre-school provision.[52]

Keeping down capital costs

Capital costs can be kept down not only by drawing on all available local resources but also by choosing less expensive options. In many instances, very small investments are needed – for instance to protect a spring or help ensure better protection of a well. Capital costs are generally higher in ille-gal or informal settlements in urban areas, but the average cost of providing a household with water piped to their house or house-plot and high qual-ity sanitation (eg connection to a shallow or small bore sewer) will generally fall in the range of US$300–600.[53] The lower end of this estimate is gener-ally achieved in places where each household helps reduce costs – for instance by helping to dig the ditches for pipes and drains – and where local organizations manage the whole process to keep to a minimum the work that needs to be done by contractors. Where safe, convenient and accessible sanitation can be provided by well designed latrines – for instance where soil conditions permit and where densities are not too high and each house plot can accommodate such a latrine, including provision for emptying it – the capital cost of much improved sanitation can be less than $100 per household – see Table 6.2.

Table 6.2 *Typical Range of Capital Costs per Household of Alternative Sanitation Systems (1990 prices)*

Type of System	US$
Twin pit pour-flush latrines	75–150
Ventilated improved pit latrine	68–175
Shallow sewerage	100–325
Small-bore sewerage	150–500
Conventional septic tanks	200–600
Conventional sewerage	600–1200

Notes: Capital costs alone cannot provide a meaningful basis for determining the cost of a system since some systems are more expensive than others to operate and maintain. What must be determined are the total discounted capital, operation and maintenance costs for each household to determine the charge that must be levied for the service and also to establish that households can afford to pay this amount.

Source: Sinnatamby, Gehan (1990), 'Low cost sanitation' in Jorge E. Hardoy et al (Eds), The Poor Die Young: Housing and Health in Third World Cities, *Earthscan, London*

The costs per household of installing site drains can often be much reduced if combined with road construction and integrated into the road design. Many programmes to upgrade illegal or informal settlements have found that there is a considerable cost saving per household served from undertaking a combination of improvements – for instance installing water pipes, sewers, drains, electricity cables and paving roads together – compared to the cost of installing each of these separately.[*] For instance, in India, the cost of a comprehensive upgrading with public standpipes, improved pit latrines, storm drains incorporated into improved (paved) roads, a lined sullage drain and overhead electricity cables costs from $38 to $60 per household per year – including capital, operation, maintenance and replacement costs.[54]

Many NGO programmes are also showing new ways of keeping down costs, especially as individual household or community efforts take over work that would otherwise be done by contractors (who often make high profits on work contracted from aid agencies or public authorities). For instance, the toilet blocks[**] developed in Bombay by *Mahila Milan*, SPARC (Society for the Promotion of Area Resource Centres) and the National Slum Dwellers Federation have demonstrated how low-income communities can build these blocks much cheaper than private contractors and also generate income from those using them to pay for the cost of cleaning and maintaining them.[55]

---

[*] One problem with many externally directed upgrading programmes has been the failure to ensure that provision would be made to repair and maintain the new infrastructure – which is linked to the failure of the implementing agencies to work with local organizations in designing and implementing the upgrading.

[**] Communal toilet blocks were preferred to individual connections by low income groups because their houses were so small that it was difficult to incorporate toilets and washing facilities within existing homes and because communal toilet blocks were much cheaper.

The South African Homeless People's Federation can build a two bedroom house through mutual self-help (although each household involved does most of the work on the house that is to be theirs) for around a third of the price that a private contractor would charge.[56] The Chilean NGO *Hogar de Cristo* developed its own construction company for prefabricated panel housing units because this greatly reduced the cost of each unit – and these are units that low-income households can assemble rapidly and are also easily upgraded.[57] These allow among the lowest-income households to obtain their own housing with part of the costs recovered through a complementary loan programme; by 1995, more than 200,000 units had been built.[58]

In addition, if low-income groups and their representative organizations are fully involved in planning and management and if achieving cost-reductions mean that either they have to pay less back or can do more with a set sum of funding, they will find ways of saving money that no contractor or external funding agency is interested in. For instance, there are examples of community organizations negotiating with municipal authorities to borrow municipal equipment to dig drainage ditches or improve internal roads during holidays with the community paying the additional costs involved such as the wages of the municipal workers who operate the equipment and the fuel costs. This can be much cheaper than hiring such equipment from a contractor. In Dar es Salaam, for example, the community organization in Kijitonyama borrowed equipment from the municipality (paying only for the fuel) in order to rationalize individual water connections and improve access to the settlement by reducing flooding.[59]

The costs of new housing can also be much reduced per unit through good site design. Part of this comes from savings on land costs through smaller building lots and less space allocated to roads or other public or semi-public space that is not needed. Part of it comes from plot sizes, shapes and layouts that keep to a minimum the costs per plot of providing piped water, site drainage, sewers (or other forms of sanitation), roads and paths – and significant savings can be achieved per household with different site designs which have exactly the same number of plots of the same size within the same land development.[60] Obviously, the cost savings that are possible through such measures must be fully discussed with low-income households so their needs and priorities in terms of plot size and shape, overall site layout and extent, size and location of public space are incorporated in the final design.

The cost of building, improving or extending housing can be much reduced if the cost of building materials, fixtures and fittings and of getting them to the house site can be reduced. These costs can represent most of the total costs for low-income households who are undertaking most of the building themselves and have acquired a land site for the house free or relatively cheaply.* Community schemes to buy building materials in bulk at wholesale prices or to make some materials themselves can bring major cost savings. In addition, having a small warehouse or store with building

---

* In urban areas, low-income households often find ways of obtaining land relatively cheaply as they occupy it illegally or purchase an illegal subdivision; however, it is also evident that illegal land markets have become highly commercialized in many cities where illegal subdividers or illegal land brokers have pushed land prices beyond what most low income households can afford.

materials within a low-income settlement managed by the community can also mean that individual households do not have to arrange transport to obtain materials (which is often expensive) and the warehouse or store can also be open in the evenings and at week-ends when much self-help work takes place and when most conventional building suppliers are closed. Developing such a building materials warehouse within Barrio San Jorge (see Box 6.7) has not only meant cheaper building materials but also that local firms selling building materials have dropped their prices and provided better services for building material delivery.[61] The Carvajal Foundation took a slightly different approach by locating a warehouse in the middle of a squatter area which allowed producers of construction materials to rent space and sell their products at wholesale prices.[62]

Costs can also be saved on house construction when materials are reused. One of the ways in which the South African Homeless People's Federation save money is through reusing old materials, and fixtures and fittings wherever possible. The same strategy has been used in Namibia and, with finance obtained through the Building Together Programme, women have been able to build one-room houses with a toilet for less than one fifth of the cost that the government would have had to pay.[63]

Inevitably, when low-income households know that their only possibility of obtaining funding for improving housing and living conditions and basic services is through schemes where there has to be repayment, they will find many ways of reducing capital costs or of doing more with a set capital sum. As a later section will describe, the constraints on the provision of such funding lie much more with external funders.

Drawing on local willingness to pay

External agencies often underestimate the amount that low-income households are prepared to pay for improved housing and basic services that provide all household members with safer, more healthy living conditions. This means that they assume that the cost per household of providing households with water piped into their home or yard and safer, more convenient, forms of sanitation are too high for low-income areas. However, many low-income households are prepared to pay a considerable proportion of their income for water piped to their yard (or into the house) and for good quality sanitation and drainage. For instance, surveys in Zimbabwe found that people were prepared to pay 2.3 times as much for yard connections as they were for standpipes.[64] It is often the case for households in which one or more member (usually women and children) has to spend considerable amounts of time fetching and carrying water – as noted earlier, it is so easy for external professionals to underestimate the time and effort needed to fetch and carry water from standpipes, or from water vendors or other water sources outside the house or yard. This is especially the case for households who are already paying a high price for water which has to be purchased from local vendors.

In many instances, especially in urban areas, the cost of installing and running a much improved piped water system can be fully repaid in a relatively short period through charging households no more than they previously paid to water vendors.[65] For instance, in Guatemala City, a community-managed well and piped water distribution system set up in *El Mesquital*, a low income settlement, cost $100 per family served and once all house connections are completed, revenues are likely to exceed costs with surplus revenue available for other community projects. The new water supply also meant households paying between 25 and 60 per cent less than they had previously paid for water from other sources.[66]

Governments and international agencies have generally proved very reluctant to provide loans to low-income households to allow them to purchase, build or extend their homes and to help cover the cost of improved water supplies, sanitation and drainage or of paying connection charges to water authorities or companies. Even where housing loans are available, they are generally provided on the assumption that the person obtaining the loan is purchasing a house. There are no smaller, shorter-term loans available for people who want to improve or extend their existing home, yet this is much the most common way through which low-income households can obtain better quality housing. The procedures that households have to go through to get a loan and the loan conditions they have to meet often disqualify most low-income households from obtaining loans. And external agencies often make assumptions about what local inhabitants can pay, based on some 'rule of thumb' – for instance, that housing costs must not exceed 25 per cent of incomes (so housing loans are restricted in size by this assumption). These can prove misleading in terms of what low-income households want and what they are prepared to pay for. Certain households are prepared to pay more than 25 per cent of their incomes for a housing loan for certain periods of their lives, if this allows them to become an owner-occupier; it may even be that they were previously paying more than this to rent accommodation. Loans for households to improve or extend their house not only increases the value of what is usually much their most valuable asset but can also permit them to increase their income – for instance by allowing income-earning activities within the home or the addition or conversion of rooms for renting out.

Despite the reluctance of most governments and international funding agencies to consider loans as a way of supporting improved housing conditions and basic service provision among low-income households, there are many examples of successful loan programmes. These can be divided into two. The first are loans provided to individual households to allow them to improve or extend their housing, including paying for improved water supply, sanitation or drainage – with these households responsible for repayments to the funding institution. The second are loans provided to community or neighbourhood organizations for settlement-wide improvements – with the local organizations having responsibility for collecting repayments from each household. There are many examples of NGOs or foundations in the South developing such loan programmes, although programmes providing loans to individual households are more common.

While the provision of loans requires considerable capital sums in advance, it can lead to self-sustaining funding systems as repayments come to fund new loans. Many NGOs have run successful housing-loan programmes both for households wanting to improve or extend their housing and for households seeking to purchase a unit or purchase land and materials and organize the construction themselves – and in so doing, have achieved very high levels of loan repayment.[67] A few have also achieved a considerable scale – for instance the Grameen Bank in Bangladesh which is best known for its loan programme for income generation also has a housing-loan programme which by May 1995 had reached over 300,000 households.[68] The Costa Rican NGO, FUPROVI, achieved high levels of cost recovery from its loan programme that has supported both new housing units and the upgrading of existing housing units.[69] By 1995, the El Salvador NGO, FUNDASAL, had supported the construction or improvement of over 25,000 housing units, much of it implemented through mutual help groups, and although it only supports low-income households, it recovers a proportion of the costs through loans.[70]

Many recent government programmes have drawn on this NGO experience to fund loans for individual housing – but also loans to fund community initiatives or community improvements in urban areas. Examples include the work of the National Fund for Low-income Housing (FONHAPO) in Mexico in the early 1980s, the Mutirao Programme's work in Fortaleza and the community initiatives supported by the Urban Community Development Office in Thailand; each has achieved or is achieving significant levels of cost recovery from low-income groups while also greatly improving housing and living conditions and basic services.[71]

Ensuring that repayment schedules and procedures are affordable and flexible and keep down costs
The extent to which relatively low-income households are able and willing to make regular payments for loans is much influenced by the extent to which repayment schedules and procedures meet their needs. The fact that so many of the housing-loan programmes for low-income households mentioned above managed to achieve very low levels of loan default show that low-income households can make regular repayments. Obviously, the overall cost of housing-loan programmes and thus the amount that needs to be charged to each person with a loan is kept down by having a very low level of loan default.

In addition, if the initial capital costs can be kept down and households can repay the costs over a number of years, the proportion of households able to pay for significant improvements in water supply, sanitation and drainage *increases dramatically*. For instance, if major improvements in the provision for water, sanitation and drainage can be achieved for between US$300–600 (as is usually the case, especially where all efforts are made to keep down capital costs) the capital cost per household may seem far beyond the means of most low-income households. But if a household can repay the capital cost over a ten year period in a single weekly or monthly payment that also covers operation and maintenance, the extent of possible cost recovery becomes much greater. Special arrangements can also be made to help those who face some crisis or unexpected problem from defaulting on their interest payments.[72]

Supporting increased incomes

PEC initiatives always try to include more stable or adequate livelihoods for low-income groups, even if the main goals of many initiatives are better environmental management or improved health. For instance, in the many illegal or informal settlements in cities that are inaccessible to garbage trucks, community-based collection systems can cost no more per person served than a conventional garbage collection service. If municipal authorities are prepared to fund community-based systems, this also means some paid employment within the community. Such community-based systems can often include the collection and sale of reusable or recyclable materials and the composting of organic wastes, which can further increase local employment generation.

However, it may be that the less direct benefits or the benefits whose economic value is less easily quantified are more important. For instance, improved housing and living conditions that translate into improved health and less injury bring not only direct cost savings and less time off work but benefits whose economic value is obvious but not easily measured. For instance, improved health and less injury means reduced costs in medicines and treatment and also less time off work for income earners and for adults who are taking care of the household members who are sick or injured. But healthier children also miss school less and learn more. Healthier children also mean less stress for parents or carers – not least as sick infants or children often have to be attended to several times during the night by adults who then also have to work long hours at arduous tasks during the day. Water supply piped into each household's yard or home can considerably reduce the domestic workload of those responsible for collecting water, washing, laundry and cooking, which may also mean more possibility of income earning.

Projects may be used to improve local skills and therefore incomes. In the case of the toilet block project developed in Bombay by *Mahila Milan*, SPARC and the National Slum Dwellers Federation, women construction workers were given additional skills and increased their wages by 200 per cent from Rs 40 (£0.87) a day to Rs 120 (£2.37).[73] In Rio de Janeiro, the Nova Hollanda settlement developed a building materials cooperative to sell materials both to members and to other residents. The municipality agreed to supply them with the raw materials they needed in return for a guaranteed number of bricks each month.

Reduced costs of repair and rehabilitation

All aid agencies and development banks and many government agencies in the South have considerable problems ensuring that public buildings and facilities and infrastructure and services are maintained. Although the debate about sustainable development has grown to encompass much more than this, part of the origin for this term was the desire of international funding agencies to ensure that what their projects had built were 'sustained' at the end of the project.[74] A considerable proportion of all project aid during the 1980s was spent on rehabilitating the roads, hospitals, higher education institutions, power stations, ports and other forms of infrastructure built with project aid in the previous decade.[75] PEC initiatives should not only have better provision for maintenance but also keep down costs as most or all maintenance and repair can be handled by local specialists.

Financial Disadvantages for Funding Agencies

From the perspective of agencies who fund projects, PEC may appear to have some financial disadvantages. It is low-key, so the capacity to absorb funds does not seem high initially. It poses serious problems in terms of administration and monitoring, given the multiplicity of small initiatives that it seeks to support. Box 6.13 contrasts the characteristics of many successful community-based projects with the characteristics which make implementation easier for external funding agencies; the difficulties in reconciling the two are obvious.

PEC projects may require a greater proportion of total funding in the early stages, when investment is directed to building human and institutional capacities. PEC may also entail investment in experimental activities and, due to its community level focus, it does not primarily stimulate production for export. However, by adopting a national PEC policy and ensuring that it multiplies beyond small pockets of success, it would be possible to stimulate production on a larger scale, renewing export opportunities.

Since support for PEC implies support to a great variety of very different kinds of initiative, and the external capital funding needed to support many initiatives will be relatively small, the costs of personnel relative to 'funding for projects' will rise as the staff of external agencies have to spend more time with the people who are developing local initiatives – including time spent on monitoring and evaluation. Costs spent on personnel which ensure sound initiatives that reflect the needs and priorities of local inhabitants and that develop within a time-frame that best meets their needs should be well spent as the success rate of projects supported increases. Furthermore, if parallel spending on infrastructure that supports PEC, such as roads, markets, water development for agriculture and for domestic use, support for sanitation and site drainage is coordinated with PEC initiatives, these can help absorb some of the personnel costs.

However, it would be naïve not to recognize the political and administrative constraints which most international funding agencies and many government agencies face in being able to support a great number of diverse projects, most of which require relatively small sums of external funding, many of which will be staff intensive relative to total costs and many of which require local structures to encourage cost recovery. Multilateral development banks may face the greatest constraints, as their whole institutional structure is set up to fund large capital projects through recipient governments. And as in all banks, one of the key measures of 'efficiency' is how low staff costs are kept relative to total lending. Most such multilateral agencies also have a high concentration of their staff in their head office, few technical staff based in the countries where most of their funding is spent and very few staff with knowledge and experience in the kind of participatory dialogue with communities that support for PEC requires. Their whole institutional framework dates from the time when the 'solution' to development was seen as development banks providing

Box 6.13 **The Most Important Aid Project Characteristics from Two Different Viewpoints**

Characteristics of many successful projects from the beneficiaries' perspective	*Characteristics of projects which are easily implemented by external funding agency*
Small scale and multi-sectoral – addressing multiple needs of poorer groups	Large scale and single sector
Implementation over many years – less of a project and more of a longer term continuous process to improve housing and living conditions	Rapid implementation (internal evaluations of staff performance in funding agencies often based on volume of funding supervised)
Substantial involvement of local people (and usually their own community organizations) in project design and implementation	Project designed by agency staff (usually in offices in Europe or North America) or by consultants from funding agency's own nation
Project implemented collaboratively with beneficiaries, their local government and certain national agencies	Project implemented by one construction company or government agency
High ratio of staff costs to total project cost	Low ratio of staff costs to total project cost
Difficult to evaluate using conventional cost-benefit analysis	Easy to evaluate
Little or no direct import of goods or services from abroad	High degree of import of goods or services from funding agency's own nation

Source: Chapter 7 of Hardoy, Jorge E. Diana Mitlin and David Satterthwaite, Environmental Problems in Third World Cities, *Earthscan, London, 1992*

the capital flows for productive investment and the infrastructure to support it, coupled with technical assistance that was the transfer of 'western' know-how – in effect the exact opposite of support for PEC. Although such agencies have recognized the need for change, their institutional structures still remain largely unchanged.

The large official bilateral agencies also face major difficulties in supporting a large multiplicity of small and continuous PEC processes. Most are also highly centralized with most of their specialist and technical staff based in their head offices. Most also have an institution that still in its form is better suited to the 1960s conception of aid as large capital sums

215

and 'technical assistance'. Most are under great political pressure to keep down their staff costs, relative to total funding flows. There still remains this perception among the government ministries or agencies that oversee aid programmes and the general public in the North that an efficient aid agency is one that keeps its staff costs to a minimum. One of the main criteria still used to measure the 'effectiveness' of official and private aid agencies is the ratio of their staff costs to project funding. Large capital projects are usually the best means to keep down staff costs. They make it much easier for a funding agency that has to disburse large sums with limited staff.

One partial solution to this – which many agencies have adopted – is to incorporate the staff costs of particular projects into the cost of the project, rather than include it separately as personnel costs. Another is to increase the proportion of staff within offices in the recipient nation – but if such staff are largely specialists from the donor country, this is also very expensive. Many of the official bilateral agencies are not permitted to hire many professional staff or senior staff from people from the recipient country. Many government agencies and most official bilateral and multilateral agencies also lack the staff 'on the ground' with the knowledge and experience of working in participatory ways with local initaitives. In addition, the rapid throughput of such staff in any country also prevents the building up of local knowledge and experience.

The lack of staff 'on the ground', the need to spend large sums of money and the need to keep down staff costs biases most funding agencies against funding PEC. Some examples have already been given as to how much low-income groups and their organizations can achieve with small amounts of external funding. But it did not do justice to the range of ways and means by which households and community organizations can keep down costs, if it is in their interests to do so. They will not strive to keep down costs if the incentive framework does not encourage them to do so. When there are possibilities of external funding to support a new initiative, if the inhabitants do not have to repay the costs they will prefer the most comprehensive (and expensive) solution implemented by external contractors. But most external funding agencies are poorly equipped to support the cheapest solutions where there is some cost recovery and where their funding is distributed around a great number of initiatives, each developed in partnership with the inhabitants.

Most agencies also lack the staff and financial and accounting structure to encourage and support cost recovery from the projects they fund. Even if loans are provided by official bilateral and multilateral agencies, this does not mean that the activity funded has to generate the cost recovery.

Most international aid agencies or multilateral banks have supported many projects that showed a very poor understanding of the environment and the complex local environmental management practices of local farmers. Box 6.14 considers the role of 'experts' in water management in Africa. As a consequence of the projects 'experts' helped design and implement, many farmers have faced increasing problems in meeting the basic needs of their households. The impacts include: crop failure from reduced downstream river flow, resettlement due to reservoir construction, lower fish

Box 6.14 **Role of 'Experts' in Water Management in Africa**

The environment of Africa is complex, unpredictable and often harsh. These are not facts which would surprise a Rendille herder in northern Kenya or an Ewe fisherman on the River Volta. They should not surprise those who presume to enter Africa to transform the environment in the name of 'development' of water resources, although, sadly they often do.

The future for African rural people must be based on the informal skills of local people, organized and directed in concerned political and practical action by those people themselves. Development is what those people will do with the resources and ideas at their disposal. Development planning must be something they control. Outsiders must come as equals to meet with local people face to face, and must seek to facilitate and not dominate.

But the development of Africa has always been driven by outsiders. This is true not simply in the sense that economic power in colonial and independent Africa have lain outside the continent but also in the power to define goals, to make plans and spend money. Indeed, the power to define the meaning of development itself has long been in the hands of strangers.

Both government and aid-agency decision makers depend on the reports of consultants. These 'experts' usually come from the First World. They have their own preconceptions, built up from their education, the views commonly accepted by their peers and the ideas that have proved acceptable to other clients on previous missions. The chief failure of outside development agencies and those that work for them has not been that they make mistakes but that they have (by and large) been so bad at learning from them. Furthermore, many of the mistakes of the past were caused by attitudes, ideas and institutions and economic structures that are still in place. Standard approaches to project planning have proved inapplicable and unsuccessful. The same approaches and institutional structures are unlikely to work much better in the future, no matter how their targets are redefined.

Much rainfall planning has been based on records of this century only. This period represents 'normality' for many of the administrators and planners whose ideas and opinions have created the official view of what is happening in Africa and who have determined the institutional memory of the modern urbanized bureaucrats of the continent. However, the last 60 years is a misleading timeframe within which to view African climate. Rainfall in the past has been much more variable that the recent record might suggest.

Most major African rivers have now been dammed. Most of these dams have been built in the last 30 years and most have been designed using very short runs of discharge data. There are serious problems using such data sets for predictive purposes. Of course, it would be ridiculous to argue that development can only take place when perfect data is available: in Africa this would mean that almost nothing would get done. It does mean that data bases must be maintained and updated and where data are limited or poor, great caution should be exercised by planners. The lack of money and skills in African hydrological organizations means that such work is rarely possible 'in-house' by someone experienced in the region and its problems. The constraints of the consultancy business mean that there is seldom opportunity for visiting 'experts' to build up the real practical experience necessary to interpret the available data property.

Source: Adams, W M (1992), Wasting the Rain: Rivers, People and Planning in Africa, *Earthscan, London*

populations, waterlogged soils and poor health due to diseases associated with standing water.

As they are currently structured, most official bilateral and multilateral agencies cannot allocate a significant proportion of their funding to PEC initiatives. The best possibilities for them doing so are either through intermediary institutions who have the staff with the knowledge and experience to work 'on the ground' or special units within the agencies that have the staff and the incentive structures that allow them to fund a multiplicity of smaller, community-directed initiatives.

Many official donor agencies and most international private voluntary organizations have turned to a much greater collaboration with national and local NGOs in the countries in which they work, to address some of the above issues. Since most international private voluntary organizations have also long had more of their staff outside their head offices and working in the recipient countries, many official donor agencies have also long channelled a proportion of their funding through the international private voluntary organizations from their own country. If support for PEC initiatives is to increase substantially, it is likely that this will involve a greater role for international private voluntary organizations (often as channels through which official bilateral agencies pass funding) and a much greater role for local NGOs or other forms of 'intermediary' institution based in the city or district where the PEC initiatives are supported.

Role of Intermediary Institutions

Local or national NGOs have had important roles in developing many PEC initiatives. They have also had a central role in writing up the case studies that have been used in this book – and in other work about PEC. Although there have been few comprehensive studies of the work that they do, the evidence suggests that such institutions may be key to the successful establishment and scaling up of many initiatives.

Donors supporting PEC have tended to work through NGOs but not exclusively so. Financial support has mainly been through direct grant assistance for specific activities, but also for core and unrestricted support on some occasions. Donor efficiency is improved and the high level of disaggregation maintained, where intermediate organizations or federations pass resources to the many smaller, more local and flexible organizations.[76]

This reliance of both official development assistance agencies and private voluntary organizations on national or local NGOs as the means through which PEC initiatives can be supported also means that the quality and scale of their support is much influenced by the quality of the support that such local and national NGOs can provide. If funding for PEC initiatives is to be increased, so too must attention be directed to ensuring that the intermediary institutions that support this can do so effectively. Many donors currently find it difficult to assess what makes an effective NGO, especially the extent to which that NGO works in participatory ways with low-income groups and their community organizations. Many donors are also reluctant to provide continuous support to PEC type initiatives through particular local or national NGOs. This means that these NGOs are dependent on negotiating project funding or funding for technical support for PEC initiatives on an ad hoc basis. This does not provide a good basis for support-NGOs being able to develop continuous programmes of support for PEC type initiatives.

There is also a particular kind of NGO or intermediary institution that has a key role in expanding support for PEC initiatives. These provide credit and technical and legal advice to PEC initiatives but very often in response to projects initiated by community organizations or groups. As such, they support self-mobilization for PEC. They are 'intermediary' in the sense that they make funding and technical, legal, financial or organizational advice available to individuals or community organizations and draw part of their capital or collateral from national governments or international funding agencies – or sometimes from other sources. An increasing number of case studies of such intermediary organizations (most of them NGOs in Latin America and Asia) show how they are reaching low-income groups with credit and technical advice for income generation, infrastructure and services and housing construction or improvement and achieving high levels of cost recovery; various examples of such institutions are given in boxes in this chapter – and were mentioned in the earlier section on financial assistance.

Donors continue to have a significant role in convening regular feedback meetings with NGOs, in making long-term financial arrangements, in promoting South–South cooperation, in networking with government agencies and NGOs, and in granting local NGOs the freedom to select and hire consultants of their choice. Through these efforts, more emphasis can be placed upon institutional development and building in-country capacity to facilitate PEC.

ACTING ON THE WIDER CONSTRAINTS

If there is to be a large expansion in PEC initiatives, the question as to why such initiatives remain the exception rather than the rule has to be considered. The section above considered the constraints on the capacity of external agencies to support such initiatives. But there are also all the external forces and factors ranged against PEC initiatives. They include the powerful companies and corporations whose interests in mining, logging and major infrastructure projects are certainly not served by giving more power and decision making to local groups. In urban areas, they usually include landowners and real-estate companies, since a considerable proportion of the low-income groups whose environmental health and development needs would be served by PEC initiatives are on land that they are occupying illegally. The whole concept of giving those living in particular localities more right to influence larger scale decisions that affect them also threatens the companies or corporations involved in large scale urban developments – or redevelopments.

Many government agencies concerned with natural resource exploitation and/or management in rural areas and land-use planning and management in urban areas are also unused to the idea that local citizen groups or community organizations have rights to influence their decisions and their mode of operation. As Friedmann and Rangan note, when introducing a series of case studies on environmental action, environmental actions are often as much about the inhabitants in a locality demanding that their voices are heard in decisions about development or environmental management; 'history reveals time and again that powerful groups can empty landscapes by rendering entire communities invisible'.[77]

There are also the international factors that can systematically undermine the capacity of the inhabitants in any particular settlement to work collectively. For instance, a community that invests in improving the productivity of local agriculture may see its efforts destroyed by climate changes caused by atmospheric warming. Similarly, these efforts may be undermined by international systems of production and consumption which, through the use or extraction of local resources for international markets, impact on local agricultural production.[78] Many local environmental problems cannot be dealt with at a local level.

Ironically, an overreliance on market forces and on state directed development are both major constraints on PEC initiatives. An overemphasis on state power and a concentration of decision making in state institutions will inevitably constrain the number, range and scope of PEC initiatives. This can be seen in: inappropriate legislation, state ownership of natural resource assets and a lack of local influence on how funds are spent. Inappropriate legislation often deems illegal the key local initiatives to improve the environment – for instance as people develop their own housing and improve water supply and drainage but not to the standards set in local bye-laws or building and infrastructure codes.

It is now recognized that state ownership of many natural assets may be inappropriate, not only encouraging rapid depletion and unsustainable use but undermining previous, community-based systems for natural resource management. Box 6.15 illustrates the effects of state ownership on forests in India. A lack of local control over how funds are spent resulted in local priorities being neglected in favour of centrally determined investment and expenditure. PEC approaches necessitate a willingness on the

---

Box 6.15 **From Community Management of Forests to State Ownership in India**

Before the advent of the modern state in India, grazing lands, forest lands and water bodies were mostly common property and village communities had an important role in their use and management. The British colonial government was the first to nationalize these resources and bring them under the management of government bureaucracies. The British initiated a policy of converting common property resources into government property resources.

The expropriation has alienated the people from their commons and initiated an informal free-for-all. Today even tribal people, who have lived in harmony with forests for centuries, are so alienated that they feel little compunction in felling a green tree to sell it for a very small return. Their justification is simply that what is the point in saving the forests, because if they do not exploit them first, the forest contractors will take out the trees and gain all the benefits themselves.

Today, nearly one third of India's land and all its water resources are owned by the government. These are government property systems, not community property systems. The result is that the village communities have lost all interest in their management or protection. And as the villagers have realized that the main objective of government management has, in most cases, been to meet urban–industrial needs, their motivation too, is to exploit these resources without any care for the future. This alienation has led to massive denudation of forests, overexploitation of grazing systems and neglect of local water systems. This will only change if the local people are given a stake in the improvement of the natural resource base by reversing the current legal structure of control over natural resources.

Source: Agarwal, Anil and Sunita Narain, 'Towards green villages; a strategy for environmentally sound and participatory rural development in India' Environment and Urbanization *Vol 4, No 1, April 1992.*

---

part of the central state to relinquish power to more locally-based decision making bodies.

The dominance of a market ideology also mitigates against a PEC approach. Market-dominated decision making tends to be short-run and often results in the degradation of natural resources and a failure to invest in resource conservation (including recycling, reuse and reclamation technologies and schemes). Most economic analysis and most economic models do not even include natural resource depletion as a cost.[79] Meanwhile, poorer groups rarely receive much benefit from economic growth because they cannot get access to the capital assets they need to prosper within the market.

Control over natural resources tends to pass to those with greatest access to capital with the majority of those living in low-income communities being excluded. In many instances, this has also meant the people who lost rights over resource use and management were the very people who had had mechanisms to ensure resource conservation and the protection of environmental capital for future generations.[80] Those who control the assets can freely move capital between a large range of different investments; as such, they are likely to maximize short-term profits rather than manage natural resources to obtain a lower but sustainable income. While there has been increasing concern about the inability of market prices to take account of present and future environment costs, there has been no agreed and widespread response to address this problem.

The possibilities for PEC type approaches becoming widespread depend, in effect, on more democratic and more decentralized systems of government. Building a national framework in support of PEC implies also supporting the capacity of local groups and community organizations to acquire more political power, and to confront the forces ranged against them. In some cases, the forces are so large that this can only be done through strategic alliances with a number of other groups sharing common concerns.

Reinforcing Poorer Groups Land Tenure or Use Rights

PEC initiatives concerned with soils, forests, pastures and fisheries cannot become widespread unless users have rights of use that are defined and protected. Stronger and less ambiguous rights of land use, management or tenure are needed for poorer groups, both women and men, and for groups whose traditional rights to use and manage common pool/property resources are being eroded. In many countries, achieving this implies the need to strengthen the rights of traditional user groups or herder associations, since government is too weak to enforce this.

Too little attention has been given to the current and potential role of community-based management systems. In many instances, traditional, community-based resource management systems protected common property resources and it is their erosion by external forces (for instance government appropriation or commercial penetration) which underlies resource degradation.[81] The diversity of commons regimes makes any general conclusions difficult but what they generally share is a degree of local control over resource use and management and a sufficient consensus among different resource users within a culture of shared responsibility to ensure resource management.

Toulmin, Scoones and Bishop note that in dryland Africa, the actual form of tenure that farmers and herders have is probably less important than the extent to which their rights are enforced when conflict arises.[82] In this region, customary land tenure probably provides sufficient incentive for farmers to invest time and money in soil and water conservation, as long as they are sure that their rights to use the land are confirmed when disputes arise. For instance, in irrigated agricultural schemes in Mali, new rules regarding tenure and responsibility for maintenance enabled tenant farmers to retain rights over their irrigated plots and the combination of increased security of land tenure and devolved responsibility to farmer groups plus rehabilitation of irrigation channels help explain the rapid increase in yields per hectare.[83] One of the key problems is that with weak systems of public administration in many poor countries, farmers and herders have no guarantee that the state will protect their rights.[84] In many instances, governments will have to take complementary action to control or halt commercial penetration into pastoral and forested lands.

Successful PEC initiatives in the urban settlements with a predominance of low-income groups often depend on these people acquiring more secure tenure. A high proportion of low-income groups in urban areas live in shelters on illegally occupied or subdivided land and insecure tenure discourages individual investment and community action to improve housing, basic services and other aspects of their residential environment.

Strengthening Control by Local Users

Not only do local people have a strong interest in ensuring the continued productivity of the resource on which their lives (and the lives of their children) depend but, in many countries (especially Africa), there are few other alternatives, given the weakness of local governments and central or state government agencies.[85] Each village or urban neighbourhood needs its own institution which brings together its members to manage its common resources and provide a forum for resolving disputes.[86] External support is often needed to stimulate and support local initiatives and to develop local management.[87] *What has been so lacking in the past is the capacity of such external support to build on local knowledge and management systems, respond to the specifics of each area's people and ecology and remain accountable and transparent to the population.*

Box 6.16 gives an example of the work of the Aga Khan Rural Support Programme in Gilgit, Pakistan, which illustrates how external support built on local knowledge and local priorities. Many other examples can be given of more successful rural and agricultural development programmes whose success is strongly linked to supporting local level decisions and organizations.[88]

The State of World Rural Poverty noted that it may be best to leave pasture management to pastoralists themselves, while bestowing rights to the rural poor to use forested land in return for adopting appropriate conservation investment, cropping patterns and farming technologies.[89] However, there are obvious political obstacles to be overcome in most countries. In discussing how to address problems in dryland Africa, Toulmin, Scoones and Bishop note that governments rarely devolve real power away from the centre and that, to date, making local communities responsible for resource management seems restricted to cases where the government wants to divest itself of certain costly obligations such as borehole maintenance or cleaning out irrigation canals.[90]

More power and responsibilities to local people is often not the whole solution. Traditional systems of common property resource management may have difficulties coping with internal and external stresses – including rising external demand for local goods or local resources and population pressures. In addition, as the interests of different members diverge – for instance as a result of new technologies and new possibilities for commercialization – communal systems of management may come under stress

Box 6.16 **External Support for Local Capacity Building – the Aga Khan Rural Support Programme in Gilgit, Pakistan**

The Aga Khan Rural Support Programme is a non-profit NGO which began work in Gilgit in 1982 with the objective of increasing the capacity of local people to identify and utilize opportunities to address their own problems. It sought to induce local capacity to plan and implement development programmes which would contribute to increased income and employment. The programme was implemented in three districts with a rugged and hilly topography with steep heavily dissected slopes. The landscape is highly irregular due to erosion and landslides. Some 750,000 people in 1030 villages live in an area covering about 70,000 square kilometres. Agriculture is the major economic activity and a wide range of farming systems are evident. Wheat, maize, millet and buckwheat are the major crops and there is very little commercialization and no specialization.

Because of local resource limitations, there is seasonal migration of able bodied men from most households during the winter within the region or down country to work for cash. The three main principles followed in the support programme were: collective management of common property regimes, developed and implemented through a participatory approach; upgrading and creation of appropriate skills by expanding the indigenous knowledge system and providing training to face the new challenges; and capital formation through group savings to undertake new ventures that the traditional subsistence economy did not allow.

Village organizations were established – broad-based coalitions of village residents whose common economic interest is best served by forming a multipurpose development organization. These were formed after a series of diagnostic dialogues undertaken by programme staff and villagers which identified projects for common benefits and considered their feasibility. Technical supervision was provided and the nature of partnership between the support programme and the villagers carefully worked out. Grants were provided for village organizations to execute an irrigation channel, develop link roads or build a storage reservoir. This became the means to create an effective organization for collective management. The work has emphasised increasing productivity and sustainability of natural resources and enhancing villagers' capability to manage supra-village resources. In considering the underlying factors which helped to make this approach effective, the long-established tradition of cooperation, the absence of administrative or political interference and the high proportion of homogenous settlements were other characteristics judged to be important.

Sources: Bajracharya, D (1992), 'Institutional imperatives for sustainable resource management in the mountains', in N S Jodha, M Banskota and Tej Partap, (Eds) Sustainable Mountain Agriculture: Perspectives and Issues *Vol 1, Oxford* and IBH Publishing, New Delhi, pp 205–234, drawing from Husain, T, A Jan and F Mahmood (1990), Village Management Systems and the Role of the Aga Khan Rural Support Programme in Northern Pakistan, *MPE Series No 10*, ICIMOD, Kathmandu; World Bank (1987), The Aga Khan Rural Support Program in Pakistan; an Interim Evaluation, *Operations Evaluations Department*, World Bank, Washington DC; and World Bank (1990), The Aga Khan Rural Support Program in Pakistan; Second Interim Evaluation, *Operations Evaluations Department*, World Bank, Washington, DC.

and break down. The social and economic basis for collective control are eroding in many instances[91] and policies must be based on a recognition of the limits and opportunities of local management.

Anil Agarwal and Sunita Narain describe the failure of the village *panchayats* in India (the lowest level of local government) to promote good natural resource management and stress the need for effective institutions within each village; one reason is that each *panchayat* often has within it several villages or hamlets and environmental management mediated through the *panchayats* often lead to inter-settlement tension.[92] The two key roles of the state suggested for dryland Africa are in providing an appropriate legal framework to permit and support local control and improving the economic incentives for desirable management practices.[93] These are roles which are also appropriate in other regions. Box 6.17 presents some conditions for successful collective action based on the author's experience with common property resource management in South India.[94]

New Incentive Frameworks

National and state level incentive frameworks need to be adjusted or changed so they reward and support PEC type initiatives and no longer support or subsidize actions that work against PEC. Thus, for agriculture, pastoralism and forestry, the incentive framework increases returns for smallholders, rewards their investments in soil and water conservation and good farming or forestry and pastoral management, and removes the explicit and implicit policy influences which encourage resource degradation. Such a framework must also permit local solutions to be developed which build on people's traditional knowledge and management practices, although also provide the methods and incentives which can help these cope with increased commercial pressures and perhaps population pressures. In urban areas, far more consideration is given by municipal authorities and funding agencies to supporting the initiatives of community or neighbourhood organizations to improve their living environment. This is especially important where resources are too limited to permit public or private utilities to provide all settlements with a basic level of water supply, sanitation, drainage and garbage collection.

Its implementation has to be within a participatory, resource-conservation oriented development strategy so that extension services and technical support are provided in ways which permit farmers and pastoralists to take an active role in developing technical and institutional solutions which

Box 6.17 Conditions for Successful Collective Action, Based on Experiences with Common Property Management in South India

Resources: The smaller and more clearly defined the boundaries of the common resources, the greater the chances of success.

Technology: The higher the costs of exclusion technology (such as fencing), the better the chances of success.

Relations between resources and users:

Location: the greater the overlap between the location of the common-pool resources and the residence of the users, the greater the chances of success.

Users' demands: the greater the demands (up to a limit) and the more vital the resource for survival, the greater the chances of success.

Users' knowledge: the more users know about sustainable yields, the greater the chance of success.

Characteristics of users:

Size: the smaller the number of users, the better the chances of success. However, there is a minimum number below which the tasks able to be performed by such a small group cease to be meaningful.

Boundaries: the more clearly defined the boundaries of the group, the better the chance of success.

Relative power of subgroups: the more powerful are those who benefit from retaining the commons and the weaker are those who favour enclosing private property, the better the chances of success.

Existing arrangements for discussion of common problems: the more concerned people are about their social reputations, the better the chance of success.

Noticeability: The more noticeable is cheating on agreements, the better the chances of success. Noticeability is a function partly of how clearly defined are the resource boundaries, how near they are to users' residencies and how large is the group of users.

Relations between users and the state: The less the State can or wishes to undermine locally based authorities and the less it can enforce private property rights effectively, the better the chances of success.

Source: Wade, R (1987), 'The management of common property resources; finding a cooperative solution', The World Bank Research Observer Vol 2, No 2, July, pp 219–234, quoted in Bajracharya, D (1992), 'Institutional imperatives for sustainable resource management in the mountains, in N.S. Jodha, M. Banskota and Tej Partap (Eds), Sustainable Mountain Agriculture: Perspectives and Issues Vol 1, Oxford and IBH Publishing, New Delhi, pp 205–234.

address their specific needs within their ecological context.[95] But this also implies something more fundamental in that it requires a greater official recognition of the validity and utility of traditional/local knowledge and institutional structures for applying it. To be effective, such a recognition cannot only be within agricultural or forestry extension officers. It must also be accepted within the education system. At present, the formal education system is often undermining or discouraging traditional knowledge rather than integrating it and indeed involving students in learning more about it.

Local Government

Local government has great potential as an enabler and supporter of PEC initiatives. It can adjust policies to the local context and (in theory) respond more quickly than national or international institutions to local needs and demands. While the interest of central government may be viewed as antagonistic to local interest groups, the relations with local government are less clear cut, especially where local governments are democratic. However, in most countries in the South, local government is weak, inefficient and lacking a secure funding base – and certainly lacking in staff with the skills and knowledge to support PEC initiatives.[96] In many instances, it remains unrepresentative. It is also common for higher levels of government to give local governments little financial independence and often deny them the right or the capacity to raise local funds for local use. Without the resources to operate effectively, the capacity of local governments to support PEC initiatives will always be limited.

Another problem is inevitably the reluctance of many local government institutions to relinquish the right to make decisions and to implement policies on their own. One of the attributes of successful PEC approaches is 'the participation of local people in all stages of planning, management and monitoring'. But officials often wish to retain their traditional control. Such officials may have been coopted by local elites and continue to support their position. On occasion, higher level officials may be convinced of the need for new approaches but local level staff still resist such changes.

National Government

A nation's legislation sets the framework within which people's right to own or use resources is defined. National government determines the balance between the rights of individual women and men, communities and the state over land ownership and rights of use – although this is often rooted in historical factors and difficult to change, not least because of the conservative nature of the legal profession and the power of the vested interests whose interests are served under current legislation. But it is also national government that determines the extent to which this legal basis is followed and applied. The government also determines whether certain areas should be protected from development and whether foreign investment to exploit natural resources should be encouraged or constrained.

In the context of PEC, it is important that the legal system is such that it supports and maintains the rights of low-income communities to obtain access to the environmental resources they require.[97] Communities who know that they are at risk of eviction or of exclusion from what were common property or open access resources in both rural and urban areas are unlikely to prioritize those improvements which bring major environmental benefits but which require major effort and/or investment. For instance, no urban community is likely to develop their own community-wide solution to problems of drainage and improved water supplies if they are threatened with eviction in the near future. Communities whose rights to occupy or use land are ambiguously defined have less reason to practise sustainable cultivation practices.

Legal frameworks should focus on the unambiguous definition of land ownership, tenancy and use rights for farmers, pastoralists and urban dwellers to provide the owners or users with the security to foster long-term investments which help in sustainable management. But such legislation and its implementation will also have to be 'pro-poor' and 'pro-users' in that, without this, it would simply reinforce the power of landowners. Legal frameworks should also ensure the implementation of appropriate regulations to prevent pollution (which so often degrades open access or common property resources to the detriment of many users) and other resource-degrading activities.

National governments' macro-economic policies have a persistent and comprehensive impact on the lives of most low-income communities. Exchange rates influence the relative prices of domestic and imported goods (including food). Taxes and subsidies affect income levels and thus the scale of expenditure on different goods. Interest rates influence the returns from investment and saving. Macro-economic policies affect the political and economic context within which low-income women and men struggle for the survival of their households. The impacts are both direct, affecting poorer groups' incomes and the costs of many goods and services and indirect, impacting on the environment from which and within which they secure their livelihoods. The major paths by which macro-economic and sectoral policies impact on the environment are summarized in Box 6.18.

Economic policies should be designed and adjusted to promote PEC. This implies: action on distorting subsidies that foster the waste of resources; targeting of subsidies to the poor in ways which address their most pressing needs and the elimination of those subsidies which primarily benefit wealthier groups (who have the political power to capture them); the application of charges to those who pollute or damage the environment; and attention to pricing policies that encourage resource-enhancing rather than degrading activities. Conventional development policies have clearly failed to promote a sustainable use of natural resources; in many cases, they have been based on the unsustainable exploitation of natural resources.

International Aspects

This chapter began by noting the importance of allowing and supporting the knowledge and capacity of local groups to act collectively in environmental management and development initiatives. The term PEC was given to the process by which local groups acquire (or recapture) the power to address their own development needs within systems of resource use and

Box 6.18 **Macro-economic and Sectoral Policies and the Environment**

Macro-economic policy

Fiscal	Government expenditure	Publicly funded agencies may protect biologically unique areas; public works (roads and dams) may encourage land uses that degrade fragile areas.
	Tax/subsidy	Multisectoral action may alter general demand conditions and thus the total consumption of resources.
Monetary	Monetary	Credit restrictions can have similar effects to tax/subsidy; credit rationing and interest rate increases may reduce demand but also make investment in conservation more expensive.
International	Exchange rate	Devaluation will increase prices of imports and raise profitability of exports; the environmental effects will depend on the resources and products affected.
	Trade	Import/export taxes and quotas will alter the price of particular commodities; the environmental effect will depend on the resources and products affected.
	Capital controls	If used to maintain overvalued currency, they will reduce the prices of imports and the profitability of exports will fall; the environmental effect will depend on the resources and products affected.

Sectoral policy

	Price controls	They may be used to stimulate or retard environmentally damaging production; the environmental effect will depend on the resources and products affected.
	Tax/subsidy	They will have indirect effects through changes in aggregate demand; they may also be used to alter the choice of inputs and outputs through changes in relative prices (eg fertilizer subsidies).

Source: Adapted from Bishop, J et al, Guidelines for Applying Environmental Economics in Developing Countries, Gatekeeper Series No 91–02, London Environmental Economic Centre, London, 1991.

environmental management that are sustainable. The importance of PEC for children and for the environment is obvious, as this improves the material circumstances and the environment of the hundreds of millions of households in which children are most at risk from environmental hazards and inadequate food intake. The importance of involving children in such initiatives is discussed in Chapter 7. But the discussion of what constrains primary environmental care takes one further and further away from children and from the environment in which they live, as the economic, social and political constraints to PEC are discussed. This was also the case with the final sections of Chapter 1, in considering the factors that influence child health. Here, as in Chapter 1, the importance of the international constraints on primary environmental care must be mentioned, although a detailed discussion of such constraints lies far beyond the scope of this book.

Earlier sections described the great difficulties that most international funding agencies have in funding a multiplicity of diverse PEC initiatives. This implies the need for quite fundamental changes in the structure of international aid – for instance through much more aid being available through foundations or public agencies located within each region or city in the South which can respond much more rapidly and appropriately to a great multiplicity of requests for funding and support from their locality than international agencies. These foundations or agencies can also better provide the technical, financial and organizational support to PEC initiatives that encourage minimum reliance on external funding.[98] Such foundations or agencies can also be far more transparent in their workings than most international funding agencies and more accountable to those living in their locality. But there are not many indications of such a move. And as Chapter 5 notes, the extent to which the international debate about sustainable development misrepresents the roles of low-income groups in environmental degradation and concentrates on 'sustainability' with little attention given to the development needs and priorities of low-income groups does not augur well for such a change. Nor too does the very low priority given by most international funding agencies to tackling the environmental problems that underlie or contribute to so much infant and child death, injury and illness. Nor does the tendency of international funding agencies to address symptoms rather than helping the parents of children at most risk to acquire more adequate livelihoods, better quality housing and access to health care.

In addition, most of the dominant international economic forces will act against PEC initiatives or destroy the possibility of local collective action for resource management or environmental enhancement, without a political and legal system within the country which gives voice and power to local groups. It is hardly coincidental that so many examples of PEC initiatives are in remote rural areas or on land of relatively poor quality or among squatters in urban areas inhabiting land that is ill-suited to commercial development. They are protected by distance and/or by the low market value of the environmental resources they manage. But political systems and legal structures are generally the means through which disputes between the inhabitants of any locality and external forces are resolved. The more a country or region is fully incorporated in the world market and the more all resources and their exploitation is monetized, the more the possibilities of PEC initiatives will depend on the extent to which political systems and legal structures provide them with the space to operate.

One of the main reasons for the high level of pressure on soils in many of the poorest countries is these countries' reliance on agricultural exports for a high proportion of their export earnings.[99] For instance, in 1988, the proportion of export earnings contributed by agricultural and natural resource commodities was 99 per cent for Ethiopia, 95 per cent for Somalia, 89 per cent for Chad and 83 percent for Kenya.[100] As noted in Chapter 1, most of the poorest countries have very little possibility of breaking out of this dependence on agricultural exports. Inevitably, this puts great pressure on soil and water resources. This reliance on natural resource exports is often combined with falling prices for these commodities on the world market (which may be linked to limited international markets because of trade barriers around the wealthiest markets) and a high external debt (so governments give priority to boosting exports).

International agencies are often considered as key elements in eroding the power of community or neighbourhood organizations within development and environmental management. But there are also examples of such agencies doing the opposite. Very often, they work with the intermediary institutions whose importance was noted earlier. Two examples, one rural, one urban, are given below. UNICEF had an important role in each, but what appears important in both instances is that there was an international agency with a local office and a constant presence in the country that was able to respond rapidly to a request for help coming direct from low-income groups. In Box 6.19, it was the residents of a village in Mauritania that requested help and did so through their local health post. It is also worth noting how the inhabitants felt confident to address other environmental and livelihood needs, once they had successfully addressed the most pressing environmental problem together.

Box 6.20 gives an example of a whole series of initiatives in informal or illegal settlements in Guatemala City.[101] Again, what became a large programme involving many different settlements and many different initiatives began as a response by UNICEF and *Médecins Sans Frontières* to a single request for help. This came from one particular squatter settlement, *El Mezquital*, which needed help with water supply after an outbreak of typhoid. In *El Mezquital*, this developed into a network of community health promoters who were elected from among the inhabitants – with one health promoter to every 50 or so families. Box 6.20 describes their work, and the other initiatives that developed in *El Mezquital* and in other informal or illegal settlements.

This is also a good illustration of the institutional framework needed to scale up from one single initiative in one settlement to a wide range of initiatives in many settlements. This became possible in 1986 when a newly elected government established a Committee for Attention to the Population of Precarious Areas in Guatemala City (COINAP). This committee brought together representatives from several ministries, the different city authorities, local universities, NGOs and aid agencies, and representatives from community organizations where projects were under-

Box 6.19 **Protecting Water Supplies from Desertification in Mauritania**

In 1989, the residents of the village of Lewreia requested UNICEF's help in protecting their only well from moving sand dunes. The well had been constructed in 1955 and was a reliable supplier of good quality water. Children, women and men had to remove sand from the well once a week, using camels, baskets and carts. As the sand dunes reached within 20 metres of the well, they realized that they needed a more effective approach. They were considering renting a bulldozer to remove the sand and level the dunes but this would cost them $15,000 – as much as digging a new well. But they had also heard about a successful low-cost initiative undertaken by people on the outskirts of Nouakchott, where a green belt had been established to protect their water source. UNICEF's help was requested through the health post that had been established in their village.

The Greenbelt project was initiated with support from various agencies and, within a year, the advance of the sand dune was halted and the weekly collective removal of sand no longer became necessary. In the second year, the project was extended to four more sites and, by 1992, the village was almost completely protected and the inhabitants had mastered the process of sand-dune fixation and the maintenance of the green belt. The cost, borne by outside agencies, was $6700 during the three years. Technical assistance was provided by the Department for the Protection of Nature and the World Lutheran Federation for training the villagers and developing the two-phase action plan to first protect the well and secondly to protect the village. UNDP paid for the materials and UNICEF supervised the programme and covered the cost of transporting the materials. The inhabitants contributed labour to establish a nursery and for reforestation and sand-dune stabilization. The project also enhanced the inhabitants' self-confidence. New projects have been initiated – including a windmill for pumping water, and additional wells are being dug, partly for drinking water but also to irrigate the green belts and increasingly for growing vegetables in small plots. Similar efforts are being developed in other villages.

Source: Bajracharya, Deepak, 'UNICEF and the challenge of sustainable livelihood; an overview', Presented at the UNICEF Preparatory Meeting for the Inter-Regional Consultation on PEC and the UNICEF Programming Process, Villa de Layva, 1993.

way, and it has had a central role in promoting and supporting a great range of initiatives, including community health promoters and pharmacies, improved water supplies managed by community organizations, house improvement and construction, community day-care centres, improved sanitation, reafforestation and education.

Box 6.20 **Community-based Initiatives in 'Precarious' Settlements in Guatemala City**

The network of health promoters: By 1993, 600 community health promoters were active in 60 illegal or informal settlements and were serving over 150,000 inhabitants. Each was elected by their neighbourhood and gave eight hours a week of voluntary service. These health promoters undertook a physical survey of the settlement, noting on a map all relevant social and geographic information. This provided project organizers with a precise idea of the resources available in a given area – for instance a health clinic, church, public water tap or shop – as well as health hazards such as garbage dumps or polluted streams.

The health promoters then worked with a technical team from the government's coordinating 'Committee for Attention to the Population of Precarious Areas in Guatemala City' (COINAP) to help identify the main causes of ill health and possible solutions that they could realistically address, drawing mainly on local resources. Each undertook house-to-house surveys to discover the specific health or social problems within their micro-zone. This formed the basis for developing a workplan and, with training and technical support to help their efforts, the health promoters helped the inhabitants prevent diarrhoeal diseases (and to rapidly treat them when they occurred). They maintained health records for all the families in their micro-zone and helped ensure that all children received vaccinations. They also helped encourage the inhabitants to use local health services and developed health education materials and community pharmacies; some community-based laboratories have also been set up to carry out simple tests on blood, urine and faeces.

Environmental improvements: As health services improved, with its strong emphasis on education, community members sought ways to address other problems, especially water supply. Two different models for an improved water supply developed: the single source tank and the well. Both combined the active involvement of a community group, reliance on technical assistance, and institutional cooperation from COINAP members.

In the first, residents requested that Empagua, Guatemala's municipal water enterprise, install a single, large water tank in the neighbourhood. From this single source, the community created a supply network to reach individual residences with UNICEF providing the funds for the pipes and other materials. Each family carried out the work necessary for their own home connection. The local community association receives one large bill from the water company and then collects fees from residents according to usage measured by individual meters. A resident, chosen by the community, was trained to manage billing and the collection of fees. Most of the fees are to cover actual costs but a portion is set aside for maintenance and the surplus will go towards other local infrastructure needs such as drains and sewers. For the community-managed well, a deep well is dug and water pumped from this is then distributed to households. The community has formed a small, private enterprise managed by local residents to operate the new water project.

Other environmental initiatives have included reforestation projects and new wood-burning stoves. The reforestation projects were initiated in three settlements with volunteer labour from the community, support from the government's forestry division and seedlings donated by the National Committee for the Environment (CONAMA). Some 20,000 rapid-growth trees have been planted with the aim of establishing a sustainable fuelwood supply. The trees also help stop soil erosion on the hillsides where many of the precarious settlements are located. Some are fruit and avocado trees that will provide produce for the community and also improve the whole neighbourhood environment. In two communities, residents working with the COINAP technical team produced a simple, low-cost composting unit, fed by household wastes.

Housing and urban improvement: A new programme was initiated in one of the settlements, *El Mezquital* to improve housing conditions and water supply and provide paved roads and a park. This is to be funded through loans provided to the residents at a monthly cost that the relatively low-income households can afford. Entitled PROUME (Programme for the Urbanization of *El Mezquital*), this receives support from the World Bank, the government of Guatemala, the community and UNICEF. With regard to housing, 1000 new homes will be built and 500 improved. Each family can choose one of five designs for its home, depending on its needs and the size of the lot. The designs allow for the construction of a second storey in later years. Loans are available for families wishing to upgrade their homes – or for constructing a new unit with the loan covering construction materials and labour. The plan also includes street-paving, the installation of drains and sewers, and the construction of a park and community centre. Each household will have to contribute labour towards these improvements and help to pay for materials.

New models for community-based day care: A young trainee teacher developed a new model for day care in one precarious settlement through inviting children between the ages of four and six into her home during the afternoon, at a time when these children would normally be playing or wandering around the settlement. With no pre-school support, they were ill-prepared when they entered school at the age of seven and often had to repeat grades. Many were on the way to becoming street children as parents, discouraged by their lack of progress at school, allowed them to drop out and put them to work – but again in work for which the youngsters were usually ill-prepared. The improved performance of the young children when they entered school was so impressive that both parents and educators developed a pre-school centre. All aspects of the day care are agreed during meetings between the staff (that include two community health promoters) and the mothers. The local technical team helped design and build furniture for the centre. The health promoters also monitor the growth and development of the children and within a year of the centre's opening, more than three quarters of the children met or surpassed standards in all areas. Fees are charged on a sliding scale, according to family income.

A different kind of day-care model was developed in another settlement where there was no space to construct a centre. A 'home day-care network' was set up, with support from UNICEF and COINAP. With the help of a local health promoter, five community women received one month's training in early childhood development. Each home day-care mother receives a small salary and her home is remodelled to provide water, toilets and appropriate outdoor space for ten children. Home day-care mothers from one community then helped to train others, using printed materials and their own experience. The same model soon began operating in other crowded settlements, so that by 1993 about 250 children were receiving care in 25 homes that are part of the network.

Source: Lair Espinosa and Oscar A. López Rivera (1994), 'UNICEF's urban basic services programme in illegal settlements in Guatemala City', Environment and Urbanization Vol 6, No 2, Oct 1994.

CONCLUDING COMMENTS

In this chapter, as in Chapter 4, little has been said specifically about children. The focus has been on ensuring a more adequate, stable and sustainable livelihood and improving environmental health for low-income groups through locally initiated and/or directed actions. Achieving this for the hundreds of millions of rural and urban households who currently lack stable and adequate livelihoods and are constantly faced with life-threatening and health-threatening environmental hazards would bring enormous benefits to their children in terms of improved nutrition and health. It would probably mean shorter working hours for adults, less pressure on children to work and to drop out of school early (though there may be differences in the way girl and boy children are treated), and more stable households (including less need for one or more adult member to migrate). Developing the capacity of local institutions and government support for the initiatives and priorities of women and men is also likely to bring benefits in improved provision of health care, education, water and sanitation and other aspects. These have obvious direct and indirect benefits for infants and children. Increasing prosperity (or simply reducing the vulnerability of low-income groups to changes in prices and incomes) and improved service provision will also lessen stresses within poorer households, which will also bring important benefits for the health and well-being of all members of such households. In areas where there is successful natural resource management in which all population groups participate and benefit, the whole basis for the life of children there is much improved when compared to the children in households that are constantly struggling for survival.

REFERENCES

1   See for instance Agarwal, Anil, Darryl d'Monte and Ujwala Samarth (Eds) (1987), *The Fight for Survival: People's Action for Environment*, Centre for Science and Environment, New Delhi; Davidson, Joan, Dorothy Myers and Manab Chakraborty (1992), *No Time to Waste: Poverty and the Global Environment*, OXFAM, Oxford; and Friedmann, John and Haripriya Rangan (1993), *In Defence of Livelihood: Comparative Studies on Environmental Action*, Kumarian Press, West Hartford.

2   See for instance Turner, Bertha (Ed) (1988), *Building Community – A Third World Case Book*, Habitat International Coalition, London; Hardoy, Jorge E and David Satterthwaite (1989), *Squatter Citizen: Life in the Urban Third World*, Earthscan, London; Douglass, Mike (1992), 'The political economy of urban poverty and environmental management in Asia: access, empowerment and community-based alternatives' *Environment and Urbanization* Vol 4, No 2, October; and Douglass, Mike and Malia Zoghlin (1994), 'Sustaining cities at the grassroots: livelihood, environment and social networks in Suan Phlu, Bangkok', *Third World Planning Review*, Vol 16, No 2, pp 171–200.

3   Pretty, J N and Irene Guijt (1992), 'Primary Environmental Care: an alternative paradigm for development assistance', *Environment and Urbanization* Vol 4 No 1, April, pp 22–36.

4   Cleary, David (1991), 'The 'Greening' of the Amazon', in David Goodman and Michael Redclift (Eds), *Environment and Development in Latin America: The Politics of Sustainability*, Manchester Univeristy Press, Manchester and New York, quoted in Friedmann and Rangan 1993, op cit.

5   Bajracharya, Deepak (1993), 'UNICEF and the challenge of sustainable livelihood; an overview', presented at the UNICEF Preparatory Meeting for the Inter-Regional Consultation on PEC and the UNICEF Programming Process, Villa de Layva.

6   Jazairy, Idriss, Mohiuddin Alamgir and Theresa Panuccio (1992), *The State of World Rural Poverty: an Inquiry into its Causes and Consequences*, IT Publications, London.

7   UNCHS (Habitat) (1996), *An Urbanizing World: Global Report on Human Settlements*, 1996, Oxford University Press, Oxford and New York.

8   Hardoy, Jorge E, Sandy Cairncross and David Satterthwaite (Eds) (1990), *The Poor Die Young: Housing and Health in Third World Cities*, Earthscan, London.

9   Douglass 1992, op cit; Hardoy, Jorge E, Diana Mitlin and David Satterthwaite (1992), *Environmental Problems in Third World Cities*, Earthscan, London.

10 Satterthwaite, David (1995), 'The scale and nature of international donor assistance to housing, basic services and other human-settlements related projects', Paper presented at the UNU/WIDER Conference on 'Human Settlements in the changing global political and economic processes', Helsinki.

11 Ibid.

12 Ibid.

13 Friedmann and Rangan 1993, op cit.

14 Douglass 1992, op cit.

15 Sarin, Madhu (1991), 'Improved stoves, women and domestic energy', *Environment and Urbanization*, Vol 3, No 2, October, p 51.

16 Pretty and Guijt 1992, op cit.

17 Bagadion, B U and F F Korten (1991), 'Developing irrigators' organisations; a learning process approach' in Cernea, M M (ed), *Putting People First*, Oxford University Press, Oxford 2nd Edition; Korten, D (1980), 'Community organization and rural development: a learning process approach', *The Public Administration Review*, Vol 40, pp 480–511.

18 Hart, Roger (1996), *Children's Participation in Sustainable Development: The Theory and Practice of Involving Young Citizens in Community Development and Environmental Care*, Children's Environments Research Group, Earthscan, London.

19 Ibid.

20 Kottak, C P (1985), 'When people don't come first: some sociological lessons from completed projects' in Cernea, M M op cit.

21 Hardoy et al 1990 and Douglass and Zoghlin 1994, op cit; Arlosoroff, S, G Tscahanneri, D Grey, W Journey, A Karp, O Langenegger and R Roche (1987), *Community Water Supply; The Handpump Option*, World Bank, Washington DC; and Arrossi, Silvina, Felix Bombarolo, Luis Coscio, Jorge E Hardoy, Diana Mitlin and David Satterthwaite (1994), *Funding Community Initiatives*, Earthscan, London.

22 Cernea, M M (1991), 'Social actors of participatory afforestation strategies' in Cernea, M M (Ed), op cit; Murphy, Denis (1990), 'Community organizations in Asia' *Environment and Urbanization* Vol 2, No 1, April, pp 51-60; Jodha, N S (1990), *Rural Common Property Resources: A Growing Crisis*, Gatekeeper SA24, IIED, London; and Rahman, M A (Ed) (1984), *Grass-roots Participation and Self-Reliance*, Oxford and IBH Publication Co, New Delhi.

23 Bunch, R (1990), *Low Input Soil Restoration in Honduras: the Cantarranas Farmer-to-Farmer Extension Programme*, Gatekeeper SA23, IIED, London; Hasan, Arif (1990), 'Community groups and NGOs in the urban field in Pakistan', *Environment and Urbanization* Vol 2, No 1, pp 74–86; Paul, S (1987), *Community Participation in Development Projects – The World Bank Experience*, World Bank Discussion Paper 6, Washington DC; and Jintrawet, A, S Smutkupt, C Wongsamun, R Katawetin and V Kerdsuk (1985), *Extension Activities for Peanuts after Rice in Ban Sum Jan, N E Thailand: A Case Study in Farmer-to-Farmer Extension Methodology*, Khon Kaen University, Khon Kaen.

24 Pretty, J N, I Guijt, I Scoones and J Thompson (1992), 'Regenerating agriculture: the agroecology of low-external input and community based development' in Holmberg J (ed), *Policies for a Small Planet*, Earthscan, London.

25 Hardoy et al 1990, op cit; Cabannes, Y (1988), 'Human settlements' in Conroy, C and M Litvinoff, (Eds), *The Greening of Aid*, Earthscan, London.

26 Furedy, Christine (1990), 'Social aspects of solid waste recovery in Asian cities' *Environmental Sanitation Reviews* No 30, ENSIC, Asian Institute of Technology Bangkok, December, pp 2–52; Furedy, Christine (1992), 'Garbage: exploring non-conventional options in Asian cities' *Environment and Urbanization* Vol 4, No 2, October; Furedy, Christine (1994), 'Socio-environmental initiatives in solid waste management in Southern cities: developing international comparisons', Paper presented at a workshop on 'Linkages in Urban Solid Waste Management', Karnataka State Council for Science and Technology, University

of Amsterdam and Bangalore Mahanagara Palike, 18–20 April, Bangalore.

27   Bunch R (1991), 'People centred agricultural improvement' in Haverkort B et al (Eds), *Joining Farmers' Experiments*, IT Publications, London; Reij, C (1988), 'The present state of soil and water conservation in the Sahel', paper for the Club du Sahel, Free University, Amsterdam.

28   Mikkelsen, Britha with Yanti Yulianti and Anton Barré (1993), 'Community involvement in water supply in West Java', *Environment and Urbanization* Vol 5, No 1, April pp 52–67.

29   Sriskandarajah, N, R J Bawden and R G Packham (1991), 'Systems agriculture; a paradigm for sustainability', *Association for Farming Systems Research Extension Newsletter*, Vol 2, No 2, pp 1–5.

30   Huby, M (1990), *Where You Can't see the Wood for the Trees*, Kenya Woodfuel Development Programme Series, the Beijer Institute, Stockholm; Mascarenhas J, P Shah, S Joseph, R Jayakaran, J Devavaram, V Ramachandran, A Fernandez, R Chambers and J N Pretty (1991), 'Participatory Rural Appraisal', RRA Notes 13, pp 1–143 IIED, London.

31   Yacoob, May and Linda M Whiteford (1995), 'An untapped resource: community-based epidemiologists for environmental health', *Environment and Urbanization*, Vol 7, No 1, pp 219–230.

32   Ibid.

33   Espinoza, Lair and Oscar A Lopez Rivera (1994), 'UNICEF's urban basic services programme in illegal settlements in Guatemala City', *Environment and Urbanization*, Vol 6, No 2, October, pp 9–29.

34   Guijt, I (1991), *Perspectives on Participation: Views from Africa*, IIED, London.

35   Singh, Neera M and Kundan K Singh (1993), 'Saving forests for posterity', *Down To Earth* 15 April, pp 25–28.

36   Moser, Caroline O N (1989), *Community Participation in Urban Projects in the Third World*, Progress in Planning, Vol, 32, No 2, Pergamon Press, Oxford; Moser, Caroline O N (1993), *Gender Planning and Development; Theory, Practice and Training*, Routledge, London and New York.

37   Leach, Melissa (1991), 'Engendered environments: understanding resource mangement in the West Africa forest zone', *IDS Bulletin*, Vol 22, No 4; Levy, Caren (1992), 'Gender and the Environment: the challenge of cross-cutting issues in development policy and planning', *Environment and Urbanization* Vol 4, No 1, April, pp 120–135.

38   Levy 1992, op cit.

39   Lee-Smith, Diana and Catalina Hinchey Trujillo (1992), 'The struggle to legitimize subsistence: Women and sustainable development', *Environment and Urbanization* Vol 4, No 1, April, pp 77–84.

40   Ibid.

41   Lee-Smith and Trujillo 1992, op cit, p 84.

42   Agarwal, Anil and Sunita Narain (1992), 'Towards green villages; a strategy for environmentally sound and participatory rural development in India', *Environment and Urbanization*, Vol 4, No 1, April, p 61.

43   This section draws heavily on Agarwal and Narain 1989, Jazairy, Alamgir and Panuccio 1992 and Lee-Smith and Hinchey Trujillo, op cit; *The Ecologist* (1992), *Whose Common Future*, Earthscan, London; Bajracharya, Deepak (1992), 'Institutional imperatives for sustainable resource management in the mountains', in N S Jodha, M Banskota and Tej Partap (Eds), *Sustainable Mountain*

Agriculture: Perspectives and Issues Vol 1, Oxford and IBH Publishing, New Delhi, pp 205–234; Toulmin, Camilla, Ian Scoones and Josh Bishop (1992), 'Drylands', in Johan Holmberg (Ed), op cit.

44 Edwards, Michael and David Hulme (1992), 'Scaling-up the development impact of NGOs: concepts and experiences', and 'Making a difference: concluding comments' discuss the different ways in which international private voluntary organizations can scale up, drawing on many case studies, in Michael Edwards and David Hulme (Eds), *Making a Difference: NGOs and Development in a Changing World*, Earthscan, London.

45 Lecomte, B J (1986), *Project Aid: Limitations and Alternatives*, Development Studies Centre, OECD, Paris; and Mascarenhas et al 1991, op cit.

46 Hudson, N (1991), *A Study of the Reasons for Success or Failure of Soil Conservation Projects*, FAO Soils Bulletin 64, Rome; Uphoff, N (1990), 'Paraprojects as new modes of international development assistance', *World Development* Vol 18, pp 1401–1411.

47 Kumar, S (1991), 'Ananthapur experiment in PRA training' in Mascarenhas J et al (Eds), 'Participatory Rural Appraisal', *RRA Notes* 13, pp 112–117 IIED, London.

48 People's Dialogue (South Africa) and SPARC/National Slum Dewllers Federation/Mahila Milan (India) (1994), *Regaining Knowledge; an Appeal to Abandon Illusions*, SPARC, Bombay.

49 Mascarenhas et al 1991, Huby 1990, Bunch 1990 and Jintrawel et al 1985, op cit; Hardoy, Ana, Jorge E Hardoy and Ricardo Schusterman (1991), 'Building community organization: the history of a squatter settlement and its own organizations in Buenos Aires' *Environment and Urbanization* Vol 3, No 2, October, pp 104–120.

50 Cotton, Andrew and Richard Franceys (1994), 'Infrastructure for the urban poor: Policy and planning issues', *Cities*, Vol 11, No 1, February, pp 15–24.

51 Rahman, Perween and Anwar Rashid (1991), 'Low Cost Sanitation Programme Maintenance/Rectification', Orangi Pilot Project; Research and Training Institute, Karachi.

52 Diana Mitlin, field visit.

53 See Cairncross, Sandy (1990), 'Water supply and the urban poor' and Sinnatamby, Gehan (1990), 'Low cost sanitation' in Jorge E Hardoy et al (Eds), op cit.

54 Cotton and Franceys 1994, op cit.

55 See Patel, Sheela and Michael Hoffmann (1993), 'Homeless International, SPARC IS13 Toilet Block Construction, Interim Report', Homeless International, Coventry; UNCHS 1996, op cit.

56 Joel Bolnick, People's Dialogue, personal communication.

57 Anzorena, Jorge (1993), 'Supporting shelter improvements for low-income groups', *Environment and Urbanization*, Vol 5, No 1, October, pp 122–131 and Anzorena, E J (1995), 'Activities of Hogar de Cristo during 1994', SELAVIP Newsletter (Journal of Low-Income Housing in Asia and the World), October, pp 39–42.

58 Ibid.

59 Diana Mitlin, field visit, 1995.

60 See Caminos, Horacio and Reinhard Goethert (1978), *Urbanization Primer*, The MIT Press, Cambridge (Mass) and London.

61 Ana Hardoy, IIED-América Latina, personal communication.

62 Cruz, Luis Fernando (1994), 'NGO Profile: Fundación Carvajal; the Carvajal Foundation', *Environment and Urbanization*, Vol 6, No 2, October, pp 175–182.

63 Lankatilleke, Lalith (1995), 'Build Together: National Housing Programme of Namibia', paper presented at a workshop on Participatory Tools and Methods in Urban Areas, IIED, London.

64 Briscoe, John and David deFerranti (1988), *Water for Rural Communities: Helping People Help Themselves*, World Bank, Washington, DC.

65 Cairncross 1990, op cit.

66 Espinosa and López Rivera 1994, op cit.

67 See for instance Arrossi and others 1994, op cit; also Vol 5, No 1 of *Environment and Urbanization* on funding community initiatives.

68 Anzorena, E J (1993), *Housing the Poor: the Asian Experience*, Asian Coalition for Housing Rights, Cebu; and Anzorena, E J (1995), 'Grameen Bank', SELAVIP Newsletter (Journal of Low-Income Housing in Asia and the World), Oct, p 3.

69 Sevilla, Manuel (1993), 'New approaches for aid agencies; FUPROVI's community based shelter programme', *Environment and Urbanization*, Vol 5, No 1, pp 111–121.

70 Arrossi and others 1994; Anzorena, E J (1995), 'FUNDASAL: 25 years of service', SELAVIP Newsletter (Journal of Low-Income Housing in Asia and the World), Oct, pp 38–41.

71 UNCHS (1996), *An Urbanizing World: The Global Report on Human Settlements 1996*, Oxford University Press, Oxford; and Asian Coalition for Housing Rights/Habitat International Coalition (1994), 'Finance and resource mobilization for low income housing and neighbourhood development: a workshop report', Pagtambayayong Foundation, Philippines.

72 See for instance Patel, Sheela and Celine D'Cruz (1993), 'The Mahila Milan crisis credit scheme; from a seed to a tree', *Environment and Urbanization*, Vol 5, No 1, pp 9–17.

73 Diana Mitlin, field visit, 1995.

74 See for instance the discussion about sustainable development in Stein, Robert E and Brian Johnson (1979), *Banking on the Biosphere?*, Lexington Books, D C Heath and Company, Lexington and Toronto.

75 Hardoy, Jorge E and David Satterthwaite (1991), 'Environmental problems in Third World cities: a global issue ignored?', *Public Administration and Development*, Vol 11, pp 341–361.

76 Arrossi and others 1994, op cit; Bebbington, A (1991), *Farmer Organizations in Ecuador: Contributions to Farmer First Research and Development*, Gatekeeper SA26, Sustainable Agriculture Programme, IIED, London.

77 Friedmann and Rangan 1993 op cit, p 16.

78 Levy 1992, op cit; Redclift, Michael (1987), *Sustainable Development: Exploring the Contradictions*, Routledge, London and New York.

79 von Amsberg, Joachim (1993), *Project Evaluation and the Depletion of Natural Capital: an Application of the Sustainability Principle*, Environment Working Paper No 56, Environment Department, World Bank, Washington, DC.

80 The Ecologist 1992, op cit.

81 See for instance the Ecologist 1992, op cit and McGranahan, Gordon (1991), 'Fuelwood, subsistence foraging and the decline of common property', *World*

Development, Vol 19, No 10, pp 1275–1287.

82   Toulmin, Scoones and Bishop 1992, op cit.

83   Jaujay, J (1990), 'The Operation and Maintenance of a Pilot Rehabilitated Zone in the Office du Niger, Mali', Irrigation Management Network Paper No 90/1c, ODI, London; and Wageningen, University of (1990), 'Design for Sustainable Farmer-Managed Irrigation Schemes in sub-Saharan Africa', Contributions to an international workshop, 5–8 February.

84   Ibid.

85   Agarwal and Narain 1989 and Toulmin, Scoones and Bishop 1992, op cit.

86   Ibid.

87   Bajracharya 1992, op cit.

88   Ibid; Agarwal and Narain 1989 and Pretty and Guijt 1992, op cit.

89   Jazairy, Alamgir and Panuccio 1992, op cit.

90   Toulmin, Scoones and Bishop 1992, op cit.

91   Lawry, S (1989), *Tenure Policy towards Common Property Natural Resources*, Land Tenure Center Paper No 34, University of Wisconsin, Madison.

92   Agarwal and Narain 1989, op cit.

93   Toulmin, Scoones and Bishop 1992, op cit.

94   Wade, R (1987), 'The management of common property resources; finding a cooperative solution', *The World Bank Research Observer* Vol 2, No 2, July, pp 219–234.

95   Bajracharya 1992 and Toulmin, Scoones and Bishop 1992, op cit; WHO (1992), *Our Planet, Our Health*, Report of the Commission on Health and Environment, Geneva.

96   UNCHS 1996, op cit.

97   See for instance Adewale, O (1992), 'The right of the individual to environmental protection: a case study of Nigeria', *Environment and Urbanization*, Vol 4, No 2, Oct, pp 176–183.

98   See Hardoy, Mitlin and Satterthwaite 1992, op cit.

99   Toulmin, Scoones and Bishop 1992, op cit.

100 Ibid.

101 Espinosa and López Rivera 1994, op cit.

7

Children as a Bridge to Sustainable Development*

INTRODUCTION

All societies need to find ways to reproduce through their children the knowledge and skills of past and present generations in using and managing environmental resources to ensure the survival of future generations. Traditionally, this took place in predominantly agricultural societies, with this knowledge being passed down from mother to daughter and father to son through *in situ* apprenticeship. In societies where change was relatively slow and agricultural practices remained largely the same from one generation to the next, this learning by demonstration from elders proved adequate. What we need now is a more conscious, self-monitoring population who can learn about traditional knowledge and practices while also being knowledgeable of outside forces of change and how to cope with them in order to maintain the integrity of the environment. This chapter will outline, with examples, some important principles for fostering in children a caring, knowledgeable and competent relationship to the environment, which will enable them to become effective stewards and in turn pass on an undegraded environment to their children.

Children of the 1990s are within a world at a point of history where many nations are not only reassessing their use of natural resources but also, in the light of the UN Convention on the Rights of the Child, rethinking the extent to which children have the rights and responsibilities to be involved in shaping their own futures and the futures of their communities. Box 7.1 highlights some of the articles within this convention that are concerned about such rights and responsibilities. Clearly, these movements to reassess the use of natural resources and the needs and rights of the child have to come together in the form of lasting programmes for children's participation in sustainable development within their communities or neighbourhoods all over the world.

---

* This chapter was drafted by Roger Hart and draws on the companion volume to this - Hart, Roger, *Children's Participation in Sustainable Development: The Theory and Practice of Involving Young Citizens in Community Development and Environmental Care*, Children's Environments Research Group, Earthscan, London, 1996.

Box 7.1 **Examples of Articles Concerned with Children's Participation in the UN Convention on the Rights of the Child**

Article 12
1. State Parties shall assure to the child who is capable of forming his or her own views the right to express those views freely in all matters affecting the child, the views of the child being given due weight in accordance with the age and maturity of the child.
2. For this purpose, the child shall in particular be provided the opportunity to be heard in any judicial and administrative proceedings affecting the child, either directly, or through a representative or an appropriate body, in a manner consistent with the procedural rules of national law.

Article 13
1. The child shall have the right to freedom of expression; this right shall include freedom to seek, receive and impart information and ideas of all kinds, regardless of frontiers, either orally, in writing or in print, in the form of art, or through any other media of the child's choice.
2. The exercise of this right may be subject to certain restrictions, but these shall only be such as are provided by law and are necessary: a. for respect of the rights and reputations of others; or b. for the protection of national security or of public order, or of public health and morals.

Article 14
1. States Parties shall respect the right of the child to freedom of thought, conscience and religion.
2. States Parties shall respect the rights and duties of the parents and, when applicable, legal guardians, to provide directions to the child in the exercise of his or her right in a manner consistent with the evolving capacities of the child.
3. Freedom to manifest one's religion or beliefs may be subject only to such implications are prescribed by law and are necessary to protect public safety, order, health or morals, or the fundamental right and freedom of others.

Article 15
1. States Parties recognize the rights of the child to freedom of association and freedom of peaceful assembly.
2. No restrictions may be placed on the exercise of these rights other than those imposed in conformity with the law and which are necessary in a democratic society in the interests of national security or public safety, public order, the protection of public health or morals or the protection of the rights and freedoms of others.

Article 17

State Parties recognize the important function performed by the mass media and shall ensure that the child has access to information and material from a diversity of national and international sources, especially those aimed at the promotion of his or her social, spiritual and moral well-being and physical and mental health. To this end, States Parties shall:

a) Encourage the mass media to disseminate information and material of social and cultural benefit to the child and in accordance with the spirit of article 29;

b) Encourage international cooperation in the production, exchange and dissemination of such information and material from a diversity of cultural, national and international sources;

c) Encourage the production and dissemination of children's books;

d) Encourage the mass media to have a particular regard to the linguistic needs of the child who belongs to a minority group or who is indigenous;

e) Encourage the development of appropriate guidelines for the protection of the child from information and material injurious to his or her well-being, bearing in mind the provisions of articles 13 and 18.

Article 23

States Parties recognize that mentally or physically disabled children should enjoy a full and decent life in conditions which ensure dignity, promote self-reliance and facilitate the child's active participation in the community.

Article 29

1. States Parties agree that the education of the child shall be directed to:

a) The development of the child's personality, talents, and mental and physical abilities to their fullest potential;

b) The development of respect for human rights and fundamental freedoms, and for the principles enshrined in the Charter of the UN;

c) The development of respect for the child's parents, his or her own cultural identity, language and values, for the national values of the country in which the child is living, the country from which he or she may originate, and for civilizations different from his or her own;

d) The preparation of the child for responsible life in a free society, in the spirit of understanding, peace, tolerance, equality of sexes and friendship among all peoples, ethnic, national and religious groups and persons of indigenous origin;

e) The development of respect for the natural environment.

2. No part of the present article or article 28 shall be construed so as to interfere with the liberty of individuals and bodies to establish and direct educational institutions, subject always to the observance of the principles set forth in paragraph 1 of the present article and to the requirements that the education given in such institutions shall

conform to such minimum standards as may be laid down by the State.

Article 31
1. State Parties recognize the right of the child to rest and leisure, to engage in play and recreational activities appropriate to the age of the child and to participate freely in cultural life and the arts.
2. State Parties shall respect and promote the right of the child to participate fully in cultural and artistic life and shall encourage the provision of appropriate and equal opportunities for cultural, artistic, recreational and leisure activity.

Beyond Social Mobilization

The UN Conference on the Human Environment in Stockholm in 1972, the first global recognition of the seriousness of environmental problems, recognized the importance of environmental education and citizen-based environmental action. But it saw this being achieved through centrally directed, 'top-down' environmental education which was to mobilize societies to act. As one of its recommendations (No 96) emphasized, environmental education was to be directed towards the general public, particularly the ordinary citizen, with a view to educating them as to the simple steps they might take, within their means, to manage and control their environment. While there have been benefits from this kind of educational approach, it is time for a deeper, more grounded involvement of citizens in the environment that builds on their knowledge and capacity and addresses their needs and priorities – as outlined in Chapter 6.

This grounded approach has not been emphasized with children. Although girls and boys in many countries have become vociferous defenders of the environment, they usually seem to be parroting the messages of the media and environmental education programmes. For example, they speak at conferences with great emotion about national and global issues, but with little apparent knowledge of their own communities and with no accounts of personal experience. Conferences are not the ideal setting for children's genuine participation, and they are mentioned here only to highlight the need to convince politicians, NGOs, international agencies and other institutions to take children's participation seriously at the local level and within PEC initiatives.

Politicians may appear to be moved by children's testimonies at conferences, but very few of them bring children's perspectives into their own agendas or encourage children's participation in environmental planning and management issues in their own residential communities. We need fewer trite examples of children speaking and singing out of how they are the future and how they alone best understand global environmental problems and more models that genuinely recognize the untapped competencies of children to take a significant role in community-based sustainable development, particularly when collaborating with adults.

GLOBAL EDUCATION FOR ALL, WITH A PURPOSE

We do not need all children of the world to become sophisticated ecologists or noisy environmental activists. We should aim, however, for all children in all cultures to become responsible and effective participants in the primary environmental care of their households and communities. The most obvious way to achieve this is to make it central to all school curricula. A number of the largest international agencies are collaborating to achieve 'Education for All' by the end of the century. This movement could be combined with the movement promoting sustainable development to create meaningful education for all, namely education related to people's livelihoods and to the care of the local community and its environment. Education for All focuses on the primary school grades which for a large majority of the world's children is all the schooling they will ever have. We urgently need to find and build upon the best models for fostering and developing livelihood skills and fostering of the environment with children from approximately 6 to 12 years of age.

Primary Schools as Centres for Sustainable Development at Community Level

Children and teenagers are taking an important role in the environmental movement within Europe and North America. Unfortunately, it is often not clear how much this is a fashion that will fade, like the fashion for environmental education of the early 1970s in the USA. The question of how girls and boys become deeply concerned about the environment is critical, but unfortunately, there is remarkably little theory and research on this question. Most research is on children's understanding of environmental education curricula; we know very little about how and why children develop a genuine concern for the environment.

Most environmental educators recognize that a substantial part of an education programme, particularly for pre-adolescent children, should involve some kind of direct action in the environment. Unfortunately, environmental educators usually assign children to work on environmental projects rather than involving them in identifying problems themselves and collaborating with them in finding solutions. This is founded in a restricted notion of the value of children's actions in environmental learning. Most educators, if asked why actions by children are important to their environmental learning, will answer that such direct experiences are necessary for their understanding. This concept is not new, stretching from the early educational philosophy of Froebel[1] through the writings of Dewey[2] and Piaget.[3] But children's actions with environments have importance beyond the purely cognitive. There is considerable theoretical reason for believing that concern for the environment is based on an affection for it and this can only come from autonomous or unmediated contact with it.[4] If it is true that children are only likely to develop a genuine, lasting sense of ecological responsibility out of a 'personal knowing' of the non-human world, we need to be concerned about the narrowing of people's everyday, spontaneous contact with environments in many countries due to rapid urbanization and, in the North, due to parents' fears of crime and traffic.[5]

Ironically, while television and other forms of electronic media enable children in many countries to have a greater understanding of global environmental issues, their intimate contact with and concern for their local environment is diminishing. This is a problem that has to be addressed in environmental planning policies and also by fundamentally transforming primary schools. Schools need to be connected with both their surrounding physical environment and with the residents of their community. With such a policy, schools can assist in the planning and management of community-based sustainable environments and may even serve as the catalysts for this.

Unfortunately, there have been few attempts by nations to foster community participation of children or youth through their public school systems.[6] Most schools in most nations remain completely isolated from their surrounding communities and their environmental problems. It is difficult to imagine how a citizenry can become interested in and committed to democratic participation except by experiencing its benefits, yet civic responsibility is still taught as a classroom subject, through texts, as with the remainder of the school curriculum. Even in the progressive educational philosophy of John Dewey and the many which have followed it, democratic experiences have rarely extended beyond the classroom; the school has served as a microcosm of society.[7] Now, with the growing global recognition of the environmental crisis, and the rush by many nations to develop environmental education programmes, the need for a genuine involvement of children in the environmental issues of their own surrounding communities must be addressed.

The main barrier is that teachers usually feel incompetent or fearful of conducting field-based activities with the children they teach. They need the help of environmental professionals from developmental and environmental NGOs and from government and planning agencies. By supporting teachers and helping them form collaborations with community-based organizations, schools could become the focus for long-term strategies for the sustainable development of their communities. Community organizations need to merge their community development and environmental goals with the curriculum goals of schools, through the joint design of programmes with teachers. The schools will also require continued in-service support for each teacher in learning how to satisfy their curriculum goals through research and action on the local environment because this is a radical departure from the traditional classroom teaching provided to teachers in most countries. Box 7.2 describes a programme in East Africa that sought to help teachers and their students to develop environmental education initiatives that were linked to the environmental issues of relevance to them and the community of which they were part. This programme also sought to actively involve the children in gathering valuable information about environmental issues and traditional knowledge.

Box 7.2 **Environmental Information for and from Children**

Since the 1979 International Year of the Child, Mazingira Institute in Nairobi has been exchanging information with primary school children about their environment. A series of illustrated learning packages on environmental issues developed for schools sought not only to provide students and teachers with material about environmental issues but also to stimulate responses from the children. Annual competitions invited children to answer questions and submit essays and drawings. Children's responses have proved not only a valuable source of information on their perceptions of environmental issues but have also contained information on traditional knowledge and action in their communities.

Since the project's inception, a series of illustrated learning packages in the form of comic books containing stories, articles, games and puzzles have been sent out to all the primary schools in Kenya. One of the most important components is an annual competition, which invites children to answer questions and to send in essays and drawings. Their responses have been used as data and the best entries receive prizes for themselves and their schools. Winning entries are published in another full colour printed package distributed to everyone who enters.

The topics on which the project has focused have varied over the years, often responding to what has been learned from the children. Major themes have included tree planting, water management, wood fuel, tree seedlings, water and sanitation, health and nutrition, health and safety, immunization, nutrition, and occupational and environmental hazards. In addition to the main topic, major subthemes such as pesticides, population and women's work, are also discussed, and these often lead to useful new information or further research. For example, a competition question revealed that 80 per cent of Kenyan children were cleaning their teeth with chewsticks from different species of plant or shrub. Follow-up research with the Kenya Medical Research Institute showed these chewsticks to be as effective as using a toothbrush, and extension packages on chewsticks were sent out to schools, health centres and teacher training colleges.

The information in the learning packages seeks to balance useful technical knowledge (for example, how combustion and carbon monoxide poisoning work, immunization principles and schedules) with what will stimulate the children to investigate, evaluate and act on their own environment. For example, the issues raised include what is good and bad about large and small families and what are traditional health practices. Certain attitudes are reinforced, including respect for elders' traditional knowledge, gender equality, support to parents in the home (especially appreciation of mothers' work load) and bringing home useful knowledge to help the family. The first competition in 1979 elicited so much information about the uses of Kenyan trees and shrubs, for fuel, fibre, food, building and medicines that a book was published. At that time, there were only about 5,000 primary schools in Kenya. Since then the number has increased to over 14,000. From 1983-86, the project was extended to Ugandan primary schools as well. Usually, each school receives ten copies of the package, necessitating print runs of between 50,000 and 250,000.

Source: Lee-Smith, Diana and Taranum Chaudhry (1990), 'Environmental information for and from children', Environment and Urbanization *Vol 2, No 2*

A GROUNDED APPROACH TO ENVIRONMENTAL EDUCATION

Most environmental action programmes with children work on the same set of orthodox issues, defined for them by the mass media and by the majority of environmental education curricula – such as garbage clean-ups, recycling projects or community mural painting. Environmental education curricula often imply that there is a clear and unquestionable set of environmental problems that have been defined by professionals, which teachers and their students should follow – and these usually ignore the realities of the living environments of people. We need to convince children that they can and should be involved themselves in the identification of problems, one of the most effective ways of achieving this is to have children begin with a critical analysis of their own daily activities in the environment of their community. In doing this, one can build gradually from a research base that the children know better than anyone else. The Convention on the Rights of the Child make it very clear that society should maximize children's opportunity to have a voice, and in particular stresses elements of children being able to speak on matters which most directly affect them. Yet how rare it is ever to involve children in the planning and design of their everyday play environments.

For example, do girls and boys have space to play? What is missing or inadequate about the quality of these play places? Is the journey to the school or community centre dangerous in any way? The girls and boys can then proceed with this kind of analysis to an investigation of the quality of environment of other members of the community. Through this grounded kind of approach, based in the everyday perceptions of community residents, one can transform the top-down kind of environmental education into a community-based type of environmental education as called for by the concept of primary environmental care.

Using this child-initiated approach with the tens of millions of children who already engage in important tasks of household food production, fuel and fodder collection and environmental management, one can quickly move into an analysis of the central issues of livelihoods and resource use by the larger community. For the more privileged children, this child-based approach to environmental action will lead to environmental action projects related more specifically to the world of childhood. Similarly, differences in the experiences and perceptions of girls and boys will lead to more gender-integrated environmental action projects that are more relevant to the felt need of girls and boys. Evaluating play and recreational needs in their community and developing planning proposals for improvement is the kind of research endeavour relevant to children in urban areas throughout the world: North and South, rich and poor. Such a project offers children the opportunity to speak out clearly about issues which they and their peers have the most obvious right to speak about.

From such research and action it is a small step for children to become involved in issues of more general concern to their community. Children aged ten and eleven in an elementary school in Knowsley, Lancashire (UK) identified dog excrement as a serious issue for them, for it was distributed throughout the streets and play spaces of their neighbourhood. With the support of teachers from a number of different classes, they developed a multi-pronged research, public awareness, planning and design project to deal with the problem. Excrement was mapped, dog owners were inter-viewed and posters were placed in shops throughout the neighbourhood. The children even developed a rapid deployment force for intercepting dog-owning abusers of their newly established standards of community care and hygiene. Once intercepted, the dog owners were made aware of the campaign and offered the opportunity to purchase one of the new 'scoopers' designed by the children in one of their science and technology classes. This resulted in a rapid turnaround of an important community public health problem with implications not only for the quality of chil-dren's play opportunities but also for their health and for the health of the larger community. More importantly, it undoubtedly provided children with an unforgettable introduction to the pleasures of finding themselves capable of having a voice and taking action to help their community.

For children to feel that they are taking a useful role in environmental improvement, it is not necessary that they physically change it. One of the most useful roles they can take is to conduct research on the quality of the environment and communicate their findings to the larger community, including community leaders, planners and politicians. Such research is frequently of much greater value to a community than some minor physi-cal improvement. And as long as the children feel that adults listen to their conclusions and engage in a dialogue, the benefits to their sense of 'owner-ship' of the community are great. Furthermore, there are extraordinary motivational benefits to children's learning when they feel that they are genuinely involved in research with a purpose.

Environmental education should not be a separate subject of the curriculum; it should be integrated into all subjects. This is possible because environmental education does not involve a new content area of the curriculum. Science, maths, geography and history, art and the languages together enable most aspects of environmental education to be covered. What is new about environmental education is the ecological perspective. This ecological perspective should not be taught as a separate subject because it is too important and is best understood as it is applied to all areas of the curriculum.

On-going environmental projects by the children can be related to each of the school subjects by the teacher, particularly if the teacher turns to environmental NGOs and knowledgeable community residents for help. Ecological thinking can then be learned in the study of each subject area. Figure 7.1 illustrates children's developing capacity to participate in the development and management of environments from the age of 6 up to the age of 14 or older. From the age of six (or even earlier), there is an interest and capacity in caring for animals or plants. As the child gets older, so can their interest and involvement be broadened – to helping with local environmental management, then working on local action research through to their involvement in community projects, community environmental action, research and monitoring. Figure 7.1 also illustrates how the child's understanding of the environment develops over time, especially the crucial area of the strong and complex links to society.

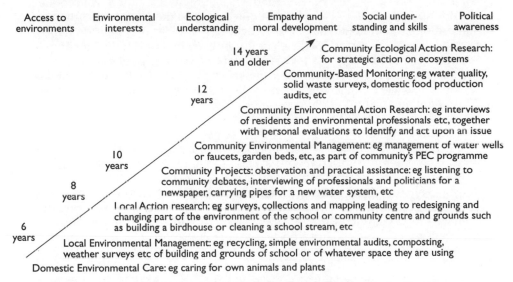

Source: Hart, Roger (1996), *Children's Participation in Sustainable Development: The Theory and Practice of Involving Young Citizens in Community Development and Environmental Care*, Earthscan, London

Figure 7.1 *Children's developing capacity to participate in the development and management of environments*

HOUSEHOLD ENVIRONMENTAL MANAGEMENT

For thousands of years, girls and boys all over the world have been involved in work for their families. As Chapter 4 described, this commonly involves work which directly impacts on the natural resources that surround them, particularly (but not exclusively) in rural areas: collecting firewood and fodder, foraging for food, helping with agricultural work (especially at times when most labour is needed on the farm) and shepherding animals. Sometimes this work is excessive and exploitative, and hence needs to be eradicated or the workload much reduced. But often it is a natural apprenticeship to the responsibilities of adulthood. In these cases, it is a most appropriate place to try and foster more ecologically responsible actions where these do not traditionally exist. For those cultures in the northern hemisphere where children's involvement in household work is a rare phenomenon, household environmental management represents an entirely new opportunity for girls and boys who are commonly denied all opportunity for meaningful engagement in work.

In recent years, children in the North have begun to serve as catalysts for responsible environmental awareness and action within their own families. This has often involved issues of conservation communicated by the school down to the family via the children, rather than encouraging dialogue between the child and the family over environmental issues. Because children usually understand the inherent wisdom of environmental conservation, they are often effective (even self-righteous) carriers of environmental messages. But there is a danger of abuse in this uncritical channel of communication. For example, school teachers in the USA who often feel starved of environmental education teaching materials, are only too happy to use materials provided by the electrical power companies. Power companies are required by law to provide a certain amount of public information on conservation. Unfortunately, the materials provided by these companies are usually biased, suggesting for example that energy wastage is a problem caused entirely by household consumers and that children learn (and teach others) to switch off lights, turn down heating systems or reduce the use of air conditioning, and use less hot shower water.

These are all valuable lessons, but only if prescribed within the larger context of energy production and a knowledge of the waste of energy in commerce, industry and transport and in the power companies themselves. Teachers should beware of programmes which require actions of their children without reflection. We need *more* than a *personal* action from children; we need to develop children's *critical* analysis and reflection on environmental issues if we are to develop a *citizenry capable of sustained, independent, environmentally responsible behaviour.*

BROADENING PRIMARY HEALTH CARE PROJECTS INTO PRIMARY ENVIRONMENTAL CARE

A natural entry point for a PEC project is through primary health care. The similarity between the names is not accidental. Primary environmental care is in many respects an extension of primary health care, with its emphasis on the most fundamental aspects of health maintenance, into the larger environment, and its emphasis on community participation. Some primary health care projects have been quietly developing the PEC concept for some time though not calling it such. One example is given in Box 7.3 below.

Box 7.3 **Project** *Saude e Alegria* **(Health and Happiness)**

Project *Saude e Alegria* is a community health project in the Brazilian Amazon with a broad vision extending its reach into community development and environmental education. The project was explained by 'Magnolio' the clown who is also the programme coordinator for cultural development and education. It reaches 20,000 people in 17 villages along the banks of the Amazon and Tapajoa river, a tributary reaching the Amazon river at the city of Santarem where the project is based. The strategy is to train health volunteers in 17 villages. At the time of the interview, there were 150 volunteers.

One of the major problems with the health of the villages is that people in their most active years (20–40 years of age) leave for the cities, resulting in an age distribution which has an uncomfortably high proportion of children under ten – 20 per cent. The primary strategy for animating the community is one which is used quite commonly in Brazil – the circus. The circus is excellent for getting the entire community to become more aware of health and community development issues. All of the professional staff and volunteers of the project become performers for the evening circuses.

Each village is visited for approximately 60 days per year – six visits with an average stay of ten days. Most of these visits involve two or three people although once a year the entire team goes to the village for four days. The teams have different programmes for different age groups:

- For babies and infants – the education of parents and girls in the psychomotor stimulation of infants;
- For 6–12 year olds – workshops on the care of small children, hygiene, the functioning of the human body, water treatment, garbage issues, and the national values of local plant material;
- For 13–18 year olds – newspaper production, radio, folklore and dance. The teams also seek to get the youth involved in community projects such as the planting of gardens and the building of a centre for community use and for sports. Through these projects, the animators seek to train the older pre-adolescents and teenagers to become monitors who will then stimulate projects themselves.

The project also seeks to introduce the concept of responsibility for the village, including environmental planning, by teaching them how much the environment has already been transformed by human action, including their own. A major vehicle for introducing ideas is to have the children study their own ontogenesis. By beginning from the child's own birth, they are able to stress to them that they enter the world with a responsibility and that from the first moment they, and their families, are transforming the earth. Efforts are made throughout the curriculum to carry it out in a participatory way. For example, the children relive the moments of their own human history by talking with their families about their birth.

Source: Hart, Roger, Children's Participation in Sustainable Development: The Theory and Practice of Involving Young Citizens in Community Development and Environmental Care, *Children's Environments Research Group, Earthscan, London, 1996*

SCHOOLS AS CENTRES FOR PRIMARY ENVIRONMENTAL CARE

For many decades, schools all over the world have included gardening in their curriculum and taught it through a garden on the school grounds. Now with the growing understanding of the need to develop new approaches to sustainable development in all communities, a few schools are beginning to ask their children to take a more active and even catalytic role. *Education Rural Andina* in the high Andes of Peru is an excellent example. All the children in the programme have their own garden beginning with their first year in school at six years of age. In this programme, they progressively learn about the diversity of crops, conditions for growth and nutritional value of crops which can be grown at the altitude of their home, which for some children is more than 12,000 feet (3660 metres) above sea level.

Their parents are encouraged to locate a small garden at home and both girls and boys bring young plants to these home gardens from propagating gardens at the school. In this way, the scene is set for each child to experiment with a diversity of crops in front of their parents. Additionally, the fathers, who in this region are primarily responsible for farming, are invited to assist the school teacher in the garden programme at the school. In this way, an internal debate is established for each father between his own practices and alternative growing methods and crops he sees being used by his children. This is truly two-way learning with the children as the experiences between tradition and innovation. Father and child help one another learn more than either knew before. In those cases where the father finds no time to assist the child with her/his own garden, at least he observes different crops and growing methods being successfully demonstrated in his own territory.

To a lesser extent, the children's mothers are drawn into the discussions through nutritional issues. In such programmes it is common for girls and boys to receive the same educational opportunities related to the environment but one cannot quickly change gender roles in environmental practice and decision making within families. Moreover, mothers and fathers can be involved in the programme, depending on their different roles in agriculture and domestic activities.

Beyond the school gardens, regrettably most community environmental educational activities in schools are designed as occasional short-term projects. The *Escualas Nuevas* (new schools) in Colombia are a remarkable exception as they require children every year to design and run community projects as a basic part of their education. With only 10 per cent in extra expenses, these new schools are now serving as a model for many countries. They incorporate many of the principles of active learning by children both individually and in small groups, thereby liberating the teacher to function as a facilitator responding as a resource to the demands of the children as they move through the curriculum themselves. In addition, these schools have developed new types of organizations to enable them to function as organized, democratic communities. So well integrated is the curriculum of these schools with the life of the community that it seems as though all of it is concerned with the environment. An example is useful, however, for revealing how schools can themselves become centres of PEC. Box 7.4 gives the example of a fish farming project developed by one *Escuela Nueva* in Colombia.

Box 7.4 **The Fish Farming Project at Hojas Anchas School, Colombia**

The fish farming project at Hojas Anchas school in Colombia was among several environmental projects, each with its student committee. The projects had emerged from interviews undertaken by the children in the community, along with walking ecological surveys of the entire town.

The fish farming project was described with great enthusiasm by the children because they seemed to be quite clear that they had developed a programme by themselves which had surprised both themselves, and the larger community in its effectiveness as both a source of income for the community and as a way of reducing damage to some of the river valleys from excessive fishing there. In this project, the school is very much functioning as an experimental station with the children as scientists experimenting with locations and types of fish. The results of this research are then shared with the community so that the fish farming programme is fully assimilated by the community as a whole. The school is experimenting with the idea of each class having a different project as their primary responsibility and at the time of my visit, the seventh grade was in charge of developing fish farming. The current coordinator of the group, 14 year old Luce Empada, explained how the project worked.

Children keep logs of the fish that are fished, and their size. After about five months, the fish are ready for consumption but their size varies greatly depending on the species. The critical variable is the altitude, so the children were experimenting with ponds on a number of different slopes. Luce explained that the 14 children in her class all took part in the project. I asked if this was all done during class time and she explained 'Oh no, we have to be alert with this project. The fish need to be kept fed very regularly so we work not only after class but also on weekends'. They tried different species of fish and discovered that tilapia fish performed well in the first small fish pond they built with help from the *junta* or local government. But they found that the ponds higher up the slopes have not worked as well. A by-product of this test has been the discovery of contamination in the ponds and the ability of the students to create clean water for this project, which has benefited residents living further down the slopes. They are now beginning in a more distant pond to experiment with four different species of fish. In agreement with the *junta* of the village, half of the fish are made available to the community and half are for the school. As with each project in the school, the elected child treasurer for this project manages the funds.

Source: Hart, Roger, 1996, op cit

REACHING THE POOREST CHILDREN

Although it might be considered difficult to teach the poorest children or the children that are in the most difficult circumstances – for instance street children – there are examples of successful environmental programmes. Box 7.5 gives the example of *El Programa Muchacho Trabajador*, a national movement in Ecuador for working children.

Box 7.5 **The Working Child Programme in Ecuador**

El Programa Muchacho Trabajador (the working child programme) is a national movement in Ecuador which uses children's rights as an organizing focus. It has a national system of centres for working children and children otherwise at risk because of poverty that are called 'Alternative Spaces.' Each has a dedicated, trained coordinator committed to empowering children to become active agents in defence of their rights and improvement of their lives. These alternative spaces are located primarily in poorer urban areas and offer opportunities for children to informally learn to defend their rights. They do this through play, learning, discussion and action founded on the principles of the UN Convention on the Rights of the Child. They learn about their histories, both individually and collectively, and through play and artistic activities develop an identity in their multi-cultural society. As many as 80 children in each alternative space are free to attend, or not, the three to five meetings a week. Locations vary depending on available space.

This programme chose the environment as its annual theme for 1993 and now has environmental projects in 21 provinces and 23 cities involving a total of 50,000 children. Many of the centres were in public schools whose space is available after school. There is the hope that schools will be persuaded to incorporate the environmental projects within their regular curriculum, which at present includes no study of the local environment. Youth units are to be trained in each city to work as promoters of environmental groups. Each city established a local support group to serve as the training programme for these youth groups.

Source: Hart, Roger, 1996, op cit

FROM LOCAL TO GLOBAL UNDERSTANDING

While this chapter has argued that we have relatively few models of environmental education programmes that are truly based in residents' own definitions of local problems, it is even more rare to find programmes that simultaneously link these local problems to global issues. Sometimes, with communities who are struggling to survive with inadequate land or access to other resources, the focus must at first be totally concerned with sustainable development locally. If the residents have been involved successfully in such a project, they are more likely to show interest in environmental issues that are shared with other communities and thereby to become concerned about wider environmental problems, including global problems.

There is a growing tendency to bring children together, often from great distances and across national boundaries, to meet in conferences. Too often this is done in a manner which is superficial and wasteful. Children who are not particularly engaged in local research or action, but who are highly articulate, are selected to speak with other equally articulate children as though they were representatives of 'children' even though they were neither elected nor see themselves as representatives of their peers in a sense that they intend to bring messages from or return from the conference with new insights for them. However, it is possible to design a conference which includes children who are deeply involved in local research and action and who are selected by their peers to represent them and their work. One example brought together children from all of the provinces of the Ecuadorian Amazon region who were working in *El Programa Muchacho Trabajador* described in Box 7.5. Immigrant and indigenous children from each region exchanged knowledge and values about their local environment and the projects they are engaged in. There was a sense that the Amazon children's conference did make a contribution to the growth of environmental understanding and the different culture's environmental perspectives and practices that could continue to be built upon after the conference and the inevitable mass media exposure was over.

'Environmental exchange' or 'linking' is an effective strategy for fostering a perspective on the environment that is grounded in the local definition of environmental problems but which seeks to understand these problems in a larger context. It does so by having children from different communities share their research with each other. In a demonstration project with schools in the states of New York, New Jersey and New England in the USA, children living in dramatically different communities corresponded with each other for a year about their research on their community environment. The experiment involved grades four through eight (9–14 year olds). The project served as a focus for teachers to integrate all subjects of the school curriculum. Only modest in-service support, in the form of weekly visits by graduate student environmental interns, was required to help the teachers see how to meet some of their particular curriculum goals through the project.

In the first exchange of letters about each other and about their respective environments, stereotypes were shattered. Then, in each classroom, local environmental study sites were identified by the children themselves through their own experiences and through interviews with community residents. These sites were locations that were slated to change or that the children thought should be changed. The children then spent the year studying these sites, projecting alternative futures for them, and assessing the positive and negative social and environmental impacts of their proposals. Each classroom created a book of their own community's environmental study sites and constructed a book of their 'twin' community's study sites through the correspondence. At the end of the year, they visited their twin communities with enough background to be led around the sites and to have informed discussion without adult mediation. The classes also made presentations to community residents, environmental planners, community leaders and local political representatives. These discussions may not often lead directly to physical changes but, more important than this, through dialogue with adults, children come to understand the environmental decision-making process in their own community and what role they might have in the future. From such projects, the most important changes occur in the minds of the children and in their increased sense of caring for their community.

The correspondence exchange process leads quite naturally to classroom discussion on both commonality and differences in their two environments, and of the different priorities the citizens of the two communities have. This provides an excellent basis for the teachers to lead the children into discussions of regional, national and global environmental problems. If the children discover that damage to trees in the park of their East Harlem twin community is coming from the same source as pollutants in their Vermont community, then they are no longer only investigating local problems.

Experiments are proceeding in many places with children's environmental exchanges using electronic technology. This may have value, particularly for international projects, in that it speeds up the exchange. But one should be aware of the seductive quality of electronic technology. It is critical that children begin with environmental issues in their local environment and that they identify these themselves. Also, electronic technology should not narrow the multi-media nature of the exchange: drawings, charts, photos and artifacts collected from the environment, not just words, should be exchanged. Finally, we must remember that so many of the communities we need to support in these tasks do not even have pencils and paper, never mind computers with modems that permit electronic exchanges.

REFERENCES

1   Froebel, F (1886), *The Education of Man* (W M Hailman, translator), Appleton, New York.

2   Dewey, J (1990), *The School and Society*, University of Chicago Press, Chicago.

3   Piaget, J (1963), *The Psychology of Intelligence* (original published in French in 1947), Littlefiels Adams, Totowa, New Jersey.

4   Hart, Roger and Louise Chawla (1982), 'The Development of children's environmental concerns' in N Watts and J Wohlwill (Eds), special issue of Zeitschrift für Umweltpolitik on Environmental Psychology, International Institute for Environment and Society, Berlin; and Chawla, L and Roger Hart (1988), The Roots of Environmental Concern: Proceedings of the 19th Conference of the Environmental Design Research Association, EDRA, Washington, DC.

5   *Children's Environment* (1992), special issue on 'Children's Changing Access to Public Spaces', Vol 9, No 2, Children's Environments Research Group, New York

6   Ward, C and A Fyson (1976), *Streetwork: The Exploding School*, Routledge and Kegan Paul, London; Hart, Roger A (1992), *Children's Participation; from Tokenism to Citizenship*, Innocenti Essays No 4, March, UNICEF International Child Development Centre, Florence.

7   Dewey, 1900, op cit.

8   Espinosa, M F (1994), 'The First Summit of Children and Youth of the Ecuadorian Amazon', *Children's Environment* Vol 11, No 3, pp 212–220.

BIBLIOGRAPHY

Adams, W M (1992), *Wasting the Rain: Rivers, People and Planning in Africa*, Earthscan, London

Adewale, O (1992), 'The right of the individual to environmental protection: a case study of Nigeria', *Environment and Urbanization*, Vol 4, No 2, pp 176–183

Agarwal, Anil (1987), 'Between need and greed – the wasting of India; the greening of India', in Anil Agarwal, Darryl d'Monte and Ujwala Samarth (eds), *The Fight for Survival: People's Action for Environment*, Centre for Science and Environment, Delhi

Agarwal, Anil (1992), 'Who will help her learn? To keep the girl at school, the environment must be improved', *Down To Earth*, Nov 15

Agarwal, Anil, Darryl d'Monte and Ujwala Samarth (eds) (1987), *The Fight for Survival: People's Action for Environment*, Centre for Science and Environment, New Delhi

Agarwal, Anil and Sunita Narain (1989), *Towards Green Villages – a Strategy for Environmentally Sound and Participatory Rural Development*, Centre for Science and Environment, Delhi, India

Agarwal, Anil and Sunita Narain (1992), 'Towards green villages; a strategy for environmentally sound and participatory rural development in India', *Environment and Urbanization*, Vol 4, No 1, pp 53–64

Alder, Graham (1995), 'Tackling poverty in Nairobi's informal settlements: developing an institutional strategy', *Environment and Urbanization*, Vol 7, No 2, pp 85–108

Alexander, C S, E M Zinzeleta, E J Mackenzie, A Vernon and R K Markowitz (1990), 'Acute gastrointestinal illness and child care arrangements', *American Journal of Epidemiology*, Vol 131, pp 124–131

Allsebrook, Annie and Anthony Swift (1989), *Broken Promise: The World of Endangered Children*, Hodder & Stoughton, London

Anand, S and M Ravallion (1993), 'Human development in poor countries: on the role of private incomes and public services', *Journal of Economic Perspectives*, Vol 7, No 1, pp 133–150

ANAWIM (1990), published by the Share and Care Apostolate for Poor Settlers, Manila, Vol IV, No 4

Anderson L J, R A Parker, R A Strikas et al (1988), 'Day–care center attendance and hospitalization for lower respiratory tract illness', *Pediatrics*, Vol 82, pp 300–308

Anzorena, E J (1993), *Housing the Poor: the Asian Experience*, Asian Coalition for Housing Rights, Cebu

Anzorena, Jorge (1993), 'Supporting shelter improvements for low-income groups', *Environment and Urbanization*, Vol 5, No 1, pp 122–131

Anzorena, E J (1995), 'Grameen Bank', SELAVIP Newsletter (Journal of Low-Income Housing in Asia and the World), Oct, p 3

Anzorena, E J (1995), 'The Urban Community Development Office (UCDO)', SELAVIP Newsletter (Journal of Low-Income Housing in Asia and the World), Oct, pp 73–76

Anzorena, E J (1995), 'Activities of Hogar de Cristo during 1994', SELAVIP Newsletter (Journal of Low-Income Housing in Asia and the World), Oct, pp 39–42

Anzorena, E J (1995), 'FUNDASAL: 25 years of service', SELAVIP Newsletter (Journal of Low-Income Housing in Asia and the World), Oct, pp 38–41

Arlosoroff, S, G Tscahanneri, D Grey, W Journey, A Karp, O Langenegger and R Roche (1987), *Community Water Supply; The Handpump Option*, World Bank, Washington, DC

Arrossi, Silvina, Felix Bombarolo, Luis Coscio, Jorge E Hardoy, Diana Mitlin and David Satterthwaite (1994), *Funding Community Initiatives*, Earthscan, London

Arulpragasam, L C (1990), 'Land reform and rural poverty in Asia', *The State of World Rural Poverty Working Paper 21*, IFAD, Rome

Asian Coalition for Housing Rights (1989), 'Evictions in Seoul, South Korea', *Environment and Urbanization*, Vol 1, No 1, pp 89–94

Asian Coalition for Housing Rights/Habitat International Coalition (1994), 'Finance and resource mobilization for low income housing and neighbourhood development: a workshop report', Pagtambayayong Foundation, Philippines

Askoy, M et al (1976), 'Types of leukaemia in a chronic benzene poisoning', *Acta haematologica*, Vol 55, pp 67–72

Audefroy, Joël (1994), 'Eviction trends worldwide – and the role of local authorities in implementing the right to housing', *Environment and Urbanization*, Vol 6, No 1, pp 8–24

Auer, C (1989), *Health Problems (especially intestinal parasitoses) of Children Living in Smokey Mountain, a Squatter Area of Manila, Philippines*, Msc Thesis, Swiss Tropical Institute, Department of Public Health and Epidemiology, Basel

Bagadion, B U and D F Korten (1991), 'Developing irrigators' organisations; a learning process approach' in Cernea, M M (ed), *Putting People First*, Oxford University Press, Oxford 2nd ed

Bairoch, Paul (1988), *Cities and Economic Development: From the Dawn of History to the Present*, Mansell, London

Bajracharya, Deepak (1992), 'Institutional imperatives for sustainable resource management in the mountains', in N S Jodha, M Banskota and Tej Partap, *Sustainable Mountain Agriculture: Perspectives and Issues*, Vol 1, Oxford and IBH Publishing, New Delhi, pp 205–234

Bajracharya, Deepak (1993), 'UNICEF and the challenge of sustainable livelihood; an overview', Presented at the UNICEF Preparatory Meeting for the Inter-Regional Consultation on PEC and the UNICEF Programming Process, Villa de Layva

Barlow, S and F M Sullivan (1982), *Reproductive Hazards of Industrial Chemicals*, Academic Press, London

Barrón, Anonieta (1994), 'Mexican rural women wage earners and macro economic policies', in Isabel Bakker (ed), *The Strategic Silence: Gender and Economic Policy*, Zed Books in association with the North–South Institute, London

Barrow, C J (1995), 'Sustainable development: concept, value and practice', *Third World Planning Review*, Vol 17, No 4, pp 369–386

Bartlett, S, forthcoming, *The Physical Environment of the Home as a Factor in Socialization*, Children's Environments Research Group, City University of New York, New York

Bebbington, A (1991), *Farmer Organizations in Ecuador: Contributions to Farmer First Research and Development*, Gatekeeper SA26, Sustainable Agriculture Programme, IIED, London

Bhatt, Chandi Prasad (1990), 'The Chipko Andolan: forest conservation based on people's power' *Environment and Urbanization*, Vol 2, No 1, pp 7–18

Bishop, J et al (1991), *Guidelines for Applying Environmental Economics in Developing Countries*, Gatekeeper Series No 91–02, London Environmental Economic Centre, London

Bolnick, Joel and Sheela Patel (1994), 'Regaining knowledge: an appeal to abandon illusions', *RRA Notes 21: Special Issue on Participatory Tools and Methods in Urban Areas*, IIED, London

Borrini, G (ed) (1991), *Lessons Learned in Community–Based Environmental Management*, ICHM, Rome

Bradley, R H, L Whiteside, D J Mundfrom, P H Casey, K J Kellerher and S K Pope (1994), 'Early indications of resilience and their relation to experiences in the home environments of low birth weight, premature children in poverty', *Child Development*, Vol 65, pp 346–360

Bradley, David J (1993), 'Environmental aspects of public health in developing countries', Proceedings of a symposium 'Ambiente, Salute e Sviluppo', Accademia Nazionale dei Lincei, Rome, pp 85–95

Bradley, David, Carolyn Stephens, Sandy Cairncross and Trudy Harpham (1991), *A Review of*

Environmental Health Impacts in Developing Country Cities, Urban Management Program Discussion Paper No 6, World Bank, UNDP and UNCHS (Habitat), Washington, DC

Braungart, Michael, Justus Engelfried, Katja Hansen and Joyce Rosenthal (1992), *Impact of Lead and Agrochemicals on Children*, Environmental Protection Encouragement Agency, Hamburg

Briceno-Leon, Roberto (1990), *La Casa Enferma: Sociologia de la Enfermedad de Chagas*, Consorcio de Ediciones, Capriles C A Caracas

Briscoe, John and David deFerranti (1988), *Water for Rural Communities: Helping People Help Themselves*, World Bank, Washington, DC

Brown, George and Tirril Harris (1978), *Social Origins of Depression: a Study of Psychiatric Disorder in Women*, Tavistock Publications, London

Brydon, Lynne and Sylvia Chant (1989), *Women in the Third World: Gender Issues in Rural and Urban Areas*, Edward Elgar, Aldershot

Budiman, Gani et al (1988), 'The nutritional and health status of children under five in the subdistrict of West Padmangan, Metropolitan Jakarta', Paper presented at a workshop on 'Population Health Systems' Interaction in Selected Urban Depressed Communities', March

Bunch, R (1990), *Low Input Soil Restoration in Honduras: the Cantarranas Farmer–to–Farmer Extension Programme*, Gatekeeper SA23, IIED, London

Bunch R (1991), 'People centred agricultural improvement' in Haverkort B et al (eds), *Joining Farmers' Experiments*, IT Publications, London

Bundey, D A P, S O P Kan and R Rose (1988) 'Age related prevalence, intensity and frequency distribution of gastrointestinal helminth infection in urban slum children from Kuala Lumpur, Malaysia' *Transactions of the Royal Society of Tropical Medicine and Hygiene*, Vol 82, pp 289–294

Cabannes, Y (1988), 'Human settlements' in Conroy, C and M Litvinoff, (eds), *The Greening of Aid*, Earthscan, London

Cairncross, Sandy (1990), 'Water supply and the urban poor', in Jorge E Hardoy, Sandy Cairncross and David Satterthwaite (Eds), *The Poor Die Young: Housing and Health in Third World Cities*, Earthscan, London, pp 109–126

Cairncross, Sandy (1992), *Sanitation and Water Supply: Practical Lessons from the Decade*, Water and Sanitation Discussion Paper Series, DP Number 9, World Bank, Washington, DC

Cairncross, Sandy and Richard G Feachem (1983), *Environmental Health Engineering in the Tropics – An Introductory Text*, John Wiley and Sons, Chichester

Cairncross, Sandy and Richard G Feachem (1993), *Environmental Health Engineering in the Tropics – An Introductory Text (Revised Edition)*, John Wiley and Sons, Chichester

Caldwell, John C and Pat Caldwell (1985), 'Education and literacy as factors in health', in Scott B Halstead, Julia A Walsh and Kenneth S Warren (Eds), *Good Health at Low Cost*, Conference Report, Rockefeller Foundation, New York, pp 181–185

Caminos, Horacio and Reinhard Goethert (1978), *Urbanization Primer*, MIT Press, Cambridge (Mass) and London

Carter, J (1993), 'The Potential Of Urban Forestry In Developing Countries: A Concept Paper', FAO, Rome

Castonguay, Gilles (1992) 'Steeling themselves with knowledge' report on the work of Cristina Laurell, *IDRC Reports*, Vol 20, No 1, pp 10–12

Cauthen, G M, A Pio and H G ten Dam (1988), *Annual Risk of Tuberculosis Infection*, WHO, Geneva

Cederblad, M (1988), 'Behavioural disorders in children from different cultures', *Acta Psychiatria Scandinavica*, Vol 78 (Sup 344), pp 85–92

Centre for Science and Environment (1986), *The State of India's Environment 1984-5: The Second Citizens' Report*, New Delhi

Cernea, M M (1991), 'Social actors of participatory afforestation strategies' in Cernea, M M (ed), *Putting People First*, Oxford University Press, Oxford, 2nd Ed

CFDA; California Department of Food and Agriculture (1990), *Summary of Illnesses and Injuries Reported by California Physicians as Potentially Related to Pesticides*, 1990 (and reports in previous years), Sacramento, California, quoted in Conway and Pretty 1991

Chambers, Robert (1989), 'Editorial introduction: vulnerability, coping and policy', in *Vulnerability: How the Poor Cope*, IDS Bulletin, Vol 20, No 2, pp 1–7

261

Chambers, Robert (1990), 'Micro-environments unobserved', *Sustainable Agriculture Programme Gatekeeper Series no 22*, IIED, London

Chambers, Robert (1995), 'Poverty and livelihoods; whose reality counts?' *Environment and Urbanization*, Vol 7, No 1, pp 173–204

Chandi Prasad Bhatt, see Bhatt, Chandi Prasad

Chawla L and Roger Hart (1988), The Roots of Environmental Concern: Proceedings of the 19th Conference of the Environmental Design Research Association, EDRA, Washington, DC

Children's Environment (1992), Special Issue on 'Children's Changing Access to Public Spaces, Vol 9, No 2, Children's Environments Research Group, New York

Cleary, David (1991), 'The 'Greening' of the Amazon', in David Goodman and Michael Redclift (eds), *Environment and Development in Latin America: The Politics of Sustainability*, Manchester Univeristy Press, Manchester and New York

Cohen, Larry and Susan Swift (1993), 'A public health approach to the violence epidemic in the United States', *Environment and Urbanization*, Vol 5, No 2, pp 50-66

Commonwealth Secretariat (1989), *Engendering Adjustment for the 1990s*, Report of the Commonwealth Export Group on Women and Structural Adjustment, London

Conway, Gordon R and Edward B Barbier (1990), *After the Green revolution: Sustainable Agriculture for Development*, Earthscan, London

Conway, Gordon R and Jules N Pretty (1991), *Unwelcome Harvest*, Earthscan, London

Cooper Weil, D E, A P Alicbusan, J F Wilson, M R Reich and D J Bradley (1990), *The Impact of Development Policies on Health: a Review of the Literature*, WHO, Geneva

Cotton, Andrew and Richard Franceys (1994), 'Infrastructure for the urban poor: Policy and planning issues', *Cities*, Vol 11, No 1, Feb, pp 15–24

Crewe, Emma (1995), 'Indoor air pollution, household health and appropriate technology; women and the indoor environment in Sri Lanka', in Bonnie Bradford and Margaret A Gwynne (eds), *Down to Earth: Community Perspectives on Health, Development and the Environment*, Kumarian Press, West Hartford, pp 94–95

Critchley, W (1991), *Looking After Our Land; New Approaches to Soil and Water Conservation in Dryland Africa*, OXFAM and IIED, London

Cruz, Luis Fernando (1994), 'NGO Profile: Fundación Carvajal; the Carvajal Foundation', *Environment and Urbanization*, Vol 6, No 2, pp 175-182

Davidson, Joan, Dorothy Myers and Manab Chakraborty (1992), *No Time to Waste: Poverty and the Global Environment*, OXFAM, Oxford

de Coura Cuentro, Stenio and Dji Malla Gadji (1990), 'The collection and management of household garbage' in Jorge E Hardoy et al (Eds), *The Poor Die Young: Housing and Health in Third World Cities*, Earthscan, London, pp 169–188

Dewey, J (1900), *The School and Society*, University of Chicago Press, Chicago

DGCS (1990), *Supporting Primary Environmental Care*, report of the PEC workshop, Siena, to OECD/DAC Working Party on Development Assistance and the Environment, Ministero degli Affari Esteri, Direzione Generale per la Cooperatione allo Sviluppo, Italy

Di Pace, Maria, Sergio Federovisky, Jorge E Hardoy, Jorge E Morello and Alfredo Stein (1992), 'Latin America', Ch 8 in Richard Stren, Rodney White and Joseph Whitney (Eds), *Sustainable Cities: Urbanization and the Environment in International Perspective*, Westview Press, Boulder, pp 205–227

Dinham, Barbara, (Ed) (1993), *The Pesticide Hazard: Global Health and Environmental Audit*, Zed Books, London

Douglas, Ian (1983), *The Urban Environment*, Edward Arnold, London

Douglass, Mike (1992), 'The political economy of urban poverty and environmental management in Asia: access, empowerment and community-based alternatives' *Environment and Urbanization*, Vol 4, No 2

Douglass, Mike and Malia Zoghlin (1994), 'Sustaining cities at the grassroots: livelihood, environment and social networks in Suan Phlu, Bangkok', *Third World Planning Review*, Vol 16, No 2, pp 171–200

Duhl, Leonard J (1990), *The Social Entrepreneurship of Change*, Pace University Press, New York

Ecologist, The (1992) *Whose Common Future: Reclaiming the Commons*, Earthscan, London

Edwards, Michael and David Hulme (1992), 'Scaling-up the development impact of NGOs: concepts and experiences', in Michael Edwards and David Hulme (Eds), *Making a Difference: NGOs and Development in a Changing World*, Earthscan, London

Edwards, Michael and David Hulme (1992), 'Making a difference: concluding comments' in Michael Edwards and David Hulme (Eds), *Making a Difference: NGOs and Development in a Changing World*, Earthscan, London

Ekblad, Solvig (1993), 'Stressful environments and their effects on quality of life in Third World cities', *Environment and Urbanization*, Vol 5, No 2, pp 125–134

Ekblad, Solvig et al (1991), *Stressors, Chinese City Dwellings and Quality of Life*, D12, Swedish Council for Building Research, Stockholm

El-Hinnawi, E (1991), 'Sustainable agricultural and rural development in the Near East', Regional Document No 4, FAO/Netherlands Conference, on Agriculture and Environment, FAO, Rome

Ennew, Judith and Brian Milne (1989), *The Next Generation; Lives of Third World Children*, Zed Books, London

Espinosa, Lair and Oscar A López Rivera (1994), 'UNICEF's urban basic services programme in illegal settlements in Guatemala City', *Environment and Urbanization*, Vol 6, No 2, pp 9–29

Espinosa, Lair and Edgar Hidalgo (1994), Una Experiencia de Participacion Comunitaria en las Areas Precarias de la Ciudad de Guatemala,UNICEF (Guatemala), Guatemala City

Espinosa, M F (1994), 'The first Summit of Children and Youth of the Ecuadorian Amazon', *Children's Environment*, Vol 11, No 3, pp 212–220

Esrey, S A and R G Feachem (1989), 'Interventions for the Control of Diarrhoeal Disease: Promotion of Food Hygiene', WHO/CDD/89.30, WHO, Geneva

European Environment Agency (1995), *Europe's Environment: the Dobris Assessment*, Copenhagen

Evans, Timothy (1989) 'The impact of permanent disability on rural households; river blindness in Guinea' in special issue of the *IDS Bulletin* on 'Vulnerability: How the Poor Cope', Vol 20, No 2, pp 41–48

Evers, Barbara (1994), 'Gender bias and macroeconomic policy: methodological comments from the Indonesian example', in Isabel Bakker (ed), *The Strategic Silence: Gender and Economic Policy*, Zed Books in association with the North–South Institute, London

FAO (1988), *An Interim Report on the State of the Forest Resources in the Developing Countries*, FAO, Rome

Fashuyi, S A (1988), 'An observation of the dynamics of intestinal helminth infections in two isolated communities in south-western Nigeria', *Tropical Geographical Medicine*, Vol 40, pp 226–232

Feder, G and D Feeney (1991), 'Land tenure and property rights: theory and implications for development policy', *World Bank Economic Review*, Vol 5, No 1, pp 135–153

Fei, H T and C Chang (1945), *Earthbound China*, University of Chicago Press, Chicago

Fonseca W, B R Kirkwood, C J Victora, S R Fuchs, J A Flores and C Misago (in press), 'Risk factors for childhood pneumonia among the urban poor in Fortaleza, Brazil: a case–control study', *WHO Bulletin*

Forrester, M E, M E Scott, D A P Bundey and M H N Golder (1988), 'Clustering of Ascaris lumbricoides and Trichuris trichuria infections within households', *Transactions of the Royal Society of Tropical Medicine and Hygiene*, Vol 82, pp 282–288

Foster, Harold D (1992), *Health, Disease and the Environment*, John Wiley and Sons, Chichester

Fox, John P, Carrie E Hall and Lila R Elveback (1970), 'Environmental factors in causation of disease', Ch 6 in *Epidemiology, Man and Disease*, Macmillan, London, pp 94–110

Freeman, D B (1991), *A City of Farmers: Informal Urban Agriculture in the Open Spaces of Nairobi, Kenya*, McGill-Queens University Press, Montreal

Friedmann, John and Haripriya Rangan (1993), *In Defence of Livelihood: Comparative Studies on Environmental Action*, Kumarian Press, West Hartford

Froebel, F (1886), *The Education of Man* (W M Hailman, translator), Appleton, New York

Furedy, Christine (1990), 'Social aspects of solid waste recovery in Asian cities' *Environmental Sanitation Reviews* No 30, ENSIC, Asian Institute of Technology Bangkok, pp 2–52

Furedy, Christine (1992), 'Garbage: exploring non-conventional options in Asian cities' *Environment and Urbanization*, Vol 4, No 2

Furedy, Christine (1994) 'Socio-environmental initiatives in solid waste management in Southern cities: developing international comparisons', Paper presented at a workshop on 'Linkages in Urban Solid Waste Management', Karnataka State Council for Science and Technology, University of Amsterdam and Bangalore Mahanagara Palike, 18–20 Apr, Bangalore

Gardner G, A L Frank and L H Taber (1984), 'Effects of social and family factors on viral respiratory infection and illness in the first year of life', *Journal of Epidemiol Community Health*, Vol 38, pp 42–48

Germain, Adrienne and Jane Ordway (1989), *Population Control and Women's Health: Balancing the Scale*, International Women's Health Coalition in cooperation with the Overseas Development Council, New York

GLC Women's Committee (1984), *GLC Survey on Women and Transport*, Vols 1–7, Greater London Council

Goldstein, Greg (1990), 'Access to life saving services in urban areas' in Hardoy, Jorge E et al (Eds) *The Poor Die Young: Housing and Health in Third World Cities*, Earthscan, London

Goonasekere, K G A and F P Amerasinghe (1987), 'Planning, design and operation of rice irrigation schemes – the impact of mosquito-borne disease hazards', in *Vector-borne Disease Control in Humans through Rice Agro Eco-system Management*, International Rice Research Institute, Los Banos

Gore, Charles (1991), *Policies and Mechanisms for Sustainable Development: the Transport Sector*, mimeo

Gradwohl, J and R Greenberg (1988), *Saving the Tropical Forests*, Earthscan, London

Grazt, N (1987), 'The effect of water development programmes on malaria and malaria vectors in Turkey', in FAO, *Effects of Agricultural Development on Vector-Borne Diseases*, Doc AGL/MISC/87.12, FAO, Rome

Greenhow, Timothy (1994), *Urban Agriculture: Can Planners Make a Difference?*, Cities Feeding People Series, Report 12, IDRC, Ottawa

GRET (1991), *La Réhabilitation des Périmètres Irriguiés*, Groupe de Recherche et d'Echanges Technologiques, Paris

Guijt, Irene (1991), *Perspectives on Participation: Views from Africa*, IIED, London

Hardoy, Ana, Jorge E Hardoy and Ricardo Schusterman (1991), 'Building community organization: the history of a squatter settlement and its own organizations in Buenos Aires' *Environment and Urbanization*, Vol 3, No 2, pp 104–120

Hardoy, Jorge E, Sandy Cairncross and David Satterthwaite (Eds) (1990), *The Poor Die Young: Housing and Health in Third World Cities*, Earthscan, London

Hardoy, Jorge E, Diana Mitlin and David Satterthwaite (1992), *Environmental Problems in Third World Cities*, Earthscan, London

Hardoy, Jorge E and David Satterthwaite (1989), *Squatter Citizen: Life in the Urban Third World*, Earthscan, London

Hardoy, Jorge E and David Satterthwaite (1991), 'Environmental problems in Third World cities: a global issue ignored?', *Public Administration and Development*, Vol 11, pp 341–361

Harpham, Trudy, Paul Garner and Charles Surjadi (1990), 'Planning for child health in a poor urban environment: the case of Jakarta, Indonesia', *Environment and Urbanization*, Vol 2, No 2, Oct, pp 77–82

Hart, Roger (1987), 'Children's participation in planning and design: theory, research and practice', in C Weinstein and T David (eds), *Spaces for Children*, Plenum, New York

Hart, Roger (1992), *Children's Participation; from Tokenism to Citizenship*, Innocenti Essays No 4, UNICEF International Child Development Centre, Florence

Hart, Roger (1996), *Children's Participation in Sustainable Development: The Theory and Practice of Involving Young Citizens in Community Development and Environmental Care*, Children's Environments Research Group, Earthscan, London

Hart, Roger and L Chawla (1982), 'The Development of children's environmental concerns', in N Watts and J Wohlwill (Eds), special issue of Zeitschrift für Umelweltpolit on Environmental Psychology, International Institute for Environment and Society, Berlin.

Hasan, Arif (1989), 'A low cost sewer system by low-income Pakistanis' in Bertha Turner (Ed), *Building Community: a Third World Case Book*, Habitat International Coalition

Hasan, Arif (1990), 'Community groups and non–government organizations in the urban field in Pakistan', *Environment and Urbanization*, Vol 2, No 1, pp 74–86

Hasan, Arif and Ameneh Azam Ali (1992), 'Environmental problems in Pakistan: their origins and development and the threats that they pose to sustainable development', *Environment and Urbanization*, Vol 4, No 1, pp 8–21

Haskins R and J Kotch (1986), 'Day care and illness: evidence, cost, and public policy', *Pediatrics, Vol 77*, pp 951–982

Haughton, Graham and Colin Hunter (1994), *Sustainable Cities*, Regional Policy and Development series, Jessica Kingsley, London

Hawkins, J N (1982), 'Shanghai: an exploratory report on food for a city', *GeoJournal*, Supplementary issue

Hecht, S B (1982), 'Agroforestry in the Amazon basin: practice, theory and limits of a promising land use', in S B Hecht (ed), *Amazonia: Agriculture and Land Use Research*, CIAT, Cali, pp 331–371

Henderson, F W and G S Giebink (1986), 'Otitis media among children in day care: epidemiology and pathogenesis' *Review of Infectious Diseases, Vol 8*, pp 533–538

Hettiarchi, S P, D G H de Silva and P Fonseka (1989), 'Geohelminth infection in an urban slum community in Galle', *Ceylon Medical Journal*, Vol 34, No 1, pp 38–39

Hibbert, Christopher (1980), *London: a Biography of a City*, Penguin Books, London

Hofmaier, V A (1991), *Efeitos de poluicao do a sobre a funcao pulmonar: un estudo de cohorte em criancas de Cubatao*, Doctoral thesis, Sao Paulo School of Public Health

Honghai, Deng (1992), 'Urban agriculture as urban food supply and environmental protection subsystems in China' Paper presented to the international workshop on 'Planning for Sustainable Urban Development', University of Wales

Howe, G M (1986), 'Does it matter where I live', *Transactions*, New Series, Institute of British Geographers, Vol 11, No 4, pp 387–411

Huby, M (1990), *Where You Can't see the Wood for the Trees*, Kenya Woodfuel Development Programme Series, the Beijer Institute, Stockholm

Hudson, N (1991), *A Study of the Reasons for Success or Failure of Soil Conservation Projects*, FAO Soils Bulletin 64, Rome

Hughes, Bob (1990), 'Children's play – a forgotten right' *Environment and Urbanization*, Vol 2, No 2, pp 58–64

Hunsley Magcbhula, Patrick (1994) 'Evictions in the new South Africa: a narrative report from Durban', *Environment and Urbanization*, Vol 6, No 1, pp 59–62

Hunter, John M (1981), 'Past explosion and future threat – exacerbation of Red Water Disease (schistosomiasis haematobium) in the Upper Region of Ghana', *Geojournal*, Vol 5, No 4, pp 305–313

Hunter, John M (1990), 'Bot-fly maggot infestation in Latin America', *Geographical Review*, Vol 80, No 4, pp 382–398

Hunter, John M, et al (1982), 'Man-made lakes and man-made diseases: towards a policy resolution', *Social Science and Medicine*, Vol 16, pp 1127–1145

Hurwitz, E S, W J Gunn, P F Pinsky et al (1991), 'Risk of respiratory illness associated with day–care attendance: a nationwide study', *Pediatrics, Vol 87*, pp 62–69

Husain, T, A Jan and F Mahmood (1990), *Village Management Systems and the Role of the Aga Khan Rural Support Programme in Northern Pakistan*, MPE Series No 10, ICIMOD, Kathmandu

Huysman, Marijk (1994), 'Waste picking as a survival strategy for women in Indian cities', *Environment and Urbanization*, Vol 6, No 2, pp 155–174

India, Government of (1990), *The Lesser Child*, Department of Women and Child Development, Ministry of Human resource Development, with assistance from UNICEF

IPCC (1990), *Climate Change: the IPCC Scientific Assessment*, J H Houghton, G J Jenkins and J J Ephraums (Eds), Cambridge University Press, Cambridge

IRC (1988), *Community Participation and Women's Involvement in Water Supply and Sanitation Projects*, International Water and Sanitation Centre, The Hague, Netherlands

Jacobs, Jane (1965), *The Death and Life of Great American Cities*, Pelican, London

Jarzebski, L S (1991), 'Case Study of the Environmental Impact of the Non-Ferrous Metals Industry in the Upper Silesian Area', Paper prepared for the WHO Commission on Health and the Environment, WHO, Geneva

Jaujay, J (1990), The Operation and Maintenance of a Pilot Rehabilitated Zone in the Office du Niger, Mali, Irrigation Management Network Paper No 90/1c, ODI, London

Jazairy, Idriss, Mohiuddin Alamgir and Theresa Panuccio (1992), *The State of World Rural Poverty: an Inquiry into its Causes and Consequences*, IT Publications, London

Jintrawet, A, S Smutkupt, C Wongsamun, R Katawetin and V Kerdsuk (1985), *Extension Activities for Peanuts after Rice in Ban Sum Jan, N E Thailand: A Case Study in Farmer–to–Farmer Extension Methodology*, Khon Kaen University, Khon Kaen

Jodha, N S (1990), *Rural Common Property Resources: A Growing Crisis*, Gatekeeper SA24, IIED, London

Johnson, Victoria, Joanna Hill and Edda Ivan-Smith (1995), *Listening to Smaller Voices: Children in an Environment of Change*, ActionAid, London

Jordan, Sara and Fritz Wagner (1993), 'Meeting women's needs and priorities for water and sanitation in cities', *Environment and Urbanization*, Vol 5, No 2, Oct, pp 135–145

Juma, C (1989), *Biological Diversity and Innovation: Conserving and Utilizing Genetic Resources in Africa*, African Centre for Technology Studies, Nairobi

Kagan, A R and L Levi (1975), 'Health and environment: psycho-social stimuli – a review', in L Levi (Ed), *Society, Stress and Disease – Childhood and Adolescence*, Oxford University Press, pp 241–260

Kalter, H and J Warkary (1983), 'Congenital malformations', *New England Medical Journal*, Vol 308

Kanji, Nazneen (1995), 'Gender, poverty and structural adjustment in Harare, Zimbabwe', *Environment and Urbanization*, Vol 7, No 1, pp 37–55

Khan, Akhter Hameed (1991), *Orangi Pilot Project Programmes*, Orangi Pilot Project, Karachi

Kirkby, Richard (1994), 'Dilemmas of urbanization: review and prospects', in Denis Dwyer (Ed), *China: The Next Decades*, Longman Scientific and Technical, Harlow, pp 128–155

Korten, David C (1980), 'Community organization and rural development: a learning process approach', *The Public Administration Review*, Vol 40, pp 480–511

Korten, David C (1990), 'Observations and Recommendations on the UNICEF Urban Child Programme', *Environment and Urbanization*, Vol 2, No, 2, Oct, pp 46–57

Kothari, Smithu (1983), 'There's blood on those matchsticks', *Economic and Political Weekly*, Vol XVIII, 2 Jul, p 1191

Kottak, C P (1985), 'When people don't come first: some sociological lessons from completed projects' in Cernea, M M (ed), *Putting People First*, Oxford University Press, Oxford

Kumar, S (1991), 'Ananthapur experiment in PRA training' in Mascarenhas J et al (Eds), 'Participatory Rural Appraisal', *RRA Notes* 13, pp 112–117 IIED, London

Kutcher, Gary P and Pasquale L Scandizzo (1981), *The Agricultural Economy of Northeast Brazil*, Johns Hopkins University Press, Baltimore

Lalonde, D (1974), *A New Perspective on the Health of Canadians*, Canadian Department of Health and Welfare, Ottawa

Lamba, Davinder (1993), *Urban Agriculture Research in East Africa: Record, Capacities and Opportunities*, Cities Feeding People Series, Report 2, IDRC, Ottawa

Lane, Charles and Jules Pretty (1990), 'Displaced pastoralists and transferred wheat technology in Tanzania', Sustainable Agriculture Programme *Gatekeeper Series* no 20, IIED, London

Lankatilleke, Lalith (1995), 'Build Together: National Housing Programme of Namibia', paper presented at a workshop on Participatory Tools and Methods in Urban Areas, IIED, London

Latapí, Augustín Escobar and Mercedes González de la Rocha (1995), 'Crisis, restructuring and urban poverty in Mexico', *Environment and Urbanization*, Vol 7, No 1, Apr, pp 57–75

Lawry, S (1989), 'Tenure Policy towards Common Property Natural Resources', Land Tenure Center Paper No 34, University of Wisconsin, Madison

Leach, Gerald (1975), *Energy and Food Production*, IIED, London

Leach, Gerald and Robin Mearns (1989), *Beyond the Woodfuel Crisis – People, Land and Trees in Africa*, Earthscan, London

Leach, Melissa (1991), 'Engendered environments: understanding resource mangement in the West Africa forest zone', *IDS Bulletin*, Vol 22, No 4

Lecomte, B J (1986), *Project Aid: Limitations and Alternatives*, Development Studies Centre, OECD, Paris

Lee–Smith, Diana and Taranum Chaudhry (1990), 'Environmental information for and from children', *Environment and Urbanization*, Vol 2, No 2, pp 27–32

Lee-Smith, Diana and Catalina Hinchey Trujillo (1992), 'The struggle to legitimize subsistence: Women and sustainable development', *Environment and Urbanization*, Vol 4, No 1, pp 77–84

Lee–Smith, Diana, Mutsembi Manundu, Davinder Lamba and P Kuria Gathuru (1987), *Urban Food Production and the Cooking Fuel Situation in Urban Kenya*, Mazingira Institute, Kenya

Lee-Wright, Peter (1990), *Child Slaves*, Earthscan, London

Leitmann, Josef (1991), 'Environmental profile of Sao Paulo', Urban Management and the Environment: Discussion Paper Series, UNDP/World Bank/UNCHS

Levy, Caren (1992), 'Gender and the Environment: the challenge of cross–cutting issues in development policy and planning', *Environment and Urbanization* Vol 4, No 1, pp 120–135

Loevinsohn, M E (1987), 'Insecticide use and increased mortality in rural central Luzon, Philippines', *The Lancet*, I, pp 1359–62, quoted in Conway and Pretty 1991

Lofti, Mahshid (1990), 'Weaning foods – new uses of traditional methods', SCN News, No 6, UN ACC/SCN, Geneva

Mabala, Richard (1995), *The Girl Child* manuscript developed for UNICEF (Tanzania), Dar es Salaam

Manciaux, M and C J Romer (1986), 'Accidents in children, adolescents and young adults: a major public health problem' *World Health Statistical Quarterly, Vol* 39, No 3, pp 227–231

Mara, Duncan and Sandy Cairncross (1990), *Guidelines for the Safe Use of Wastewater and Excreta in Agriculture and Aquaculture*, WHO, Geneva

Marcondes Cupertino, Maria Amelia (1990), 'The employment of minors in Brazil', *Environment and Urbanization*, Vol 2, No 2, Oct, pp 71–76

Mascarenhas J, P Shah, S Joseph, R Jayakaran, J Devavaram, V Ramachandran, A Fernandez, R Chambers and J N Pretty (1991), 'Participatory Rural Appraisal', *RRA Notes* 13, pp 1–143 IIED, London

Mason, John B and S R Gillespie (1990), 'Policies to improve nutrition: what was done in the 1980s', *SCN News*, No 6, UN ACC/SCN, Geneva, pp 7–20

Matte, T D, J P Figueroa, S Ostrowski, G Burr et al (1989), 'Lead poisoning among household members exposed to lead-acid battery repair shops in Kingston, Jamaica (West Indies)' *International Journal of Epidemiology*, Vol 18, pp 874–881

Maxwell, D G and S Zziwa (1992), *Urban Farming in Africa: The Case of Kampala, Uganda*, ACTS Press, Nairobi

Maxwell, D G and S Zziwa (1993), 'Urban agriculture in Kampala: indigenous adaptive response to the economic crisis', *Ecology of Food and Nutrition*, Vol 29, pp 91–109

Mbiba, Beacon (1994), 'Institutional responses to uncontrolled urban cultivation in Harare; prohibitive or accomodative', *Environment and Urbanization*, Vol 6, No 1, pp 188–201

Mbiba, Beacon (1995), *Urban Agriculture in Zimbabwe*, Avebury, Aldershot

McGranahan, Gordon (1991), 'Fuelwood, subsistence foraging and the decline of common property', *World Development*, Vol 19, No 10, pp 1275–1287

McGranahan, Gordon, Jacob Songsore, Marianne Kjellén, Pedro Jacobi and Charles Surjadi (1995), 'Sustainability, poverty and urban environmental transitions', Mimeo

Mikkelsen, Britha with Yanti Yulianti and Anton Barré (1993), 'Community involvement in water supply in West Java', *Environment and Urbanization*, Vol 5, No 1, pp 52–67

Mitlin, Diana and David Satterthwaite, *Cities and Sustainable Development*, background paper for Global Forum '94, Manchester

Moctezuma, Pedro (1990), 'Mexico's urban popular movements: a conversation with Pedro Moctezuma' by Julio Davila, *Environment and Urbanization*, Vol 2, No 1, pp 35–50

Moser, Caroline O N (1987), 'Women, human settlements and housing: a conceptual framework for analysis and policy-making', in Caroline O N Moser and Linda Peake (Eds), *Women, Housing and Human Settlements*, Tavistock Publications, London and New York, pp 12–32

Moser, Caroline O N (1989), *Community Participation in Urban Projects in the Third World*, *Progress in Planning*, Vol, 32, No 2, Pergamon Press, Oxford

Moser, Caroline O N (1993), *Gender Planning and Development; Theory, Practice and Training*, Routledge, London and New York

Moser, Caroline O N, Alicia J Herbert and Roza E Makonnen (1993), *Urban Poverty in the Context of Structural Adjustment; Recent Evidence and Policy Responses*, TWU Discussion Paper DP #4, Urban Development Division, World Bank, Washington, DC

Moser, Caroline O N and Linda Peake (Eds) (1987), *Women, Human Settlements and Housing*, Tavistock Publications, New York and London

Mougeot, Luc J M (1994), *Urban Food production: Evolution*, Official Support and Significance, Cities Feeding People Series, Report 8, IDRC, Ottawa

Mueller, Charles C, (1995) 'Environmental problems of a development style: the degradation from urban poverty in Brazil', *Environment and Urbanization*, Vol 7, No 2, pp 68–84

Murphy, Denis (1990), 'Community organizations in Asia', *Environment and Urbanization*, Vol 2, No 1, pp 51–60

Myers, Robert (1991), *The Twelve Who Survive: Strengthening Programmes of Early Child Development in the Third World*, Routledge, London and New York

Needleman, Herbert L, Alan Schell, David Bellinger, Alan Leviton and Elizabeth N Allred (1991), 'The long-term effects of exposure to low doses on lead in childhood: an eleven year follow up report' *The New England Journal of Medicine*, Vol 322, No 2, pp 83–88

Newman, Oscar (1972), *Defensible Space: Crime Prevention through Urban Design*, MacMillan, New York

Newman, Peter W G and Jeffrey R Kenworthy (1989), *Cities and Automobile Dependence: an International Sourcebook*, Gower Technical, Aldershot

Nieuwenhuys, Olga (1994), *Chidren's Lifeworlds: Gender, Welfare and Labour in the Developing World*, Routledge, London

Nishioka, Shuzo, Yuichi Noriguchi and Sombo Yamamura (1990), 'Megalopolis and climate change: the case of Tokyo' in James McCulloch (Ed), *Cities and Global Climate Change*, Climate Institute, Washington, DC, pp 108–133

Odero, W (1994), 'Road traffic accidents in Kenya', Paper presented at the Urban Health Conference, London School of Hygiene and Tropical Medicine, 6–8 Dec

OECD (1995), OECD in *Figures: Statistics on the Member Countries*, 1995 edition, Paris

Oldeman, L R, R T A Hakkeling and W G Sombroek (1991), *World Map of the Status of Human-Induced Soil Degradation*, International Soil Reference and Information Centre, Wageningen

Omer, Mohamed I A (1990), 'Child health in the spontaneous settlements around Khartoum', *Environment and Urbanization*, Vol 2, No 2, pp 65–70

PAHO (1988), 'Research on Health Profiles: Brazil 1984', *Epidemiological Bulletin of the Pan American Health Organization*, Vol 9, No 2, pp 6–13

Parry, Martin, 'The urban economy', presentation at *Cities and Climate Change*, a conference at the Royal Geographical Society, 31 Mar, 1992

Patel, Sheela (1990), 'Street children, hotels boys and children of pavement dwellers and construction workers in Bombay: how they meet their daily needs', *Environment and Urbanization*, Vol 2, No 2, pp 9–26

Patel, Sheela and Celine D'Cruz (1993), 'The Mahila Milan crisis credit scheme; from a seed to a tree', *Environment and Urbanization*, Vol 5, No 1, pp 9–17

Patel, Sheela and Michael Hoffmann (1993), 'Homeless International, SPARC IS13 Toilet Block Construction, Interim Report', Homeless International, Coventry

Paul, S (1987), *Community Participation in Development Projects – The World Bank Experience*, World Bank Discussion Paper 6, Washington, DC

People's Dialogue (South Africa) and SPARC/National Slum Dewllers Federation/Mahila Milan (India) (1994), *Regaining Knowledge; an Appeal to Abandon Illusions*, SPARC, Bombay

Pepall, Jennifer (1992), 'Occupational poisoning' reporting on the work of Mohamad M Amr in *IDRC Reports*, Vol 20, No 1, Ottawa, Apr, p 15

Peterman, P (1981), 'Parenting and environmental considerations', *American Journal of*

Autopsychiatry, Vol 5, No 2, pp 351–355

Phantumvanit, Dhira and Wanai Liengcharernsit (1989), 'Coming to terms with Bangkok's environmental problems', *Environment and Urbanization*, Vol 1, No 1, pp 31–39

Piaget, J (1963), *The Psychology of Intelligence* (original pub in French in 1947), Littlefield Adams, Totowa, New Jersey

Ping, Li (1991) 'Eco–farming on Huaibei Plain', *Beijing Review*, Vol 34, No 28, pp 8–16

Pio, A (1986), 'Acute respiratory infections in children in developing countries: an international point of view', *Pediatric Infectious Disease Journal*, Vol 5, No 2, 1986, pp 179–183

Poore, Duncan (1989), *No Timber without Trees*, Earthscan, London

Pretty, Jules N (1995), 'Participatory learning for sustainable agriculture', World Development, Vol 23, No 8, pp 1247–1263

Pretty, J N and Irene Guijt (1992), 'Primary environmental care: an alternative paradigm for development assistance', *Environment and Urbanization*Vol 4 No 1

Pretty, J N, I Guijt, I Scoones and J Thompson (1992), 'Regenerating agriculture: the agroecology of low–external input and community based development' in Holmberg J (ed), *Policies for a Small Planet*, Earthscan, London

Pretty, J N and R Sandbrook (1991), *Operationalising Sustainable Development at the Community Level: Primary Environmental Care*, Report to the DAC Working Party on Development Assistance and the Environment

Prudencio, J (1994), *Institutional Assessment for Research Initiative on Urban Agriculture (Latin America and Caribbean)*, Draft consultancy report (mimeo), La Paz

Pryer, Jane (1993), 'The impact of adult ill-health on household income and nutrition in Khulna, Bangladesh', *Environment and Urbanization*, Vol 5, No 2, pp 35–49

Rabinovitch, Jonas (1992), 'Curitiba: towards sustainable urban development', *Environment and Urbanization*, Vol 4, No 2, pp 62–77

Rahman, M A (ed) (1984), *Grass-roots Participation and Self-Reliance*, Oxford and IBH Publication Co, New Delhi

Rahman, Perween and Anwar Rashid (1991), 'Low Cost Sanitation Programme Maintenance/Rectification', Orangi Pilot Project; Research and Training Institute, Karachi

Ramaswamy, V et al (1992), 'Radiative forcing of climate from halocarbon-induced global stratospheric ozone loss', *Nature*, Vol 355, No 6363, pp 810–812, quoted in World Resources Institute 1994

Redclift, Michael (1987), *Sustainable Development: Exploring the Contradictions*, Routledge, London and New York

Rees, William E (1992) 'Ecological footprints and appropriated carrying capacity: what urban economics leaves out', *Environment and Urbanization*, Vol 4, No 2, pp 121–130

Reichenheim, M and T Harpham (1989), 'Child accidents and associated risk factors in a Brazilian squatter settlement' Health Policy and Planning, Vol 4, No 2, pp 162–167

Reij, C (1988), 'The present state of soil and water conservation in the Sahel', paper for the Club du Sahel, Free University, Amsterdam

Revi, Aromar et al (1992), *BMTPC: Technology Action Plan for Rural Housing (1991–2001)*, TARU: The Action Research Unit for Development, India

Rogan, W J, et al (1988), 'Congenital poisoning by polychlorinated biphenyls and their contaminants in Taiwan', *Science*, Vol 241, p 334

Romieu, Isabelle et al (1990), 'Urban air pollution in Latin America and the Caribbean: Health perspectives', *World Health Statistics Quarterly*, Vol 23, No 2, pp 153–167

Rosenbaum, Martin (1993), *Children and the Environment*, National Children's Bureau, London

Ross, A C (1992), 'Vitamin A status: relationship to immunity and the antibody response', *Proceedings of the Society of Experimental Biology and Medicine*, Vol 200, pp 303–320

Rossi-Espagnet, A, G B Goldstein and I Tabibzadeh (1991), 'Urbanization and health in developing countries; a challenge for health for all', *World Health Statistical Quarterly*, Vol 44, No 4, pp 186–244

Rothenburg, Stephen J, Lourdes Schnaas-Arrieta, Irving A Perez-Guerrero et al (1989), 'Evaluacion del riesgo potencial de la exposition perinatal al plombo en el Valle de Mexico', Perinatologia y Reproduccion Humana, Vol 3, No 1, pp 49–56

Sapir, D (1990), *Infectious Disease Epidemics and Urbanization: a Critical Review of the Issues*, Paper prepared for the WHO Commission on Health and Environment, Division of Environmental Health, WHO, Geneva

Sarin, Madhu (1991), 'Improved stoves, women and domestic energy', *Environment and Urbanization*, Vol 3, No 2, Oct, pp 51–56

Satterthwaite, David (1993), 'The social and environmental impacts associated with rapid urbanization', Paper presented to the Expert Group Meeting on Population, Distribution and Migration, UN Population Division, Santa Cruz, Jan

Satterthwaite, David (1995), 'The underestimation of poverty and its health consequences', *Third World Planning Review*, Vol 17, No 4, Nov, pp iii–xii

Satterthwaite, David (1995), 'The scale and nature of international donor assistance to housing, basic services and other human-settlements related projects', Paper presented at the UNU/WIDER Conference on 'Human Settlements in the changing global political and economic processes', Helsinki

Schaeffer, B (1990), 'Home and health – on solid foundations?', *World Health Forum*, Vol 11, pp 38–45

Schofield, C J, R Briceno-Leon, N Kolstrup, D J T Webb and G B White (1990), 'The role of house design in limiting vector-borne disease' in Hardoy, Jorge E et al (Eds) *The Poor Die Young: Housing and Health in Third World Cities*, Earthscan, London

Scoones, Ian, Mary Melnyk and Jules N Pretty (1992), *The Hidden Harvest; Wild Foods and Agricultural Systems – a Literature Review and Annotated Bibliography*, Sustainable Agriculture Programme, IIED London

Scott, M J (1994), Draft paper on Human Settlements – impacts/adaptation, IPCC Working Group II, WMO and UNEP

Sen, Amartya (1994), *Beyond Liberalization: Social Opportunity and Human Capability*, Development Economics Research Programme DEP No 58, London School of Economics, London

Serageldin, Ismail (1993), 'Making development sustainable', *Finance and Development*, Vol 30, No 4, pp 6–10

Serageldin, Ismail (1995), *Sustainability and the Wealth of Nations: First Steps in an Ongoing Journey*, Paper presented at the Third Annual World Bank Conference on Environmentally Sustainable Development

Sevilla, Manuel (1993), 'New approaches for aid agencies; FUPROVI's community based shelter programme', *Environment and Urbanization*, Vol 5, No 1, pp 111–121

Sharp, C (1984), 'Environmental design and child maltreatment', in D Durke and D Campbell (eds), *The Challenge of Diversity*, Proceedings of the 15th Annual Conference of the Environmental Design Research Association, Washington, DC

Shrimpton, Roger (1993), 'Zinc deficiency – is it widespread but under-recognized?', *SCN News*, No 9, pp 24–27

Shrivastav, P P (1982), 'City for the Citizen or Citizen for the City: the Search for an Appropriate Strategy for Slums and Housing the Urban Poor in Developing Countries – the Case of Delhi', *Habitat International*, Vol 6, No 1/2, pp 197–207

Singh, Neera M and Kundan K Singh (1993), 'Saving forests for posterity', *Down To Earth*, 15 Apr, pp 25-28

Sinnatamby, Gehan (1990), 'Low cost sanitation' in Jorge E Hardoy et al (Eds), *The Poor Die Young: Housing and Health in Third World Cities*, Earthscan, London

Skerfvig, S (1988), 'Mercury in women exposed to methyl mercury through fish consumption, and in their new-born babies and breast milk', *Bulletin of Environmental Contamination Toxicology*, Vol 41

Smil, Vaclav (1984), *The Bad Earth: Environmental Degradation in China*, M E Sharpe, New York and Zed Press, London

Smit, Jac and Joe Nasr (1992), 'Urban agriculture for sustainable cities: using wastes and idle land and water bodies as resources' *Environment and Urbanization*, Vol 4, No 2, pp 141–152

Smith, K R (1988), 'Air pollution: assessing total exposure in developing countries', *Environment*, Vol 30, No 10, pp 28–35

Smith, D K (1989), *Natural Disaster Reduction: How Meteorological and Hydrological Services can Help*, Report No 722, World Meteorological Organization, Geneva, quoted in UNEP 1993

Sommers, Paul and Jac Smit (1994), *Promoting Urban Agriculture: a Strategy Framework for Planners in North America, Europe and Asia*, Cities Feeding People Series, Report 9, IDRC, Ottawa

Songsore, Jacob and Gordon McGranahan (1993), 'Environment, wealth and health; towards an analysis of intra-urban differentials within Greater Accra Metropolitan Area, Ghana', *Environment and Urbanization*, Vol 5, No 2, pp 10–24

Sriskandarajah, N, R J Bawden and R G Packham (1991), 'Systems agriculture; a paradigm for sustainability', *Association for Farming Systems Research Extension Newsletter*, Vol 2, No 2, pp 1–5

Stanton, B, D R Silimperi, K Khatun et al (1989), 'Parasitic, bacterial and viral pathogens isolated from diarrhoeal and routine stool specimens of urban Bangladeshi children', *Journal of Tropical Medicine and Hygiene*, Vol 92, pp 46–55

Stein, Robert E and Brian Johnson (1979), *Banking on the Biosphere?*, Lexington Books, D C Heath and Company, Lexington and Toronto

Stephens, Carolyn, Ian Timaeus, Marco Akerman, Sebastian Avle, Paulo Borlina Maia, Paulo Campanerio, Ben Doe, Luisiana Lush, Doris Tetteh and Trudy Harpham (1994), *Environment and Health in Development Countries: an Analysis of Intra-urban Differentials Using Existing Data*, London School of Hygiene and Tropical Medicine, London

Stewart, Sarah (1994), *Colombian Flowers: The Gift of Love and Poison*, Christian Aid

Surjadi, Charles (1993), 'Respiratory diseases of mothers and children and environmental factors among households in Jakarta', *Environment and Urbanization*, Vol 5, No 2, pp 78–86

TARU for Development (1994), *Giving Children back their Childhood? Habitat and the World of a Child*, Prepared for Plan International, TARU, Delhi

Thaxton, Ralph (1981), 'The peasants of Yaocun: memories of exploitation, injustice and liberation in a Chinese village', *Journal of Peasant Studies*, Vol 9, No 1, pp 3–46

The People's Dialogue (South Africa) and SPARC/National Slum Dewllers Federation/Mahila Milan (India) (1994), *Regaining Knowledge; an Appeal to Abandon Illusions*, SPARC, Bombay

The Ecologist (1992), *Whose Common Future*, Earthscan, London

Tiffen, Mary (1989), *Guidelines for the Incorporation of Health Safeguards into Irrigation Projects through Intersectoral Cooperation with Special Reference to Vector-borne Diseases*, Unpublished WHO Document, WHO, Geneva

Tiffen, Mary and Michael Mortimore (1992), 'Environment, population growth and productivity in Kenya; a case study of Machakos District', *Development Policy Review*, Vol 10, pp 359–387

Timberlake, Lloyd and Laura Thomas (1990), *When the Bough Breaks : Our Children, Our Environment*, Earthscan, London

Tolba, Mostafa K, Osama A El-Kholy, E El-Hinnawi, M W Holdgate, D F McMichael and R E Munn (1992), *The World Environment 1972–1992; Two Decades of Challenge*, Chapman and Hall on behalf of UNEP, London

Toucher, L (1981), 'Mortalidad de la 4 anos de edad: tendencias y causas; notas de poblacion', *Revista Latinoamericana de Demografia*, Vol 26, No 9, pp 27-54

Toulmin, Camilla (1990), 'Drylands and Human Settlements', Internal paper, IIED

Toulmin, Camilla (1995), *The Desertification Convention: the Strategic Agenda for the EU*, EC Aid and Development Briefing Paper No 1, IIED, London

Toulmin, Camilla, Ian Scoones and Josh Bishop (1992), 'Drylands' in Johan Holmberg (Ed), *Policies for a Small Planet*, Earthscan, London

Turner, John F C (1976), *Housing By People – Towards Autonomy in Building Environments*, Ideas in Progress, Marion Boyars, London

Turner, John F C and Robert Fichter (Eds) (1971), *Freedom to Build*, Macmillan, New York and London

Turner, Bertha (Ed) (1988), *Building Community – A Third World Case Book*, Habitat International Coalition, London

UNCHS (1996), *An Urbanizing World: Global Report on Human Settlements 1996*, Oxford University Press, Oxford

UNDP (1991), *Human Development Report 1991*, UNDP, Oxford University Press, Oxford and New York

UNDP (1994), *Human Development Report 1994*, UNDP, Oxford University Press, Oxford and New York

UNEP (1985), *Radiation: Doses, Effects, Risks*, UNEP, Nairobi

UNEP (1990), *Children and the Environment; the State of the Environment 1990*, UNEP, Nairobi

UNEP (1991), *Environmental Data Report, 1991–2*, GEMS Monitoring and Assessment Research Centre, Blackwell, Oxford and Massachusetts

UNEP (1991), *Environmental Effects of Ozone Depletion: 1991 Update*, UNEP, Nairobi

UNEP (1993), *Environmental Data Report, 1993–94*, GEMS Monitoring and Assessment Research Centre, Blackwell, Oxford and Massachusetts

UNEP and WHO (1988), *Assessment of Urban Air Quality*, Global Environment Monitoring Service, UNEP and WHO

UNEP and WHO (1992), *Urban Air Pollution in Megacities of the World*, Published on behalf of WHO, and UNEP, Blackwell, Oxford

UNICEF (1986), 'Children in especially difficult circumstances', Document based on the Executive Board Resolutions E/ICEF/1986/CRP 33, and 37 and distributed as CF/PD/PRO-1986-004, New York

UNICEF (1986), *State of the World's Children 1986*, Oxford University Press, Oxford and New York

UNICEF (1991), Report of the Area-Based Programming Seminar, Vol I, Harare, Zimbabwe, 2–4 Apr 1991, UNICEF, New York

UNICEF (1991), *The State of the World's Children 1991*, Oxford University Press, Oxford

UNICEF (1992), *Environment, Development and the Child*, Environment Section, Programme Division, UNICEF, New York

UNICEF (1992), *Children and Agenda 21*, Oct, UNICEF, Geneva

UNICEF (1995), *The State of the World's Children 1995*, Oxford University Press, Oxford and New York

UNICEF and UNEP (1990), *Children and the Environment*, The State of the Environment 1990; UNEP and UNICEF, E 90 XX USA 2, Geneva

UNICEF and WHO (1984), Primary Health Care in Urban Areas: Reaching the Urban Poor in Developing Countries – A State of the Art Report, SHS/84.4

United Nations (1995), *World Urbanization prospects: the 1994 Revision*, Population Division, the Department for Economic and Social Information and Policy Analysis, UN, New York

Uphoff, N (1990), 'Paraprojects as new modes of international development assistance', *World Development*, Vol 18, pp 1401–1411

Utting, Peter (1991), *The Social Origins and Impact of Deforestation in Central America*, UNRISD Discussion Paper No 24, Geneva

Victora C G, S C Fuchs, J A C Flores, W Fonseca and B Kirkwood (1994), 'Risk factors for pneumonia among children in a Brazilian metropolitan area', *Pediatrics, Vol 93*, pp 977–985

von Amsberg, Joachim (1993), *Project Evaluation and the Depletion of Natural Capital: an Application of the Sustainability Principle*, Environment Working Paper No 56, Environment Department, World Bank, Washington, DC

Wade, R (1987), 'The management of common property resources; finding a cooperative solution', *The World Bank Research Observer*, Vol 2, No 2, July, pp 219–234

Wageningen, University of (1990), Design for Sustainable Farmer-Managed Irrigation Schemes in sub-Saharan Africa, Contributions to an international workshop, 5–8 Feb

Wald, E R, N Guerra and C Byers (1991), 'Frequency and severity of infections in day care: three year follow–up', *Journal of Pediatrics*, Vol 118, pp 509–514

Wald, E R, N Guerra and C Byers (1991), 'Upper respiratory tract infections in young children: duration of and frequency of complications', *Pediatrics*, Vol 87, pp 129–133

Waller, Robert E (1991), 'Field investigations of air' in W W Holland, R Detels and G Knox (Eds), *Oxford Textbook of Public Health*, Vol 2 (2nd ed), Oxford University Press, Oxford and New York, pp 435–450

Walsh, Julia A (1988), *Establishing Health Priorities in the Developing World*, UNDP, Adams Publishing Group

Ward, Barbara (1974), *The Cocoyoc Declaration* adopted by the participants of the UNEP/UNCTAD symposium on 'Pattern of Resource Use, Environment and Development

Strategies' in 1974 that was drafted by Barbara Ward and republished in *World Development*, Vol 3, Nos 2 and 3, Feb–Mar 1975

Ward, Barbara (1976), 'The inner and the outer limits', The Clifford Clark Memorial Lectures 1976, *Canadian Public Administration*, Vol 19, No 3, Autumn, pp 385–416

Ward, Barbara (1979), *Progress for a Small Planet*, Penguin – repub by Earthscan, London

Ward, Barbara and René Dubos (1972), *Only One Earth: The Care and Maintenance of a Small Planet*, Andre Deutsch, London

Ward, C and A Fyson (1976), *Streetwork: The Exploding School*, Routledge and Kegan Paul, London

Warner, D B and L Laugeri (1991), 'Health for all: the legacy of the water decade' *Water International*, Vol 16, pp 135–141

WCED (1987), *Our Common Future*, Oxford University Press, Oxford and New York

West, K P Jnr, G R Howard and A Sommer (1989), 'Vitamin A and infection: public health implications', *Annual Review of Nutrition*, Vol 9, pp 63–86

White, G F, D J Bradley and A U White (1972), *Drawers of Water: Domestic Water Use in East Africa*, University of Chicago Press, Chicago

Whitehead, Ann (1992), 'Gender–Aware Planning in Agricultural Production', Module 7 of *Gender and Third World Development*, Institute of Development Studies, University of Sussex

WHO (1984), *The Role of Food Safety in Health and Development*, WHO Technical Report Series, No 705; Report of a joint FAO/WHO Expert Committee on Food Safety, WHO, Geneva

WHO (1986), *Intersectoral Action for Health – The Role of Intersectoral Cooperation in National Strategies for Health for All*, Background Document for the Technical Discussions, 39th World, Health Assembly, May, Geneva

WHO (1989), *Programme Report 1988*, Programme for the Control of Acute Respiratory Infections, WHO Document WHO/ARI/89.3, Geneva

WHO (1990), *Environmental Health in Urban Development*, Report of a WHO Expert Committee, WHO, Geneva

WHO (1990), *Public Health Impact of Pesticides used in Agriculture*, WHO, Geneva

WHO (1991), *Global Estimates for Health Situation Assessments and Projections 1990*, Division of Epidemiological Surveillance and Health Situation and Trend Analysis, WHO, WHO/HST/90.2, Geneva

WHO (1992), 'World malaria situation 1990', Division of Control of Tropical Diseases, WHO, *World Health Statistics Quarterly*, Vol 45, No 2/3, pp 257–266

WHO (1992), *Our Planet, Our Health*, Report of the Commission on Health and Environment, Geneva

WHO (1992), *Report of the Panel on Industry*, WHO Commission on Health and Environment, WHO/EHE/92.4, WHO, Geneva

WHO (1992), *Reproductive Health: a Key to a Brighter Future*, WHO Special Programme of Research Development and Research Training in Human Reproduction, Geneva

WHO (1995), *The World Health Report 1995: Bridging the Gaps*, WHO, Geneva

WHO (1996), *Creating Healthy Cities in the 21st Century*, Background Paper prepared for the Dialogue on Health in Human Settlements for Habitat II, WHO, Geneva

WHO and UNICEF (1993), *Water Supply and Sanitation Sector Monitoring Report 1993*, Water Supply and Sanitation Collaborative Council, WHO and UNICEF, Geneva

WHO and UNICEF (1994), *Water Supply and Sanitation Sector Monitoring Report 1994*, Water Supply and Sanitation Collaborative Council, WHO and UNICEF, Geneva

WHO, UNICEF and the International Council for the Control of Iodine Deficiency Disorders, (1993), Global Prevalence of Iodine Deficiency Disorders, quoted in UNICEF (1995), *The State of the World's Children 1995*, Oxford University Press, Oxford and New York

Winpenny, J T (1991), *Values for the Environment: A Guide to Economic Appraisal*, HMSO, London

WMO/UNEP (1990), *Scientific Assessment of Climate Change*, Report prepared for the Intergovernmental Panel on Climate Change by Working Group I, World Meteorological Organization, Geneva, and UNEP, Nairobi

Wohl, Anthony S (1983), *Endangered Lives: Public Health in Victorian Britain*, Methuen, London

Woodroffe, Caroline, Myer Glickman, Maggie Barker and Chris Power (1993), *Children, Teenagers and Health: The Key Data*, Open University Press, Buckingham

Woodward A, R M Douglas, N M H Graham and H Miles (1991), 'Acute respiratory illness in Adelaide children – the influence of child care', *Medical Journal of Aust*, Vol 154, pp 805–808

World Bank (1987), *The Aga Khan Rural Support Program in Pakistan; an Interim Evaluation*, Operations Evaluations Department, World Bank, Washington, DC

World Bank (1988), *World Development Report 1988*, Oxford University Press, Oxford

World Bank (1990), *The Aga Khan Rural Support Program in Pakistan; Second Interim Evaluation*, Operations Evaluations Department, World Bank, Washington, DC

World Bank (1990), *World Development Report – 1990; Poverty*, Oxford University Press, Oxford

World Bank (1992), *World Development Report 1992: Development and the Environment*, Oxford University Press, Oxford and New York

World Bank (1993), *World Development Report 1993; Investing in Health*, Oxford University Press, Oxford

Wratten, Ellen (1995), 'Conceptualizing urban poverty', *Environment and Urbanization*, Vol 7, No 1, pp 11–36

WRI (1990), *World Resources 1990–91: a Guide to the Global Environment*, Oxford University Press, Oxford

WRI (1992), *World Resources 1991–92: a Guide to the Global Environment: Toward Sustainable Development*, Oxford University Press, Oxford

WRI (1994), *World Resources 1994–95: A Guide to the Gloal Environment: People and the Environment*, Oxford University Press, Oxford

Yacoob, May and Linda M Whiteford (1995), 'An untapped resource: community-based epidemiologists for environmental health', *Environment and Urbanization*, Vol 7, No 1, pp 219–230

Yeung, Yue-Man (1985), *Urban Agriculture in Asia*, Food-Energy Nexus Programme, UN University, Tokyo

Zhongmin, Yan (1988), 'Shanghai: the growth and shifting emphasis of China's largest city' in Victor F S Sit (Ed), *Chinese Cities: the Growth of the Metropolis since 1949*, Oxford University Press, Hong Kong, pp 94–127

INDEX